Osler's
Textbook Revisited

reprint of selected
sections with
commentaries

edited by

A. M̄cGehee Harvey (signature)

A. McGehee Harvey
Professor of Medicine and Chairman
Department of Medicine

and

Victor A. McKusick (signature)

Victor A. McKusick
Professor of Medicine
Department of Medicine

Johns Hopkins University
School of Medicine
Baltimore, Maryland

APPLETON-CENTURY-CROFTS   New York
Division of Meredith Publishing Company

Osler's
Textbook Revisited

"OSLER IS IN LABOR; A BOOK IS BORN."

(From collection of William II. Welch
Medical Library, Johns Hopkins University;
also reproduced in Cushing's *Life of Sir William Osler*.)

acknowledgments

We are indebted to Dr. Owsei Temkin, William H. Welch Professor of the History of Medicine, Johns Hopkins University, for helpful suggestions. Dr. Samuel P. Asper and Dr. Philip F. Wagley, Baltimore, and Dr. William B. Bean, Iowa City, read most of the new material with valuable recommendations.

contributors

ROBERT AUSTRIAN, M. D. John Herr Musser Professor of Research Medicine, The University of Pennsylvania School of Medicine, Philadelphia.

WILLIAM B. BEAN, M. D. Professor and Head, Department of Internal Medicine, College of Medicine, University of Iowa, Iowa City.

WILLIAM B. CASTLE, M. D. Francis Weld Peabody Faculty Professor of Medicine, Harvard University; Honorary Director, Thorndike Memorial Laboratory; Consulting Physician, Second and Fourth (Harvard) Medical Services, Boston City Hospital.

DAVID B. CLARK, M. D. Professor of Neurology, Department of Neurology, College of Medicine, University of Kentucky Medical Center, Lexington.

WILLIAM DOCK, M. D. Chief of Medical Service, Veterans Administration Hospital, Brooklyn.

FRANCIS D. W. LUKENS, M. D. Professor of Medicine and Director Emeritus, George S. Cox Institute, University of Pennsylvania, Philadelphia; Chief of Staff, Veterans Administration Hospital, Pittsburgh, Pennsylvania.

MACLYN McCARTY, M. D. Vice President and Physician-in-Chief, The Rockefeller University, New York.

J. HOWARD MEANS, M. D. Jackson Professor of Medicine Emeritus, Harvard Medical School; Chief of Medical Services, Emeritus, Massachusetts General Hospital, Boston, Massachusetts.

contributors

WILLIAM D. ROBINSON, M. D. Professor and Chairman, Department of Internal Medicine, The University of Michigan Medical Center, Ann Arbor.

MAURICE B. STRAUSS, M. D. Chief of Medical Service, Veterans Administration Hospital, Boston, Massachusetts.

GEORGE W. THORN, M. D. Hersey Professor of the Theory and Practice of Physics, Harvard Medical School; Physician-in-Chief, Peter Bent Brigham Hospital, Boston, Massachusetts.

THOMAS B. TURNER, M. D. Professor of Microbiology and Dean of the Medical Faculty, The Johns Hopkins University, Baltimore.

CECIL J. WATSON, M. D. Distinguished Service Professor, University of Minnesota School of Medicine; Director of University of Minnesota Unit, Northwestern Hospital, Minneapolis.

THEODORE E. WOODWARD, M. D. Professor and Head, Department of Medicine, University of Maryland School of Medicine, Baltimore.

JAMES B. WYNGAARDEN, M. D. Chief of Medical Services, Hospital of the University of Pennsylvania; Frank Wistar Thomas Professor of Medicine, Chairman, Department of Medicine, University of Pennsylvania School of Medicine, Philadelphia.

C. GORDON ZUBROD, M. D. Scientific Director for Chemotherapy, National Cancer Institute, Bethesda, Maryland.

preface As is detailed later, Osler's Principles and Practice of Medicine played a leading role in the training of at least two generations of physicians and had an influence far beyond the direct one on medical practice. Thus Osler's book was a landmark in the medical literature, and reprinting it in part is of itself valuable. Here we have undertaken, however, both to reprint selected sections and to present commentaries by contemporary experts who have evaluated Osler's presentation and surveyed developments in each area since Osler. The historical résumé with which Osler introduced each section reflected his intense interest in, and sense for, history. Combining these with a review of developments since Osler's book results, we believe, in a useful treatment of the history of important aspects of internal medicine.

The seventh edition (1909) has been selected for use in this reprint because it was the last Osler did unaided. It represents the apogee of his textbook. The inaccuracies of earlier editions had been largely corrected, and the important advances between 1892 (when the first edition was published) and 1909 were incorporated.

A. McGehee Harvey
Victor A. McKusick

Reprints from Osler's Textbook

commentaries

Osler's
Textbook Revisited

introduction

From September 1890 to January 1892, Sir William Osler devoted most of his time to writing *The Principles and Practice of Medicine*. He was then 41 years old and Professor of Medicine in the Johns Hopkins University and Physician-in-Chief in the Johns Hopkins Hospital, which had opened its doors in May 1889. Relatively uninterrupted periods for writing were available to him because the hospital was operating smoothly and he had competent assistants, including Lafleur, his first resident, and Thayer, his second. Furthermore, the medical school was not yet opened because of the financial difficulties resulting from the failure of dividend payments by the Baltimore and Ohio Railroad, in which much of the endowment of the Johns Hopkins University was invested. Thus, his teaching responsibilities were lighter than might otherwise have been the case.

For some time Osler had recognized a clear need for a fresh endeavor in the textbook field. In 1881 he commented on "the paucity of American textbooks of medicine and the modesty of the sixty-five professors of 'Theory and Practice' who for nearly twenty years had left the field in possession of foreign authors, with whom Wood and Flint alone competed." In the 1880s four American textbooks of medicine appeared, those of Robert Bartholow (Philadelphia) in 1880, Alonzo B. Palmer (Michigan) in 1882, Nathan Smith Davis (Chicago) in 1884, and Alfred L. Loomis (New York) also in 1884. In reviewing these publications Osler displayed his dissatisfaction with them and his own germinating ideas of what a textbook of medicine should be like. For example, Davis' book, consisting essentially of 92 lectures which the author had "been in the habit of giving in the Chicago Medical College . . . illustrated the difficulty a teacher has in escaping from the bonds in which a routine course, delivered year after year, tends to inclose him. They bear the impress of the thoughts and professional opinions of thirty years ago. . . ." Osler decried Davis' objections to etiological or anatomical methods of classification, which according to Davis "lead to the grouping together of diseases the most dissimilar in their nature." Davis' book failed, furthermore, to incorporate the latest discoveries on the bacterial etiology of disease. Osler wrote: "That the evidence for a specific typhoid germ has no existence except in the human imagination is the burden of the lecture on etiology. . . ." Osler characterized Davis' therapeutics as polypharmacy. Loomis' work had advantages, in Osler's opinion: "It is systematic, the lecture form has been obliterated, it is well arranged and fully illustrated." Osler expressed regrets that "we do not feel the author's personality so strongly" as in Davis' book.

For over 40 years, in England and elsewhere in the English-reading world, Sir Thomas Watson's famous *Practice*, first published in 1843, had held first place in the textbook field. John S. Bristowe of St.

1

Introduction

Thomas's Hospital, London, produced a textbook which was also very popular, as indicated by the fact that five editions were called for in a period of seven years (1877-1884). Bristowe's work perhaps came closest to Osler's ideal. Later editions incorporated "recent views on infective organisms." "While to many an objection to this work is in the scanty details of treatment, yet there is much force in what the author says in the preface, that a man is more likely to make a thoughtful physician and benefit his patient by adapting drugs and methods to the exigencies of cases, than by following 'the stereotyped procedure of some predecessor.' He hesitates — many do not — to force his 'own routine and trivialities of practice upon students,' and contents himself with inculcating general principles 'and pointing out the specific virtues of certain drugs.' " Osler's view on treatment coincided with Bristowe's and led to his reputation as a therapeutic nihilist.

Parturit Osler, nascitur liber

On the flyleaf of his interleafed copy of the first edition, Osler penned the following statement of why and how the textbook was written (Cushing I, p. 340f):

"On several occasions in Philadelphia, I was asked by Lea Bros. to prepare a work on Diagnosis, and had half promised one; indeed, I had prepared a couple of chapters, but continually procrastinated on the plea that up to the 40th year a man was fit for better things than textbooks. Time went on and as I crossed this date I began to feel that the energy and persistence necessary for the task were lacking. In September 1890 I returned from a four months' trip in Europe, shook myself, and towards the end of the month began a work on Practice. I had nearly finished the chapter on Typhoid Fever when Dr. Granger, Messrs. Appleton's agent, came from New York to ask me to prepare a Text-book on Medicine. We haggled for a few weeks about terms and finally, selling my brains to the devil, I signed the contract. My intention had been to publish the work myself and have Lippincott or Blakiston (both of whom offered) handle the book, but the bait of a guaranteed circulation of 10,000 copies in two years and fifteen hundred dollars on the date of publication was too glittering, and I was hooked. October, November and December were not very satisfactory months, and January 1st, 1891, saw the infectious diseases scarcely completed. I then got well into harness. Three mornings of each week I stayed at home and dictated from 8 a.m. to 1 p.m. On the alternate days I dictated after the morning Hospital visit, beginning about 11:30 a.m. The spare hours of the afternoon were devoted to correction and reference work. Early in May I gave up

2

the house, 209 Monument St., and went to my rooms at the Hospital. The routine there was: — 8 a.m. to 1 p.m. dictation; 2 p.m. visit to the private patients and special cases in the wards, after which revision, etc. After 5 p.m. I saw my outside cases; dinner at the club about 6:30, loafed until 9:30, bed at 10 p.m., up at 7 a.m. I had arranged to send MS. by 1st of July and on that date I forwarded five sections, but the publishers did not begin to print until the middle of August. The first two weeks of August I spent in Toronto, and then with the same routine I practically finished the MS. by about October the 15th. During the summer the entire MS. was carefully revised for the press by Mr. Powell of the English Department of the University. The last three months of 1891 were devoted to proof reading. In January I made out the index, and in the entire work nothing so wearied me as the verifying of every reference. Without the help of Lafleur and Thayer, who took the ward work off my hands, I never could have finished in so short a time. My other assistants also rendered much aid in looking up references and special points. During the writing of the work I lost only one afternoon through transient indisposition, and never a night's rest. Between September, 1890, and January, 1892, I gained nearly eight pounds in weight."

In addition to the above quote, Cushing (I, p. 349) provided more intimate details of the writing. Moving into the famous domed building of the Johns Hopkins Hospital on May 1, 1891, Osler worked continuously on the book until the middle of October, taking only a brief breather in August. Each of the four Hopkins chief residents, in medicine, surgery, gynecology, and pathology, had a separate study and bedroom on the second floor. Hunter Robb, Kelly's resident, had the largest and quietest suite situated at the end of the corridor at the northwest corner of the building. Osler appropriated the study for a hideaway where he "camped out for the next six months."

Robb later recalled the pleasant sessions with Osler when he would interrupt his dictation "to rush into my room, and ask me to match quarters with him, or we would engage in an exchange of yarns. It was great treat for me; and except when he would court inspiration by kicking my waste-paper basket about the room, I thoroughly enjoyed his visits." Robb cured Osler of the waste-basket habit by filling it with carefully concealed bricks.

The room where the *Practice* was written was still occupied by the gynecology resident, in the direct line of descent from Robb, until 1953, when the combination of demands for administrative offices and the trend for residents to have families dictated its conversion. It is doubtful that its present occupants appreciate the hallowed ground on which they work. The mantelpiece shown in the frontispiece has now been removed.

Introduction

Transfer of authorship

As the years passed and Osler left Hopkins for Oxford he began to give thought to the disposition of the authorship of his textbook. On April 6, 1908, when he was in the throes of preparing the seventh edition, he wrote to Lewellys F. Barker, his successor in the Chair at Hopkins:

"I want an hour's chat with you about the Text-book. This new edition, due October 1908, will not be a very serious revision, as they will not break up the plates, but in the next edition we can do as we like. It would be nice if you and Thayer came in with me as joint authors. It would be possible, I think, to arrange to have the work kept up as a Johns Hopkins Hospital Text-book of Medicine. I think some arrangement could be made with the publishers and some plan devised by which the head of the Medical Department would have *ex-officio* rights in it. In the IXth edition I would probably go out altogether, and the book would appear from you and Thayer — perhaps, I retaining a small financial interest."

The proposal seems to have had a cool reception from Barker and Thayer* because with the eighth edition Thomas McCrae, a former Osler resident and later Professor of Medicine at Jefferson Medical College, joined in the textbook. After Osler's death and until his own death in 1935, McCrae continued the book (the ninth through the twelfth editions), taking sole responsibility. Henry A. Christian (1876–1951), Professor of Medicine in Harvard Medical School and Physician-in-Chief of the Peter Bent Brigham Hospital, took over the editorship with the thirteenth edition (1938). The last edition, the sixteenth, appeared in 1947. It continued as a "one man book" throughout.

Influence of the Principles and Practice

It has been said that in his textbook Osler "succeeded in making a scientific treatise literature." Cushing remarked: "Some one, some day, could well write a volume devoted to a study of the successive editions of this famous work which continues to exercise an enormous in-

*It appears, however, that Barker did not give an unqualified "no," because in January 1910 after a painful bout of urinary calculi, Osler wrote again to Barker proposing the idea of a Hopkins textbook. "Naturally, I have a strong sentiment about the book, but I know quite well that the life and success of a work depends [sic] upon the life of the man, and it is quite to the interests of the publishers as well as my own, to make provision for a gradual or immediate transfer of editorial control."

fluence on students of medicine — even those beyond English-reading countries through its many translations" (French, 1908; German, 1909; Chinese,
1910 and 1921; Spanish, 1915).

Osler's textbook is credited with a major role in direct-
ing Rockefeller philanthropy into the field of research and education in
medicine and public health (Corner, 1964). The establishment of the Rockefeller Institute now called Rockefeller University (1901) and of the Rockefeller Foundation (1913), large contributions to the Harvard Medical School,
aid to the Johns Hopkins Hospital in a period of financial difficulty resulting
from the Baltimore fire of 1904, financing of the full-time system at Hopkins,
and founding of the Johns Hopkins School of Hygiene and Public Health
(1918) and the Johns Hopkins Institute of the History of Medicine (1929)
are tangible results of the influence of the book.

The influence of Osler's textbook on Rockefeller philanthropy operated through the agency of a layman, Frederick T. Gates, a
Baptist minister, who was one of John D. Rockefeller's main advisors. While
vacationing in the Catskills in the summer of 1897, Gates read Osler's second
edition. Below is Gates' account of the background, the effects the book
had on its reader, and the course of action it prompted (Cushing I, p 454f):

"In the early summer of 1897 my interest in medicine
was awakened by a . . . Minneapolis boy* who in his loneliness in New York
used often to spend his weekends with us in Montclair. His deceased father
had been a homeopathic physician but he himself was studying in the regular
school. I determined as a result of my talks with this enthusiastic young
student to make myself more intelligent on the whole subject of medicine,
and at his suggestion I bought a copy of Dr. Osler's *Principles and Practice
of Medicine.* . . . I read the whole book without skipping any of it. I speak of
this not to commemorate my industry or intelligence but to testify to Osler's
charm, for it is one of the very few scientific books that are possessed of high
literary quality. There was a fascination about the style itself that led me on,
and having once started I found a hook in my nose that pulled me from page
to page, and chapter to chapter, until the whole of about a thousand large
and closely printed pages brought me to the end.

"But there were other things besides its style that attracted and intensified my interest. . . . To the layman student, like me,
demanding cures, and specifics, he had no word of comfort whatever. In
fact, I saw clearly from the work of this thoroughly enlightened, able and

---

*Elon O. Huntington (1870–1926), student at College of Physicians and Surgeons, had
been in Gates' congregation in Minneapolis. He received his M.D. degree from Colum-
bia in 1896 and was subsequently a medical officer in the U.S. Navy.

Introduction

honest man, perhaps the foremost practitioner in the world, that medicine had — with a few exceptions — no cures, and that about all that medicine up to 1897 could do was to suggest some measure of relief, how to nurse the sick, and to alleviate in some degree the suffering. Beyond this, medicine as a cure had not progressed. I found further that a large number of the most common diseases, especially of the young and middle-aged, were infectious or contagious, caused by infinitesimal germs that are breathed in with the atmosphere, or are imparted by contact or are taken in with the food or drink or communicated by the incision of insects in the skin. I learned that of these germs, only a very few had been identified and isolated. I made a list — and it was a very long one at that time, much longer than it is now — of the germs which we might reasonably hope to discover but which as yet had never been, with certainty, identified; and I made a longer list of the infectious or contagious diseases for which there had been as yet no cure at all discovered.

"When I laid down this book I had begun to realize how woefully neglected in all civilized countries and perhaps most of all in this country, had been the scientific study of medicine. . . . It became clear to me that medicine could hardly hope to become a science until it should be endowed, and qualified men could give themselves to uninterrupted study and investigation, on ample salary, entirely independent of practice. . . . Here was an opportunity for Mr. Rockefeller to become a pioneer. This idea took possession of me. The more I thought of it the more interested I became. I knew nothing of the cost of research; I did not realize its enormous difficulty; the only thing I saw was the overwhelming and universal need and the infinite promise, world-wide, universal, eternal. Filled with these thoughts and enthusiasms, I returned from my vacation July 24th. I brought my Osler into the office at No. 26 Broadway, and there I dictated for Mr. Rockefeller's eye a memorandum in which I aimed to show to him the actual condition of medicine in the United States and the world as disclosed by Dr. Osler's book. I enumerated the infectious diseases and pointed out how few of the germs had yet been discovered and how great the field of discovery; how few specifics had yet been found and how appalling was the unremedied suffering. I pointed to the Koch Institute in Berlin. I pointed out the fact, first stated by Huxley I think, that the results in dollars or francs of Pasteur's discoveries about anthrax and on the diseases of fermentation and of the silkworm had saved for the French nation a sum far in excess of the entire cost of the Franco-German War. I remember insisting in this or some subsequent memoranda that even if the proposed institute should fail to discover anything, the mere fact that he, Mr. Rockefeller, had established such an institution of research, if he were to consent to do so, would result in

6

other institutes of a similar kind, or at least other funds for research being established, until research in this country would be conducted on a great scale; and that out of the multitudes of workers we might be sure in the end of abundant rewards, even though those rewards did not come directly from the institute which he might found.

"These considerations took root in the mind of Mr. Rockefeller and, later, his son. Eminent physicians were consulted as to the feasibility of the project, a competent agent was employed to secure the counsel of specialists on research, and out of wide consultation the Rockefeller Institute of Medical Research, came into being. It had its origin in Dr. Osler's perfectly frank disclosure of the very narrow limitations of ascertained truth in medicine as it existed in 1897 [sic]."

The scientific climate

The first edition of Osler's *Practice* appeared in 1892; the seventh edition, which was the last Osler prepared alone, and the one from which excerpts are reprinted In this volume, appeared in 1909. It is useful to review the climate of scientific medicine in which the first edition was prepared and the advances which occurred in the 17 years between the first and seventh editions. Tables 1 and 2 list outstanding advances in the 17 years before and the 17 years after 1892. Table 3 lists works done in Osler's clinic and elsewhere at Johns Hopkins during his tenure as Professor of Medicine.

Organization of the text

Osler introduced a system for the description of disease which has been followed by many subsequent textbooks of medicine. It began with a definition, followed by a historical note, and discussions, in order, of etiology, transmission (for infectious diseases), morbid anatomy, symptoms, diagnosis, prognosis, prophylaxis, and treatment. Coming near the end of the morphological era in medicine and at the dawn of the physiological era, Osler's textbook was firmly based on morbid anatomy. It reflects its author's extensive experience in the autopsy room. The historical sections reflect Osler's interest and orientation. They remain a most useful part of the book. Together with the historical comments which accompany each reprinted section in this book, they provide a concise but rather complete history of the development of our understanding of those diseases selected for inclusion in this reprint.

Table 1. Selected Advances in Medicine*
1875-1892

1875. Sir Thomas Barlowe described infantile scurvy.
Weir Mitchell introduced rest cure for psychiatric disorders.
Hughlings Jackson described unilateral convulsions (Jacksonian epilepsy).*

1876. Johns Hopkins University founded.
Koch grew anthrax bacillus on artificial media.

1877. Pasteur discovered bacillus of malignant edema.
Ernst von Bergmann introduced corrosive sublimate (mercuric chloride) antisepsis.

1878. Erb described myasthenia gravis.

1879. Neisser discovered gonococcus.
Nitze introduced cystoscopy.

1880. Pasteur isolated streptococcus, staphylococcus, and pneumococcus.
Eberth isolated typhoid bacillus.

1881. Lavern discovered parasite of malaria.
Koch introduced plate cultures.
Wernicke described acute hemorrhagic polioencephalitis.

1882. Koch discovered tubercle bacillus.
Langenbuch excised gallbladder.
Quincke described angioneurotic edema.

1883. Edwin Klebs discovered diphtheria bacillus.
Pasteur vaccinated against anthrax.

1884. Koch discovered cholera bacillus.
Nicolaier discovered tetanus bacillus.
Ludwig Knorr prepared antipyrine.

1885. Ewald and Boas introduced test-meal.
Halsted introduced conduction (block) anesthesia.

1886. Marie described acromegaly as a pituitary disorder.
Charcot and Marie in Paris and Tooth in England described peroneal muscular atrophy.

1887. Bruce discovered coccus of Malta fever (brucellosis).
Weichselbaum discovered meningococcus.

1888. Institut Pasteur founded.

1889. Johns Hopkins Hospital opened.
Von Mering and Minkowski produced experimental pancreatic diabetes.

1890. Behring treated diphtheria with antitoxin.
Koch introduced tuberculin.
Marie described hypertrophic pulmonary osteoarthropathy.

1891. Quincke introduced lumbar puncture.

_____

*Adapted from Garrison's *History of Medicine*. Some of the dates are approximate.

Table 2. Selected Advances in Medicine*
1892-1909

1892. First edition of Osler's *The Principles and Practice of Medicine* appeared.

1893. Freud developed psychoanalysis.
Marie described hereditary cerebellar ataxia.
Johns Hopkins Medical School opened.

1894. Bruce discovered trypanosome.
Banti described "splenic anemia."
Baumann discovered iodine in thyroid hormone.
Yersin discovered causative organism in bubonic plague.

1895. Roentgen discovered x-rays.
Nobel prizes initiated.

1896. Widal and Sicard introduced agglutination test for typhoid.
Riva-Rocci introduced a new form of sphygmomanometer.
Still described juvenile rheumatoid arthritis.

1879. Shiga discovered dysentery bacillus.

1898. Löffler and Frosch investigated filtrable viruses.
The Curies discovered radium.
Theobald Smith differentiated the human and bovine tubercle bacilli.
Banti described splenomegalic anemia.
Marie described rheumatoid spondylosis.

1899. Reed and Carroll established the mosquito transmission of yellow fever.

1900. Mendelism rediscovered simultaneously and independently by Correns, Tschermak, and DeVries.
Minkowski and Chauffard described spherocytic hemolytic anemia.

1901. DeVries stated mutation theory.
Landsteiner discovered ABO blood groups.
Takamine isolated epinephrine.
Rockefeller Institute opened.

1902. Sutton (and later Boveri) presented evidence for the chromosomal theory of heredity.

1903. Metchnikoff inoculated apes with syphilis.
Einthoven invented string galvanometer for electrocardiography and other physiological recording.
Bruce showed sleeping sickness (trypanosomiasis) is transmitted by tsetse fly.
Von Pirquet and Schick identified serum sickness with anaphylaxis.

1904. Chiari recognized the syphilitic nature of aortitis.

1905. Schaudinn discovered parasites of syphilis.
Einhorn discovered novocaine.

1906. Bordet and Gengou discovered bacillus of whooping cough.

1907. Wassermann introduced serological test for syphilis.

1908. Von Pirquet introduced skin test for tuberculosis.
Garrod summarized his important studies on inborn errors of metabolism.
Buerger described thromboangiitis obliterans.

1909. Ehrlich introduced salvarsan for syphilis.

---

*Adapted from Garrison's *History of Medicine*. Some of the dates are approximate.

Table 3. Work in Osler's Clinic and Elsewhere at Johns Hopkins 1889-1905

1889–1902.	Studies of malaria by W. S. Thayer and others.
1890–1891.	Studies of amebic dysentery by William T. Councilman and Henri T. Lafleur.
1892.	Welch and Nuttall identified gas bacillus (*Clostridium welchii*). Halsted ligated first part of subclavian artery for aneurysm.
1896.	Demonstration of gonococcus in gonococcal endocarditis and septicemia by W.S. Thayer and George Blumer. Demonstration of causative organism in blastomycosis by Thomas C. Gilchrist.
1897.	Demonstration of eosinophilia in trichinosis by Thomas R. Brown, then a medical student. Description of familial cretinism by Osler. Abel's work on epinephrine.
1898.	Demonstration of causative organism in sporotrichosis by Benjamin R. Schenck.
1901.	Description of hereditary hemorrhagic telangiectasia by Osler,
1902.	Demonstration of characteristic histological changes of Hodgkin's disease by Dorothy Reed.
1903.	Study of pneumothorax by Charles P. Emerson.

Table 4. TABLES OF CONTENTS

1st edition	*7th edition*
	Diseases due to animal parasites
Specific infectious diseases	Specific infectious diseases
	The intoxications and sun-stroke
Constitutional diseases	Constitutional diseases
Diseases of the digestive system	Diseases of the digestive system
Diseases of the respiratory system	Diseases of the respiratory system
Diseases of the circulatory system	
	Diseases of the kidneys
Diseases of the blood and ductless glands	Diseases of the blood and ductless glands
	Diseases of the circulatory system
Diseases of the nervous system	Diseases of the nervous system
Diseases of the muscles	Diseases of the muscles
The intoxications; sun-stroke; obesity	
Diseases due to animal parasites	

Introduction

The order of the several sections of the first and seventh editions is compared in Table 4.

In the first edition obesity was discussed in the same section as alcoholism and morphia habit. The rationale for this is contained in Osler's statement (p. 1020): "A very important factor is overeating, a vice which is more prevalent and only a little behind overdrinking in its disastrous effects. A majority of persons over forty years of age habitually eat too much."

In the first edition, Osler considered as constitutional diseases rheumatic fever, the several forms of arthritis including gout, diabetes mellitus and diabetes insipidus, rickets, scurvy, purpura, and hemophilia. By the seventh edition obesity had been moved to "The Constitutional Diseases"; purpura, hemophilia, and scurvy had been transferred to "The Diseases of Blood and Ductless Glands," and rheumatic fever appeared among the specific infectious diseases.

Neither edition contained a separate section on nutritional deficiencies. Beriberi was in 1909 still listed as a specific infectious disease and pellagra as an intoxication "due to the use of altered maize" (p. 384). Allergic diseases were not separated as a major category of disease. Inborn errors of metabolism, even in the 1909 edition, which postdated Garrod, were not referred to as such. Alkaptonuria, which as Garrod stated in his Croonian lectures of 1908 was the best known of the inborn errors of metabolism, was discussed under "Diseases of the Kidneys" as an anomaly of the urinary secretion. This is another indication of the limited impact which Garrod's important concept made on the biology and medicine of his day.

Strange bedfellows are found in the section on diseases of the blood and ductless glands of both the first and seventh edition. "Diseases of the Suprarenal Bodies" was sandwiched between "Status Lymphaticus" and "Diseases of the Spleen." Diseases of the pituitary (except for diabetes insipidus, discussed as a constitutional disorder) and of the parathyroid glands are nowhere discussed, indicating the relatively recent origin of knowledge of the physiology and pathology of these organs.

Other comments

Specific bibliographic references are lacking from Osler's textbook. Contributors to various aspects of clinical knowledge are referred to by name, but usually no information is given on place of publication. Present-day students make greater use of the periodical literature, and a textbook without references would be viewed as undesirably authoritarian.

11

Introduction

To a considerable extent the change is attributable to the present ready access to good medical libraries. Osler contributed in no small part to the development of medical libraries through his support of the library of the Medical and Chirurgical Faculty of Maryland as a model. In Osler's day references in his textbook would have served little useful function because to most of his readers the original sources would not have been available.

Among Osler's extensive clinical writings, many people undoubtedly have favorites which will not be found here. Some, with good reason, may prefer one or another of Osler's monographs, e.g., Cerebral Palsies of Children (1889), Abdominal Tumors (1894), Chorea (1894), Angina Pectoris (1897), Cancer of the Stomach (1900). Some may regret that other sections of his textbook have not been printed here. A number of memorable passages could not be reprinted for lack of space. For example, Sidney Burwell in naming the Pickwickian syndrome took his cue from Osler's section on obesity (1909, p. 431):

"An extraordinary phenomenon in excessively fat young persons is an uncontrollable tendency to sleep — like the fat boy in Pickwick. I have seen one instance of it. Caton has reported a case. Sainton (*Narcolpesie et Obésité*, Rev. Neurologique, 1901) regards it as auto-toxic in origin."

A.M.H.

V.A.M.

REFERENCES

Corner, G.W. A History of the Rockefeller Institute 1901-1953. Origins and Growth. New York, Rockefeller Institute Press, 1964.

Cushing, H. The Life of Sir William Osler. Oxford, Clarendon Press, 1925.

Pratt, J.H. A Year with Osler, 1896-1897. Notes taken at His Clinics in the Johns Hopkins Hospital. Baltimore, Johns Hopkins Press, 1949.

THE PRINCIPLES AND PRACTICE OF MEDICINE

DESIGNED FOR THE USE OF PRACTITIONERS
AND STUDENTS OF MEDICINE

BY

WILLIAM OSLER, M.D.

FELLOW OF THE ROYAL SOCIETY; FELLOW OF THE ROYAL COLLEGE OF PHYSICIANS,
LONDON; REGIUS PROFESSOR OF MEDICINE, OXFORD UNIVERSITY; HONORARY PRO-
FESSOR OF MEDICINE, JOHNS HOPKINS UNIVERSITY, BALTIMORE; FORMERLY
PROFESSOR OF THE INSTITUTE OF MEDICINE, MCGILL UNIVERSITY,
MONTREAL, AND PROFESSOR OF CLINICAL MEDICINE IN THE
UNIVERSITY OF PENNSYLVANIA, PHILADELPHIA

SEVENTH EDITION, THOROUGHLY REVISED

NEW YORK AND LONDON
D. APPLETON AND COMPANY
1909

SPECIFIC INFECTIOUS DISEASES.

I. TYPHOID FEVER.

Definition.—A general infection caused by bacillus typhosus, characterized anatomically by hyperplasia and ulceration of the intestinal lymph-follicles, swelling of the mesenteric glands and spleen, and parenchymatous
changes in the other organs. There are cases in which the local changes are
slight or absent, and there are others with intense localization of the poison
in the lungs, spleen, kidneys, or cerebro-spinal system. Clinically the disease
is marked by fever, a rose-colored eruption, diarrhœa, abdominal tenderness,
tympanites, and enlargement of the spleen; but these symptoms are extremely
inconstant, and even the fever varies in its character.

Historical Note.—Huxham, in his remarkable Essay on Fevers, had
" taken notice of the very great difference there is between the *putrid malignant* and the *slow nervous fever.*" In 1813 Pierre Bretonneau, of Tours,
distinguished " dothiénentérite " as a separate disease; and Petit and Serres
described entero-mesenteric fever. In 1829 Louis' great work appeared, in
which the name " typhoid " was given to the fever. At this period typhoid
fever alone prevailed in Paris and many European cities, and it was universally believed to be identical with the continued fever of Great Britain, where
in reality typhoid and typhus coexisted. The intestinal lesion was regarded
as an accidental occurrence in the course of ordinary typhus. Louis' students returning to their homes in different countries had opportunities for
studying the prevalent fevers in the thorough and systematic manner of their
master. Among these were certain young American physicians, to one of
whom, Gerhard, of Philadelphia, is due the great honor of having first
clearly laid down the differences between the two diseases. His papers in
the American Journal of the Medical Sciences, 1837, are the first which
give a full and satisfactory account of their clinical and anatomical distinc-
tions. The studies of James Jackson, Sr. and Jr., of Enoch Hale and of
George C. Shattuck, of Boston, and of Alfred Stillé and Austin Flint made
the subject very familiar in American medicine. In 1842 Elisha Bartlett's
work appeared, in which, for the first time in a systematic treatise, typhoid
and typhus fever were separately considered with admirable clearness. In
Great Britain the recognition of the difference between the two diseases was
very slow, and was due largely to A. P. Stewart, and, finally, to the careful
studies of Jenner between 1849 and 1850.

Etiology.—GENERAL PREVALENCE.—Typhoid fever prevails especially in
temperate climates, in which it constitutes the most common continued fever.

Widely distributed throughout all parts of the world, it probably presents everywhere the same essential characteristics, and is everywhere an index of the sanitary intelligence of a community. *Imperfect sewerage* and *contaminated water-supply* are two special conditions favoring the distribution of the bacilli; *filth, overcrowding,* and *bad ventilation* are accessories in lowering the resistance of the individuals exposed. While from an infected person the disease may be spread by *fingers, food,* and *flies.*

In *England and Wales* in 1906 the disease was fatal to 3,169 persons, a mortality of 92 per million of living persons. It destroys more lives in proportion to population in towns than in the country. The rate was lower in 1906 than in any year but one since 1869. Compared with the quinquennial average, there was a very marked reduction (Tatham).

In *India* the disease is very prevalent; no race or creed is exempt, and 80 per cent of the cases of continued fever lasting three weeks prove to be enteric (L. Rogers).

In the *United States* typhoid fever continues to be disgracefully prevalent. From 1900 to 1904 the death rate in the registration areas was 33.8 per 100,000. It is estimated that from 35,000 to 40,000 persons die of it every year, so that at a moderate estimate nearly one half million people are attacked annually. It is more prevalent in country districts than in cities, and, as Fulton has shown, the propagation is largely from the country to the town. What is needed both in Canada and the United States is a realization by the public that certain primary laws of health must be obeyed.

In *Germany* the larger cities have comparatively little typhoid fever. The story of Hamburg, as told by Reincke (Lancet, i, 1904), should be read by all interested in the disease. During the past twenty-five years the death rate from enteric in Prussia has been reduced from an average of over 6 to less than 2 per 10,000 of the population. It is still very prevalent in some of the country districts.

Typhoid fever has been one of the great scourges of the armies, and kills and maims more than powder and shot. The story of the recent wars forms a sad chapter in human inefficiency.

In the Spanish-American War the report of the Commission (Reed, Vaughan, and Shakespeare) shows that one fifth of the soldiers in the national encampments had typhoid fever—among 107,973 men there were 20,738 cases, with 1,580 deaths. In 90 per cent of the volunteer regiments the disease broke out within eight weeks after going into camp. In the opinion of the Commission the most important factors were camp pollution, flies as carriers of contagion, and the contamination through the air in the form of dust.

In the South African War the British army, 557,653 officers and men, had 57,684 cases of enteric fever, with 8,225 deaths (Simpson), while only 7,582 men died of wounds received in battle. As in America, the disease was essentially one of the standing camps; troops constantly on the move were rarely much affected. While contaminated water was no doubt an important factor, as it always is in camp pollution, yet certain of the conditions in Africa were peculiar. Fæcal and urinary contamination must have been very common, as in the cooking, performed in the open air, sand " entered largely into every article of food." As there was a perfect plague of flies, they were without doubt a very important factor in the infection of both food and drink.

On the other hand, the Japanese and Russian War demonstrated the remarkable efficiency of modern hygiene, if carried out in an intelligent manner. The Japanese returns are not yet published, but no great war has ever been conducted with such forethought for the preservation of the fighting unit, and in consequence the mortality from typhoid fever and dysentery was exceptionally low.

Season.—Almost without exception the disease is everywhere more prevalent in the autumn, hence the old popular name autumnal fever. The exhaustive study of this question by Sedgwick and Winslow shows everywhere a striking parallelism between the monthly variations in temperature and the prevalence of the disease. In a few cities, notably Paris, Philadelphia, Chicago, and Dresden, the curves are irregular, showing, in addition to the usual summer rise, two secondary maxima in the winter and spring, and these authors suggest that epidemics at these seasons are characteristic of cities whose water-supply is most subject to pollution. In their opinion " the most reasonable explanation of the seasonal variations of typhoid fever is a direct effect of the temperature upon the persistence in nature of the germs which proceed from previous victims of the disease."

Of 1,500 cases at the Johns Hopkins Hospital (upon the study of which this section is based), 840 were in August, September, and October.

Sex.—Males and females are equally liable to the disease, but males are much more frequently admitted into hospitals, 2.4 to 1 in our series.

Age.—Typhoid fever is a disease of youth and early adult life. The greatest susceptibility is between the ages of fifteen and twenty-five. Of 1,500 cases treated in my wards at the Johns Hopkins Hospital there were under fifteen years of age, 231; between fifteen and twenty, 253; between twenty and thirty, 680; between thirty and forty, 227; between forty and fifty, 88; between fifty and sixty, 8; above sixty, 11; age not given, 1. Cases are rare over sixty, although Manges believes that they are more common than the records show. As the course is often atypical the diagnosis may be uncertain and the disease not recognized until autopsy. It is not very infrequent in childhood, but infants are rarely attacked. Murchison saw a case at the sixth month. There is no evidence that the disease is congenital even in cases in which the mother has contracted it late in pregnancy.

Immunity.—Not all exposed to the infection take the disease. Some families seem more susceptible than others. One attack usually protects. Two attacks have been described within a year. " Of 2,000 cases of enteric fever at the Hamburg General Hospital, only 14 persons were affected twice and only 1 person three times" (Dreschfeld). It is well known that usually within a short time after recovery the immune substances disappear from the blood, yet in most cases the relative immunity lasts a long time, frequently for life. An experimental explanation for this fact has been given in the demonstration that animals which have once reacted to the typhoid infection, react in throwing out immune substances more quickly and in larger amounts when danger again threatens (Cole).

BACILLUS TYPHOSUS.—The researches of Eberth, Koch, Gaffky, and others have shown that there is a special micro-organism *constantly* associated with typhoid fever. (*a*) *General Characters.*—It is a rather short, thick, flagel-

19

lated, motile bacillus, with rounded ends, in one of which, sometimes in both (particularly in cultures), there can be seen a glistening round body, at one time believed to be a spore; but these polar structures are probably only areas of degenerated protoplasm. It grows readily on various nutritive media, and can now be differentiated from *Bacillus coli,* with which, and with certain other bacilli, it is apt to be confounded. This organism now fulfills all the requirements of Koch's law—it is constantly present, and it grows outside the body in a specific manner; the third requirement, the production of the disease experimentally, has been successfully met by Grünbaum, of Leeds, who has produced the disease in chimpanzees. The bacilli or their toxins inoculated in large quantities into the blood of rabbits are pathogenic, and in some instances ulcerative and necrotic lesions in the intestine may be produced. But similar intestinal lesions may be caused by other bacteria, including *Bacillus coli.*

Cultures are killed within ten minutes by a temperature of 60° C. They may live for eighteen weeks at −5° C., although most die within two weeks, and all within twenty-two weeks (Park). The typhoid bacillus resists ordinary drying for months, unless in very thin layers, when it is killed in five to fifteen days. The direct rays of the sun completely destroy them in from four to ten hours' exposure. Bouillon cultures are destroyed by carbolic acid, 1 to 200, and by corrosive sublimate, 1 to 2,500.

(*b*) *Distribution in the Body.*—During recent years our ideas in regard to the distribution of the typhoid bacilli have been much modified, owing to the demonstration that in practically all cases the bacilli enter the circulating blood and are carried throughout the body. During life they may be demonstrated in the circulating blood in a large proportion of cases, in 75 per cent of 604 collected cases (Coleman and Buxton). They occur in the urine in from 25 to 30 per cent of the cases. They may be isolated from the stools in practically all cases at some stage. They are probably always present in the rose spots. They are reported to have been cultivated from the sweat, and they undoubtedly occur with considerable frequency in the sputum (Richardson, Rau, and others). At autopsy they are found widely distributed, most numerous and constant usually in the mesenteric glands, spleen, and gall-bladder, but are found in almost all organs, even the muscles, uterus, and lungs (von Drigalski). Cultures made from the intestines at autopsy (according to Jürgens, and also von Drigalski) show that they are very few or can not be cultivated from the rectum up to the cæcum, but above this they increase in number, being very numerous in the duodenum and jejunum, and practically constant in cultures made from the mucous membrane of the stomach. They are also present in the œsophagus and frequently on the tongue and tonsils. From endocardial vegetations, from meningeal and pleural exudates and from foci of suppuration in various parts of the body, the bacilli have also been isolated. A most important and remarkable fact is that at times they may be present in the stools of persons who show no symptoms of typhoid fever, but who have lived in very close association with typhoid-fever patients. This is especially true of children.

(*c*) *The Bacilli Outside the Body.*—In sterile water the bacilli retain their vitality for weeks, but under ordinary conditions, in competition with saprophytes, disappear within a few days. The question of the longevity of the typhoid bacillus in water is of great importance, and has been much discussed in connection with the supposed pollution of the waters of the Mississippi by the Chicago drainage canal. The experiments of E. O. Jordan would indicate that the vitality was retained as a rule not longer than three days after infection. Whether an increase can occur in water is not finally settled. Their detection in the water is difficult, and although they undoubtedly have been found, many such discoveries previously reported are not certain on account of the inaccurate differentiation of the typhoid bacillus and varieties of the intestinal bacillus closely resembling it. Both Prudden and Ernst have found it in water filters.

There are cities deriving their ice supply from polluted streams with low death rates from typhoid fever. Sedgwick and Winslow conclude from their careful study that very few typhoid germs survive in ice. The Ogdensburg epidemic in 1902–'03 was apparently due to infection from ice. Typhoid bacilli were grown from frozen material in it (Hutchins and Wheeler).

In *milk* the bacilli undergo rapid development without changing its appearance. They may persist for three months in sour milk, and may live for several days in butter made from infected cream.

Robertson has shown that under entirely natural conditions typhoid bacilli may live in the upper layers of the soil for eleven months. Von Drigalski says if stools which contain typhoid bacilli are kept at room temperature the *B. typhosus* disappears in a few days.

The direct infection by dust of exposed food-stuffs, such as milk, is very probable. The bacilli retain their vitality for many weeks; in garden earth twenty-one days, in filter-sand eighty-two days, in dust of the street thirty days, on linen sixty to seventy days, on wood thirty-two days; on thread kept under suitable conditions for a year.

MODES OF CONVEYANCE.—(*a*) *Contagion.*—Direct aerial transmission does not seem probable. Each case should be regarded as a possible source of infection, and in houses, hospitals, schools, and barracks a widespread epidemic may arise from it. Fingers, food, and flies are the chief means of local propagation. It is impossible for a nurse to avoid finger contamination, and without scrupulous care the germs may be widely distributed in a ward or throughout a house. Cotton or rubber gloves are used in some institutions. Even with special precautions and an unusually large proportion of nurses to patients, we have not been able to avoid " house " infection at the Johns Hopkins Hospital. T. B. Futcher has analyzed the 31 cases contracted in the hospital among our first 1,500 cases; physicians, 5 * among a total of 288; nurses, 15 of a total of 407; patients, 8 out of a total of 47,956 admissions; 4 of these occurred in a small ward epidemic. Two orderlies were infected while caring for typhoid patients, and one woman in charge of a supply room, where she only handled clean linen. Newman concludes from his study of enteric in London that direct personal infection, and infection through food are the two common channels for its propagation.

(*b*) *Infection of water* is the most common source of wide-spread epidemics, many of which have been shown to originate in the contamination

---

* Only three of these were in attendance on typhoid cases. Two of the five died—Oppenheimer and Ochsner.

of a well or a spring. A very striking one occurred at Plymouth, Pa., in 1885, which was investigated by Shakespeare. The town, with a population of 8,000, was in part supplied with drinking-water from a reservoir fed by a mountain stream. During January, February, and March, in a cottage by the side of and at a distance of from 60 to 80 feet from this stream, a man was ill with typhoid fever. The attendants were in the habit at night of throwing out the evacuations on the ground toward the stream. During these months the ground was frozen and covered with snow. In the latter part of March and early in April there was considerable rainfall and a thaw, in which a large part of the three months' accumulation of discharges was washed into a brook, not 60 feet distant. At the very time of this thaw the patient had numerous and copious discharges. About the 10th of April cases of typhoid fever broke out in the town, appearing for a time at the rate of fifty a day. In all about 1,200 people were attacked. An immense majority of all the cases were in the part of the town which received water from the infected reservoir.

The experience of Maidstone in 1897 illustrates the wide-spread and serious character of an epidemic when the water-supply becomes badly contaminated. The outbreak began about the middle of September, and within the first two weeks 509 cases were reported. By October 27th there were 1,748 cases, and by November 17th 1,848 cases. In all, in a population of 35,000, about 1,900 persons were attacked.

(c) *Typhoid Carriers.*—The bacilli may persist for years in the bile passages and intestines of persons in good health. They have been found by Young in the urinary bladder, and by Hunner in the gall-bladder, ten and twenty years after the fever, and there have been cases of typhoid bone lesion from which the bacilli were isolated many years after the primary attack. Within the past few years the work of Strassburg observers has called attention to a group of chronic typhoid carriers of the first importance in the spread of the disease. One woman, a baker, had typhoid fever ten years previously. The bacilli were found in large numbers in her stools. Every new employee in the bakery sooner or later became seriously ill with typhoid-like symptoms, and in two persons the disease proved fatal. Several localized epidemics have been traced to these carriers, particularly in asylums, as determined by the Strassburg observers. Ledingham, in one of the Scotch asylums at which since 1893 small outbreaks of typhoid fever had occurred, reported 31 cases with 9 fatal. Nothing abnormal could be determined in the water or in the milk. Three typhoid carriers were detected. Soper reports an instance in which a cook, apparently in perfect health, but in whose stools bacilli had been present in large numbers, had been responsible for the occurrence of typhoid in seven households in five years. Apparently there is no limit to the length of time in which the bacilli may remain in the bile passages and pass into the stools. Dean reports a case of a carrier of twenty-nine years' standing, and instances of even longer duration are recorded.

(d) *Infection of Food.*—Milk may be the source of infection. One of the most thoroughly studied epidemics due to this cause was that investigated by Ballard in Islington. The milk may be contaminated by infected water used in cleaning the cans. The milk epidemics have been collected by Ernest Hart and by Kober.

The germs may be conveyed in ice, salads of various sorts, etc. The danger of eating celery and other uncooked vegetables, which have grown in soil on which infected material has been used as a fertilizer, must not be forgotten.

Oysters.—Much attention has been paid of late years to the oyster as a source of infection. In several epidemics, such as that in Middletown, reported by Conn, that in Naples, by Lavis, and in the outbreak which occurred at Winchester, the chain of circumstantial evidence seems complete. Most suggestive sporadic cases have also been recorded by Broadbent and others. Foote showed that oysters taken from the feeding-grounds in rivers contain a larger number of micro-organisms of all sorts than those from the sea. Chantemesse found typhoid bacilli in oysters which had lain in infected sea-water, even after they had been transferred to and kept in fresh water for a time. C. W. Field, working in the laboratories of the Department of Health, New York (1904), confirms the observations of both Foote and Chantemesse, but he could not determine that the bacilli were able to multiply within the oysters. Mosny, in his report to the French Government (1900), admits the possibility of oyster infection, but he thinks that the oyster plays a very small *rôle* in relation to the total morbidity of the disease. Mussels have also been found contaminated with typhoid bacilli, and it is stated that dried fish have carried the infection.

(*e*) *Flies.*—The importance of flies in the transmission of the disease was brought out very strongly in the Spanish-American War in 1898. The Report of the Commission (Reed, Vaughan, and Shakespeare) states that "flies were undoubtedly the most active agents in the spread of typhoid fever. Flies alternately visited and fed on the infected fæcal matter and the food in the mess-tent. . . . Typhoid fever was much less frequent among members of messes who had their mess-tents screened than it was among those who took no such precautions." In the South African War there was a perfect plague of flies, particularly in the enteric fever tents, and among the army surgeons the opinion was universal that they had a great deal to do with the dissemination of the disease. Firth and Horrocks demonstrated the readiness with which flies, after feeding on typhoid stools or fresh cultures of typhoid bacilli, could infect sterile media. One of the most interesting studies on the question was made in the Chicago epidemic of 1902 by Alice Hamilton. Flies caught in two undrained privies, on the fences of two yards, on the walls of two houses, and in the room of a typhoid-fever patient, were used to inoculate eighteen tubes, and from five of these tubes typhoid bacilli were isolated.

(*f*) *Contamination of the Soil.*—Filth, bad sewers, or cesspools can not in themselves cause typhoid fever, but they furnish the conditions suitable for the preservation of the bacillus, and possibly for its propagation.

Dust may be an important factor, though it has been shown that the bacilli die very quickly when desiccated. In the dust storms during the South African War the food was often covered with dust. Possibly, too, as Barringer suggests, the dust on the railway tracks may become contaminated. Men working on the tracks are very liable to infection.

MODES OF INFECTION.—While the bacillus has its primary seat of action in the lymphatic tissues of the intestines, the fever is very largely due to its growth in the internal organs. As Maclagan very well puts it, the action is dual, one a local specific action of the parasite on the glands of the intestines, and a general action of the organism on the blood and tissues. A single bacillus in ten days, as he says, might produce a billion, and the incubation represents the period during which the bacilli are being reproduced.

We may recognize the following groups: 1. *Ordinary typhoid fever with marked enteric lesions.* An immense majority of all the cases are of this character; and while the spleen and mesenteric glands are involved the lymphatic apparatus of the intestinal walls bears the brunt of the attack. 2. *Cases in which the intestinal lesions are very slight,* and may be found only after a very careful search. In reviewing the cases of " typhoid fever without intestinal lesions," Opie and Bassett call attention to the fact that in many negative cases slight lesions really did exist, while in others death occurred so late that the lesions might have healed. In some cases the disease is a general septicæmia with symptoms of severe intoxication and high fever and delirium. In others the main lesions may be in organs—liver, gall-bladder, pleura, meninges, or even the endocardium. 3. *Cases in which the typhoid bacillus enters the body without causing any lesion of the intestine.* In a number of the earlier cases reported as such the demonstration of the typhoid bacillus was inconclusive. In others the intestine showed tuberculous ulcers, through which the organisms may have entered. But after excluding all these, a few cases remain in which the demonstration of the typhoid bacillus was conclusive, cases in which death occurred early, and yet after a very careful search no intestinal lesions could be found. There were 4 cases in this series. Undoubtedly the intestinal lesions may be so slight as not to be recognizable at autopsy. There is no conclusive evidence that typhoid bacilli ever enter the body except through the intestinal tract. 4. *Mixed infections.* It is well to distinguish, as Dreschfeld points out, between double infections, as with bacillus tuberculosis, the diphtheria bacillus, and the plasmodia of Laveran, in which two different diseases are present and can be readily distinguished, and the true mixed or secondary infections, in which the conditions induced by one organism favor the growth of other pathogenic forms; thus in the ordinary typhoid-fever cases secondary infection with the colon bacillus, the streptococcus, staphylococcus, or the pneumococcus, is quite common. 5. *Para-typhoid infections.* In 1898 Gwyn reported a remarkable case from my clinic, which presented all of the clinical features of typhoid fever, but in which no serum reaction with *B. typhosus* was present. From the blood of this patient he isolated in pure culture a bacillus, differing from *B. typhosus*, but having properties intermediate between *B. typhosus* and *B. coli.* This organism resembled one which was isolated in 1897 by Widal from an œsophageal abscess, and which he called a para-colon bacillus. In 1900 Cushing reported from the Johns Hopkins Hospital the cultivation of a similar organism from a costo-chondral abscess following an attack resembling typhoid fever. These organisms belong in a group which also contains *B. enteritidis*, described as the cause of meat poisoning, and also several varieties causing diseases in animals. Since 1900, following the introduction of more accurate bacteriological methods, similar organisms have been cultivated from numerous cases (now many hundreds) clinically like mild typhoid. Enlargement of the spleen has been quite constantly present, while rose spots have been frequently seen, and intestinal symptoms, even hæmorrhages, have occurred, but perforation has not been met with. Many cases have a very brief but acute course, resembling food poisoning. The sequelæ of ordinary typhoid fever may occur, and the para-typhoid organism has been isolated from the lesions of osteomyelitis, an inflamed testis, and a chondrosternal abscess. In the ordinary work of a medical clinic the cases are not very common. There were only 8 in the last 500 cases in my series. There have been about 15 autopsies (Birt), usually with enteric lesions. There is nothing in the clinical or anatomical features to differentiate it from ordinary typhoid, and for practical purposes they may be considered the same disease. The question is a bacteriological one, and the diagnosis rests upon the cultural peculiarities of the organism isolated from the blood or stools, and upon the agglutination tests. 6. *Local infections.* The typhoid bacillus may cause a local abscess, cystitis, or cholecystitis without evidence of a general infection. 7. *Terminal typhoid infections.* In rare instances the bacillus causes a fatal infection towards the end of other diseases. The subjects may, of course, be typhoid carriers. In two cases of malignant disease at the Johns Hopkins Hospital the bacilli were isolated from the blood, and there were no intestinal lesions.

Products of the Growth of the Bacilli.—Brieger isolated from cultures a poison belonging to the group of ptomaines—typhotoxin. Later he and Fraenkel isolated a poison belonging to the group of toxalbumins. According to Pfeiffer, the chief poison belongs to the intracellular group of toxins. Sidney Martin has isolated a poison which is in the nature of a secretion, but does not differ from that contained within the bacterial cell. Injected into animals it causes lowering of temperature, diarrhœa, loss of weight, and degeneration of the myocardium. Its chemical nature is not known. Similar, but weaker, poisons may also be isolated from cultures of *Bacillus coli* and other members of this group. No toxins have yet been isolated which cause changes in animals at all comparable to typhoid fever in human beings. Macfadyen and Rowland, by mechanically breaking up the bacilli after they had been frozen by means of liquid air obtained toxins, which injected into monkeys had both antitoxic and antibacterial properties.

Morbid Anatomy.—INTESTINES.—A catarrhal condition exists throughout the small and large bowel. Specific changes occur in the lymphoid elements, chiefly at the lower end of the ileum. The alterations which occur are most conveniently described in four stages:

1. *Hyperplasia,* which involves the glands of Peyer in the jejunum and ileum, and to a variable extent those in the large intestine. The follicles are swollen, grayish-white, and the patches may project 3 to 5 mm., or may be still more prominent. The solitary glands, which range in size from a pin's head to a pea, are usually deeply imbedded in the submucosa, but project to a variable extent. Occasionally they are very prominent, and may be almost pedunculated. Microscopical examination shows at the outset a condition of hyperæmia of the follicles. Later there is a great increase and accumulation of cells of the lymph-tissue which may even infiltrate the adjacent mucosa and the muscularis; and the blood-vessels are more or less compressed, which gives the whitish, anæmic appearance to the follicles. The cells have all the characters of ordinary lymph-corpuscles. Some of them,

however, are larger, epithelioid, and contain several nuclei. Occasionally cells containing red blood-corpuscles are seen. This so-called medullary infiltration, which is always more intense toward the lower end of the ileum, reaches its height from the eighth to the tenth day and then undergoes one of two changes, *resolution* or *necrosis*. Death very rarely takes place at this stage. Resolution is accomplished by a fatty and granular change in the cells, which are destroyed and absorbed. A curious condition of the patches is produced at this stage, in which they have a reticulated appearance, the *plaques à surface réticulée*. The swollen follicles in the patch undergo resolution and shrink more rapidly than the surrounding framework, or what is more probable the follicles alone, owing to the intense hyperplasia, become necrotic and disintegrate, leaving the little pits. In this process superficial hæmorrhages may result, and small ulcers may originate by the fusion of these superficial losses of substance.

Except histologically there is nothing distinctive in the hyperplasia of the lymph-follicles; but apart from enteric we rarely see in adults a marked affection of these glands with fever. In children, however, it is not uncommon when death has occurred from intestinal affections, and it is also met with in measles, diphtheria, and scarlet fever.

2. *Necrosis and Sloughing.*—When the hyperplasia of the lymph-follicles reaches a certain grade, resolution is no longer possible. The blood-vessels become choked, there is a condition of anæmic necrosis, and sloughs form which must be separated and thrown off. The necrosis is probably due in great part to the direct action of the bacilli. According to Mallory, there occurs a proliferation of endothelial cells due to the action of a toxin. These cells are phagocytic in character, and the swelling of the intestinal lymphoid tissue is due almost entirely to their formation. The necrosis, he thinks, is due to the occlusion of the veins and capillaries by fibrinous thrombi, which owe their origin to degeneration of phagocytic cells beneath the lining endothelium of the vessels. The process may be superficial, affecting only the upper part of the mucous coat, or it may extend to and involve the submucosa. The "slough" may sometimes lie upon the Peyer's patch, scarcely involving more than the epithelium (Marchand). It is always more intense toward the ileo-cæcal valve, and in very severe cases the greater part of the mucosa of the last foot of the ileum may be converted into a brownish-black eschar. The necrotic area in the solitary glands forms a yellowish cap which often involves only the most prominent point of a follicle. The extent of the necrosis is very variable. It may pass deep into the muscular coat, reaching to or even perforating the peritonæum.

3. *Ulceration.*—The separation of the necrotic tissue—the sloughing—is gradually effected from the edges inward, and results in the formation of an ulcer, the size and extent of which are directly proportionate to the amount of necrosis. If this be superficial, the entire thickness of the mucosa may not be involved and the loss of substance may be small and shallow. More commonly the slough in separating exposes the submucosa and muscularis, particularly the latter, which forms the floor of a majority of all typhoid ulcers. It is not common for an entire Peyer's patch to slough away, and a perfectly ovoid ulcer opposite to the mesentery is rarely seen. Irregularly oval and rounded forms are most common. A large patch may

present three or four ulcers divided by septa of mucous membrane. The terminal 6 or 8 inches of the mucous membrane of the ileum may form a large ulcer, in which are here and there islands of mucosa. The edges of the ulcer are usually swollen, soft, sometimes congested, and often undermined. At a late period the ulcers near the valve may have very irregular sinuous borders. The base of a typhoid ulcer is smooth and clean, being usually formed of the submucosa or of the muscularis.

There may be large ulcers near the valve and swollen hyperæmic patches of Peyer in the upper part of the ileum.

4. *Healing.*—This begins with the development of a thin granulation tissue which covers the base. Occasionally an appearance is seen as if an ulcer had healed in one place and was extending in another. The mucosa gradually extends from the edge, and a new growth of epithelium is formed. The glandular elements are reformed; the healed ulcer is somewhat depressed and is usually pigmented. In death during relapse healing ulcers may be seen in some patches with fresh ulcers in others.

We may say, indeed, that healing begins with the separation of the sloughs, as, when resolution is impossible, the removal of the necrosed part is the first step in the process of repair. In fatal cases, we seldom meet with evidences of cicatrization, as the majority of deaths occur before this stage is reached. It is remarkable that no matter how extensive the ulceration has been, healing is never associated with stricture, and typhoid fever does not appear as one of the causes of intestinal obstruction. Within a very short time all traces of the old ulcers disappear.

LARGE INTESTINE.—The cæcum and colon are affected in about one third of the cases.. Sometimes the solitary glands are greatly enlarged. The ulcers are usually larger in the cæcum than in the colon.

PERFORATION OF THE BOWEL.—*Incidence at Autopsy.*—J. A. Scott's figures, embracing 9,713 cases from recent English, Canadian, and American sources, give 351 deaths from perforation among 1,037 deaths from all causes, a percentage of 33.8 of the deaths and 3.6 of the cases. The German statistics give a much lower proportion of deaths from perforation; Munich in 2,000 autopsies, 5.7 per cent from perforation; Basle in 2,000 autopsies, 1.3 per cent from perforation; Hamburg in 3,686 autopsies, 1.2 per cent from perforation (Hector Mackenzie, Lancet, 1903). At the Johns Hopkins Hospital among 1,500 cases of typhoid fever there were 43 with perforation. Twenty of these were operated upon, with 7 recoveries. One other case died of the toxæmia on the eighth day after operation. At the Pennsylvania Hospital there were 50 cases of perforation among 1,948 cases. Chomel remarks that "the accident is sometimes the result of ulceration, sometimes of a true eschar, and sometimes it is produced by the distention of the intestine, causing the rupture of tissues weakened by disease." As a rule, sloughs are adherent about the site of perforation. The site is usually in the ileum, 232 times in Hector Mackenzie's collection of 264 cases; the jejunum twice, the large intestine 22 times, and the appendix 9 times in his series. As a rule, the perforation occurs within twelve inches of the ileo-cæcal valve. There may be two or three separate perforations. J. A. Scott describes two distinct varieties: first, the more common single, circular, pin-point in size, due to the extension of a necrotic process through the base of a small ulcer.

The second variety, produced by a large area of tissue becoming necrotic, ranges in size from the finger-tip to 3 cm. in diameter.

Death from hæmorrhage occurred in 99 of the Munich cases, and in 12 of 137 deaths in my 1,500 cases. The bleeding seems to result directly from the separation of the sloughs. I was not able in any instance to find the bleeding vessel. In one case only a single patch had sloughed, and a firm clot was adherent to it. The bleeding may also come from the soft swollen edges of the patch.

The *mesenteric glands* show hyperæmia and subsequently become greatly swollen. Spots of necrosis are common. In several of my cases suppuration had occurred, and in one a large abscess of the mesentery was present. The rupture of a softened or suppurating mesenteric gland, of which there are only five or six cases in the literature, may cause either fatal hæmorrhage or peritonitis. LeConte has successfully operated upon the latter condition. The bunch of glands in the mesentery, at the lower end of the ileum, is especially involved. The retroperitoneal glands are also swollen.

The *spleen* is invariably enlarged in the early stages of the disease. In 11 of my series it exceeded 20 ounces (600 grams) in weight, in one 900 grams. The tissue is soft, even diffluent. Infarction is not infrequent. Rupture may occur spontaneously or as a result of injury. In the Munich autopsies there were 5 instances of rupture of the spleen, one of which resulted from a gangrenous abscess.

The *bone-marrow* shows changes very similar to those in the lymphoid tissues, and there may be foci of necrosis (Longcope).

The *liver* shows signs of parenchymatous degeneration. Early in the disease it is hyperæmic, and in a majority of instances it is swollen, somewhat pale, on section turbid, and microscopically the cells are very granular and loaded with fat. Nodular areas (microscopic) occur in many cases, as described by Hanford. Reed, in Welch's laboratory, could not determine any relation between the groups of bacilli and these areas (Studies II). Some of the nodules are lymphoid, others are necrotic. In 12 of the Munich autopsies liver abscess was found, and in 3, acute yellow atrophy. In 2 of this series liver abscess occurred. Pylephlebitis may follow abscess of the mesentery or perforation of the appendix. Affections of the gall-bladder are not uncommon, and are fully described under the clinical features.

KIDNEYS.—Cloudy swelling, with granular degeneration of the cells of the convoluted tubules, less commonly an acute nephritis, may be present. Rayer, Wagner, and others described the occurrence of numerous small areas infiltrated with round cells, which may have the appearance of lymphomata, or may pass on to softening and suppuration, producing the so-called *miliary abscesses*, of which there were 7 cases in this series. The typhoid bacilli have been found in these areas. They may also be found in the urine. The kidneys in cases of typhoid bacilluria may show no changes other than cloudy swelling. Diphtheritic inflammation of the pelvis of the kidney may occur. It was present in 3 of my cases, in one of which the tips of the papillæ were also affected. Catarrh of the bladder is not uncommon. Diphtheritic inflammation of this viscus may also occur. Orchitis is occasionally met with.

RESPIRATORY ORGANS.—Ulceration of the larynx occurs in a certain number of cases; in the Munich series it was noted 107 times. It may come on at the same time as the ulceration in the ileum. It occurs in the posterior wall, at the insertion of the cords, at the base of the epiglottis, and on the ary-epiglottidean folds. The cartilages are very apt to become involved. In the later periods catarrhal and diphtheritic ulcers may be present.

Œdema of the glottis was present in 20 of the Munich cases, in 8 of which tracheotomy was performed. Diphtheritis of the pharynx and larynx is not very uncommon. It occurred in a most extensive form in 2 of my cases. Lobar pneumonia may be found early in the disease (see PNEUMO-TYPHUS), or it may be a late event. Hypostatic congestion and the condition of the lung spoken of as splenization are very common. Gangrene of the lung occurred in 40 cases in the Munich series; abscess of the lung in 14; hæmorrhagic infarction in 129. Pleurisy is not a very common event. Fibrinous pleurisy occurred in about 6 per cent of the Munich cases, and empyema in nearly 2 per cent.

CHANGES IN THE CIRCULATORY SYSTEM.—*Heart Lesions.*—*Endocarditis,* while not a common complication, is probably more frequent than is generally supposed. It was present without·being suspected in three out of 101 autopsies in this series, while in three other cases of my series the clinical symptoms suggested its presence. The typhoid bacilli have been found in the vegetations. *Pericarditis* was present in 14 cases of the Munich autopsies. *Myocarditis* is not very infrequent. In protracted cases the muscle-fibre is usually soft, flabby, and of a pale yellowish-brown color. The softening may be extreme, though rarely of the grade described by Stokes in typhus fever, in which, when held apex up by the vessels, the organ collapsed over the hand, forming a mushroom-like cap. Microscopically, the fibres may show little or no change, even when the impulse of the heart has been extremely feeble. A granular parenchymatous degeneration is common. Fatty degeneration may be present, particularly in long-standing cases with anæmia. The hyaline change is not common. The segmenting myocarditis, in which the cement substance is softened so that the muscles separate, has also been found, but probably as a post-mortem change.

Lesions of the Blood-vessels.—Changes in the arteries are not infrequent. In 21 of 52 cases in our series, in which there were notes on the state of the aorta, fresh endarteritis was present, and in 13 of 62 cases in which the condition of the coronary arteries was noted similar changes were found (Thayer). Arteritis of a peripheral vessel with thrombus formation is not uncommon. Bacilli have been found in the thrombi. The artery may be blocked by a thrombus of cardiac origin—an embolus—but in the great majority of instances they are autochthonous and due to arteritis, obliterating or partial. Thrombosis in the veins is very much more frequent than in the arteries, but is not such a serious event. It is most frequent in the femoral, and in the left more often than the right. The consequences are fully considered under the *symptoms.*

NERVOUS SYSTEM.—There are very few obvious changes met with. Meningitis is extremely rare. It occurred in only 11 of the 2,000 Munich cases. The exudation may be either serous, sero-fibrinous, or purulent, and typhoid bacilli have been isolated. Five cases of serous and one of purulent meningitis occurred in our series (Cole). Optic neuritis, which occurs sometimes in typhoid fever, has not, so far as I know, been described in connection with

29

the meningitis. The anatomical lesion of the aphasia—seen not infrequently in children—is not known, possibly it is an encephalitis. Parenchymatous changes have been met with in the peripheral nerves, and appear to be not very uncommon, even when there have been no symptoms of neuritis.

The *voluntary muscles* show, in certain instances, the changes described by Zenker, which occur, however, in all long-standing febrile affections, and are not peculiar to typhoid fever. The muscle substance within the sarcolemma undergoes either a granular degeneration or a hyaline transformation. The abdominal muscles, the adductors of the thighs, and the pectorals are most commonly involved. Rupture of a rectus abdominis has been found post mortem. Hæmorrhage may occur. Abscesses may develop in the muscles during convalescence.

Symptoms.—In a disease so complex as typhoid fever it will be well first to give a general description, and then to study more fully the symptoms, complications, and sequelæ according to the individual organs.

GENERAL DESCRIPTION.—The period of incubation lasts from " eight to fourteen days, sometimes twenty-three " (Clinical Society), during which there are feelings of lassitude and inaptitude for work. The onset is rarely abrupt. In the 1,500 cases there occurred at onset chills in 334, headache in 1,117, anorexia in 825, diarrhœa (without purgation) in 516, epistaxis in 323, abdominal pain in 443, constipation in 249, pain in right iliac fossa in 10. The patient at last takes to his bed, from which event, in a majority of cases, the definite onset of the disease may be dated. During the *first week* there is, in some cases (but by no means in all, as has long been taught), a steady rise in the fever, the evening record rising a degree or a degree and a half higher each day, reaching 103° or 104°. The pulse is rapid, from 100 to 110, full in volume, but of low tension and often dicrotic; the tongue is coated and white; the abdomen is slightly distended and tender. Unless the fever is high there is no delirium, but the patient complains of headache, and there may be mental confusion and wandering at night. The bowels may be constipated, or there may be two or three loose movements daily. ·Toward the end of the week the spleen becomes enlarged and the rash appears in the form of rose-colored spots, seen first on the skin of the abdomen. Cough and bronchitic symptoms are not uncommon at the outset.

In the *second week*, in cases of moderate severity, the symptoms become aggravated; the fever remains high and the morning remission is slight. The pulse is rapid and loses its dicrotic character. There is no longer headache, but there are mental torpor and dulness. The face looks heavy; the lips are dry; the tongue, in severe cases, becomes dry also. The abdominal symptoms, if present—diarrhœa, tympanites, and tenderness—become aggravated. Death may occur during this week, with pronounced nervous symptoms, or, toward the end of it, from hæmorrhage or perforation. In mild cases the temperature declines, and by the fourteenth day may be normal.

In the *third week*, in cases of moderate severity, the pulse ranges from 110 to 130; the temperature now shows marked morning remissions, and there is a gradual decline in the fever. The loss of flesh is now more noticeable, and the weakness is pronounced. Diarrhœa and meteorism may now occur for the first time. Unfavorable symptoms at this stage are the pulmonary complications, increasing feebleness of the heart, and pronounced delirium with muscular tremor. Special dangers are perforation and hæmorrhage.

With the *fourth week*, in a majority of instances, convalescence begins. The temperature gradually reaches the normal point, the diarrhœa stops, the tongue cleans, and the desire for food returns. In severe cases the fourth and even the fifth week may present an aggravated picture of the third; the patient grows weaker, the pulse is more rapid and feeble, the tongue dry, and the abdomen distended. He lies in a condition of profound stupor, with low muttering delirium and subsultus tendinum, and passes the fæces and urine involuntarily. Heart-failure and secondary complications are the chief dangers of this period.

In the *fifth and sixth weeks* protracted cases may still show irregular fever, and convalescence may not set in until after the fortieth day. In this period we meet with relapses in the milder forms or slight recrudescence of the fever. At this time, too, occur many of the complications and sequelæ.

SPECIAL FEATURES AND SYMPTOMS.—*Mode of Onset.*—As a rule, the symptoms come on insidiously, and the patient is unable to fix definitely the time at which he began to feel ill. The following are the most important deviations from this common course:

(*a*) *Onset with Pronounced, sometimes Sudden, Nervous Manifestations.* —Headache, of a severe and intractable nature, is by no means an infrequent initial symptom. Again, a severe facial neuralgia may for a few days put the practitioner off his guard. In cases in which the patients have kept about and, as they say, fought the disease, the very first manifestation may be pronounced delirium. Such patients may even leave home and wander about for days. In rare cases the disease sets in with the most intense cerebrospinal symptoms, simulating meningitis—severe headache, photophobia, retraction of the head, twitching of the muscles, and even convulsions. Occasionally drowsiness, stupor, and signs of basilar meningitis may exist for ten days or more before the characteristic symptoms develop; the onset may be with mania.

(*b*) *With Pronounced Pulmonary Symptoms.*—The initial bronchial catarrh may be of great severity and obscure the other features of the disease. More striking still are those cases in which the disease sets in with a single chill, with pain in the side and all the characteristic features of lobar pneumonia, or of acute pleurisy; or tuberculosis is suspected.

(*c*) *With Intense Gastro-intestinal Symptoms.*—The incessant vomiting and pain may lead to a suspicion of poisoning, or the case may be sent to the surgical wards for appendicitis.

(*d*) *With symptoms of an acute nephritis,* smoky or bloody urine, with much albumin and tube-casts.

(*e*) *Ambulatory Form.*—Deserving of especial mention are those cases of typhoid fever in which the patient keeps about and attempts to do work, or perhaps takes a long journey to his home. He may come under observation for the first time with a temperature of 104° or 105°, and with the rash well out. Many of these cases run a severe course, and in general hospitals they contribute largely to the total mortality. Finally, there are rare instances in which typhoid is unsuspected until perforation, or a profuse hæmorrhage from the bowels occurs.

FACIAL ASPECT.—Early in the disease the cheeks are flushed and the eyes bright. Toward the end of the first week the expression becomes more listless, and when the disease is well established the patient has a dull and heavy look. There is never the rapid anæmia of malarial fever, and the color of the lips and cheeks may be retained even to the third week.

FEVER.—(a) *Regular Course.* (Chart II.)—In the stage of invasion the fever rises steadily during the first five or six days. The evening temperature is about a degree or a degree and a half higher than the morning remission, so that a temperature of 104° or 105° is not uncommon by the end of the first week. Having reached the fastigium or height, the fever then persists with very slight daily remissions. The fever may be singularly persistent and but little influenced by bathing or other measures. At the end of the second and throughout the third week the temperature becomes more distinctly remittent. The difference between the morning or evening record may be 3° or 4°, and the morning temperature may even be normal. It falls by lysis, and the temperature is not considered normal until the evening record is at 98.2°.

(b) Variations from the typical temperature curve are common. We do not always see the gradual step-like ascent in the early stage; the cases do not often come under observation at this time. When the disease sets in with a chill, or in children with a convulsion, the temperature may rise at once to 103° or 104°. In many cases defervescence occurs at the end of the second week and the temperature may fall rapidly, reaching the normal within twelve or twenty hours. An inverse type of temperature, high in the morning and low in the evening, is occasionally seen but has no especial significance.

Sudden falls in the temperature may occur; thus, as shown in Chart IV, a drop of 6.4° may follow an intestinal hæmorrhage, and the fall may be very apparent even before the blood has appeared in the stools. Sometimes during the anæmia which follows a severe hæmorrhage from the bowels there are remarkable oscillations in the temperature. Hyperpyrexia is rare. In only 58 of 1,500 cases did the fever rise above 106°. Before death the fever may rise; the highest I have known was 109.5°.

(c) *Post-typhoid Variations.* (1) *Recrudescences.*—After a normal temperature of perhaps five or six days, the fever may rise suddenly to 102° or 103°, without constitutional disturbance, furring of the tongue, or abdominal symptoms. After persisting for from two to four days the temperature falls. Of 1,500 cases, 92 presented these post-typhoid elevations, brief notes of which are given in the Studies on Typhoid Fever. Constipation, errors in diet, or excitement may cause them. These attacks are a frequent source of anxiety to the practitioner. They are very common, and it is not always possible to say upon what they depend. As a rule, if the rise in temperature is the result of the onset of a complication, such as pleurisy or thrombosis, there is an increase in the leucocytes. Naturally one suspects at the outset a relapse, but there is an absence of the step-like ascent, and as a rule the fever falls after lasting a few days.

(2) *The Sub-febrile Stage of Convalescence.*—In children, in very nervous patients, and in cases with anæmia, the evening temperature may keep up for weeks after the tongue has cleaned and the appetite has returned. This may usually be disregarded, and is often best treated by allowing the

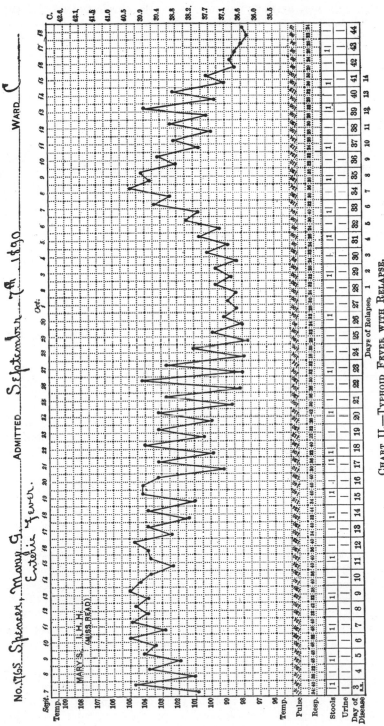

CHART II.—TYPHOID FEVER WITH RELAPSE.

33

patient to get up, and by stopping the use of the thermometer. Of course it is important not to overlook any latent complications.

(3) *Hypothermia.*—Low temperatures in typhoid fever are common, following the tubs, or spontaneously in the third and fourth week in the periods of marked remissions, and following hæmorrhage. An interesting form is the persistent hypothermia of convalescence. For ten days or more, particularly in the protracted cases with great emaciation, the temperature may be 96.5° or 97°. It is of no special significance.

(d) *The Fever of the Relapse.*—This is a repetition in many instances of the original fever, a gradual ascent and maintenance for a few days at a certain height and then a gradual decline. It is shorter than the original pyrexia, and rarely continues more than two or three weeks. (Chart II.)

(e) *Afebrile Typhoid.*—There are cases described in which the chief features of the disease have been present without the existence of fever. They are extremely rare in this country. I have seen a case, afebrile at the thirteenth day, and in which the rose spots and other features persisted till the twenty-eighth day.

(f) *Chills* occur (a) sometimes with the fever of onset; (b) occasionally at intervals throughout the course of the disease, and followed by sweats (so-called sudoral form); (c) with the advent of complications, pleurisy, pneumonia, otitis media, periostitis, etc.; (d) with active antipyretic treatment by the coal-tar remedies; (e) occasionally during the period of defervescence without relation to any complication or sequel, probably due to a septic infection; (f) according to Herringham, chills may result from constipation. There are cases in which throughout the latter half of the disease chills recur with great severity. (See Chills in Typhoid Fever, Studies II.)

SKIN.—The characteristic rash of the disease consists of hyperæmic spots, which appear from the seventh to the tenth day, usually at first upon the abdomen. They are slightly raised, flattened papules, which can be felt distinctly by the finger, of a rose-red color, disappearing on pressure, and ranging in diameter from 2 to 4 mm. They were present in 93.2 per cent of the white patients and 20.6 per cent of the colored. They come out in successive crops, and after persisting for two or three days they disappear, occasionally leaving a brownish stain. The spots may be present upon the back, and not upon the abdomen. The eruption may be very abundant over the whole skin of the trunk, and on the extremities. There were 81 in which they occurred on the arms, 17 on the forearms, 43 on the thighs, legs 15, face 5, hands 3. The cases with very abundant eruption are not necessarily more severe. As already noted, the typhoid bacilli have been found in the spots. Of variations in the rash, frequently the spots are capped by small vesicles. Cases that have not been carefully sponged may show sweat vesicles, either miliary or sudaminal. In 38 cases in my series there were purpuric spots. Three of the cases were true hæmorrhagic typhoid fever. The rash may not appear until the relapse. In 21 cases in our series the rose spots came out after the patient was afebrile.

A branny desquamation is not rare in children, and common in adults after hydrotherapy. Occasionally the skin peels off in large flakes.

Among other skin lesions in typhoid fever the following may be mentioned:

Erythema.—It is not very uncommon in the first week of the disease to find a diffuse erythematous blush—E. typhosum. Formerly we thought this might be due to quinine.

The *tache cérébrale,* a red line with white borders, is readily produced by drawing the nail over the skin, a vaso-motor phenomenon of no special significance. Sometimes the skin may have a peculiar mottled pink and white appearance. E. exudativum, E. nodosum, and urticaria may be present.

Herpes.—Herpes is certainly rare in typhoid fever in comparison with its great frequency in malarial fever and in pneumonia. It was noted in 20 of our 1,500 cases, usually on the lips.

The *taches bleuâtres—Peliomata—Maculæ cerulæ.*—These are pale-blue or steel-gray spots, subcuticular, from 4 to 10 mm. in diameter, of irregular outline and most abundant about the chest, abdomen, and thighs. They sometimes give a very striking appearance to the skin. They are due to lice (see PEDICULOSIS).

Skin Gangrene.—In children noma may occur; as reported by McFarland in the Philadelphia epidemic of 1898 there were many cases with multiple areas of gangrene of the skin. The nose, ears, and genitals may be attacked.

Sweats.—At the height of the fever the skin is usually dry. Profuse sweating is rare, but it is not very uncommon to see the abdomen or chest moist with perspiration, particularly in the reaction which follows the bath. Sweats in some instances constitute a striking feature of the disease. They may occasionally be associated with chilly sensations or actual chills. Jaccoud and others in France have especially described this *sudoral* form of typhoid fever. There may be recurring paroxysms of chill, fever, and sweats (even several in twenty-four hours), and the case may be mistaken for one of intermittent fever. The fever toward the end of the second week and during the third week may be intermittent. The characteristic rash is usually present, and, if absent, the negative condition of the blood is sufficient to exclude malaria. The sweating may occur chiefly in the third and fourth weeks.

Œdema of the skin occurs: 1. As the result of vascular obstruction, most commonly of a vein, as in thrombosis of the femoral vein. 2. In connection with nephritis, very rarely. 3. In association with the anæmia and cachexia. A yellow color of the palms of the hands and of the soles of the feet is not uncommon. *The hair* falls out after the attack, but complete baldness is rare. I have once seen permanent baldness. The nutrition of the nails suffers, and during and after convalescence transverse ridges may occur. A peculiar *odor* is exhaled from the skin in some cases. Whether due to a cutaneous exhalation or not, there certainly is a very distinctive smell connected with many patients. Nathan Smith describes it as of a " semi-cadaverous, musty character."

Lineæ atrophicæ.—Lines of atrophy may appear on the skin of the abdomen and lateral aspects of the thighs, similar to those seen after pregnancy. They have been attributed to neuritis, and Duckworth has reported a case in which the skin adjacent to them was hyperæsthetic.

Bed-sores are not uncommon in protracted cases, with great emaciation. As a rule, they result from pressure and are seen upon the sacrum, more rarely the ilia, the shoulders, and the heels. These are less common, I think, since the introduction of hydrotherapy. Scrupulous care and watchfulness do much for their prevention, but it is to be remembered that in cases with profound involvement of the nerve centres acute bed-sores of the back and heels may occur with very slight pressure, and with astonishing rapidity.

Boils constitute a common and troublesome sequel of the disease. They appear to be more frequent after hydrotherapy.

CIRCULATORY SYSTEM.—The *blood* presents important changes. The following statements are based on studies which W. S. Thayer has made in my wards (Studies I and III): During the first two weeks there may be little or no change in the blood. Profuse sweats or copious diarrhœa may, as Hayem has shown, cause the corpuscles—as in the collapse stage of cholera —to rise above normal. In the third week a fall usually takes place in corpuscles and hæmoglobin, and the number may sink rapidly even to 1,300,000 per c. mm., gradually rising to normal during convalescence. When the patient first gets up, there may be a slight fall in the number of corpuscles. The average maximum loss is about 1,000,000 to the c. mm.

The amount of hæmoglobin is always reduced, and usually in a greater relative proportion than the number of red corpuscles, and during recovery the normal color standard is reached at a later period. Leucopenia— hypoleucocytosis—is present throughout the course. Cold baths increase temporarily the number of leucocytes in the peripheral circulation. The absence of leucocytosis may be at times of real diagnostic value in distinguishing typhoid fever from various septic fevers and acute inflammatory processes. The polymorphonuclear leucocytes are normal in number, while the lymphocytes are relatively increased. When an acute inflammatory process occurs in typhoid fever the leucocytes show an increase in the polynuclear forms, and this may be of great diagnostic moment.

The accompanying blood-chart shows these changes well. (Chart III.)

The post-typhoid anæmia may reach an extreme grade. In one of my cases the blood-corpuscles sank to 1,300,000 per c. mm. and the hæmoglobin to about 20 per cent. These severe grades of anæmia are not common in my experience. In the Munich statistics there were 54 cases with general and extreme anæmia.

Of changes in the blood plasma very little is known.

The *pulse* in typhoid fever presents no special characters. It is increased in rapidity, but not always in proportion to the height of the fever, and this may be a very special feature in the early stages. As a rule, in the first week it is above 100, full in volume and often dicrotic. There is no acute disease with which, in the early stage, a dicrotic pulse is so frequently associated. Even with high fever the pulse may not be greatly accelerated. As the disease progresses the pulse becomes more rapid, feebler, and small. In 6 per cent of our cases the pulse rate rose above 140 (Thayer). In the extreme prostration of severe cases it may reach 150 or more, and is a mere undulation—the so-called running pulse. The lowered arterial pressure is manifest in the dusky lividity of the skin and coldness of the hands and feet.

During convalescence the pulse gradually returns to normal, and occasionally becomes very slow. After no other acute fever do we so frequently meet with bradycardia. I have counted the pulse as low as 30, and instances are on record of still fewer beats to the minute. Tachycardia, while

less common, may be a very troublesome and persistent feature of convalescence.

Blood Pressure.—This is usually from 115–125 m. m. Hg. (Riva-Rocci
instrument) in systole. The diastolic pressure has the normal relationship
to the systolic, and averages 85–100 m. m. Hg. There is a gradual fall during
the course to about 100–110 m. m. Hg. at the beginning of apyrexia. In two

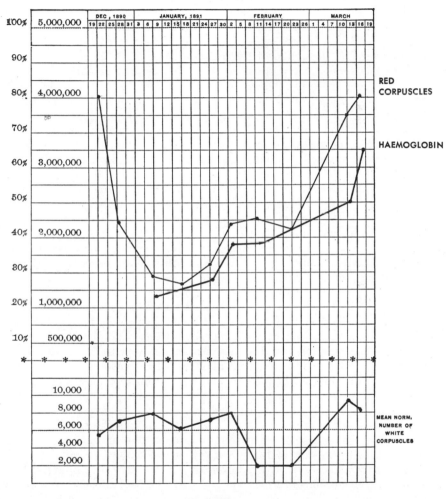

CHART III.

or three weeks later the pressure has usually returned to normal. Hæmorrhage usually produces a marked fall both in the systolic and diastolic pressure. In some cases of perforation there is a sharp rise in systolic pressure.
Tubs and ice sponges usually cause a rise of 10–20 m. m. Hg.

The *heart-sounds* may be normal throughout the course. In severe cases,
the first sound becomes feeble and there is often to be heard, at the apex and
along the left sternal margin, a soft systolic murmur, which was present in

22 per cent of our cases. Absence of the first sound is rare. Gallop rhythm is not uncommon. In the extreme feebleness of the graver forms, the first and second sound become very similar, and the long pause is much shortened (embryocardia).

Of cardiac complications, *pericarditis* is rare and has been met with chiefly in children and in association with pneumonia. It was present in three of my series and occurred in only 14 of the 2,000 Munich post mortems. *Endocarditis* was found post mortem in three cases, and the physical signs suggested its presence in three other cases in the series. *Myocarditis* is more common, and is indicated by a progressive weakening of the heart-sound and enfeeblement of the action of the organ.

Complications in the Arteries.—Arteritis with thrombus formation occurred in four cases in the series, one in the branches of the middle cerebral, two in the femoral, and one in the brachial. In one case gangrene of the leg followed. I saw a similar case with Roddick, in Montreal, in which obliteration of the left femoral artery occurred on the sixteenth day, and of the vessel on the right side on the twentieth day, with gangrene of both feet. Pain, tenderness, and swelling occur over the artery, with diminution of disappearance of the pulsations and coldness and blueness of the extremity. In two of the cases these symptoms gradually disappeared, and the pulsation returned not only in the peripheral, but in the affected vessels (Thayer). Keen refers to 46 cases of arterial gangrene, of which 8 were bilateral, 19 on the right side, and 19 on the left.

Thrombi in the Veins.—In our series there were 41 instances, distributed in the following veins: femoral 23, popliteal 5, iliac 5, veins of the calf 5, internal saphenous 3, pulmonary artery alone 1, pulmonary artery and common iliac 1, axillary vein 1 (Thayer). I saw one case in the right circumflex iliac vein. Femoral thrombosis is the most common, and almost invariably in the left vessel, due, as Liebermeister suggests, to the fact that the left iliac vein is crossed by the right iliac artery, and the blood flow is not so free. The symptoms of this complication are very definite—the fever may increase or recur. Chills occurred in 11 of all the cases. Pain and swelling at the site are constantly present, and the thrombotic mass can be felt, not always at first, nor is it well to feel for it. Swelling of the leg follows as a rule, but it is rarely so extreme, and never, I think, so painful as the puerperal phlegmasia alba dolens. In the iliac thrombosis the pain may be severe and lead to the suspicion of perforation, as in one of our cases. Leucocytosis is usually present, in 12 cases it rose above 10,000. Five of the 39 cases died, 2 only as a result of the thrombus; in the case of axillary thrombosis from pulmonary embolism, in one embolism of the inferior cava and right auricle from the dislocation of a piece of thrombus from the left iliac vein. Thayer examined 16 of the patients at varying periods after convalescence, and found in every case more or less disability from the varices and persistent swelling. In some cases, however, the recovery is complete.

DIGESTIVE SYSTEM.—Loss of appetite is early, and, as a rule, the relish for food is not regained until convalescence. Thirst is constant, and should be fully and freely gratified. Even when the mind becomes benumbed and the patient no longer asks for water, it should be freely given. The *tongue* presents the changes inevitable in a prolonged fever. Early in the disease it is moist, swollen, and coated with a thin white fur, which, as the fever progresses, becomes denser. It may remain moist throughout. It is small in size and tends to be red at the edges and tip. In severe cases, particularly those with delirium, the tongue becomes very dry, partly owing to the fact that such patients breathe with the mouth open. It may be covered with a brown or brownish-black fur, or with crusts between which are cracks and fissures. Acute glossitis occurred in one case at the onset of the relapse. In these cases the teeth and lips may be covered with a dark brownish matter called *sordes*—a mixture of food, epithelial *débris,* and micro-organisms. By keeping the mouth and tongue clean from the outset the fissures, which are extremely painful, may be prevented. During convalescence the tongue gradually becomes clean, and the fur is thrown off, almost imperceptibly or occasionally in flakes.

The secretion of saliva is often diminished; salivation is rare.

Parotitis was present in 45 of the 2,000 Munich cases. It occurred in 14 cases in my series; of these, 5 died. It is most frequent in the third week in very severe cases. Extensive sloughing may follow in the tissues of the neck. Usually unilateral, and in a majority of cases going on to suppuration, it is regarded as a very fatal complication, but recovery has followed in eight of my cases. It undoubtedly may arise from extension of inflammation along Steno's duct. This is probably not so serious a form as when it arises from metastatic inflammation. In four cases the submaxillary glands were involved alone, in one a cellulitis of the neck extended from the gland and proved fatal. Parotitis may occur after the fever has subsided. A remarkable localized sweating in the parotid region is an occasional sequel of the abscess.

The *pharynx* may be the seat of slight catarrh. Sometimes the fauces are deeply congested. Membranous pharyngitis, a serious and fatal complication, may come on in the third week. Difficulty in swallowing may result from ulcers of the œsophagus, and in one of our cases stricture followed.* Thyroiditis may occur with abscess formation.

The *gastric symptoms* are extremely variable. Nausea and vomiting are not common. There are instances, however, in which vomiting, resisting all measures, is a marked feature from the outset, and may directly cause death from exhaustion. Vomiting does not often occur in the second and third weeks, unless associated with some serious complication. Ulcers have been found in the stomach. Hæmatemesis occurred in 4 of our cases.

Intestinal Symptoms.—Diarrhœa is a very variable symptom, occurring in from 20 to 30 per cent of the cases. Of 1,500 cases, 516 had diarrhœa before entering, 260 during their stay in hospital. The small percentage may be due to the fact that we use no purges or intestinal antiseptics. Its absence must not be taken as an indication that the intestinal lesions are of slight extent. I have seen, on several occasions, the most extensive infiltration and ulceration of the Peyer's glands of the small intestine, with the colon filled with solid fæces. The diarrhœa is caused less by the ulcers than by the associated catarrh, and, as in.tuberculosis, it is probable that when this is in the large intestine the discharges are more frequent. It is most common toward

---

* Mitchell, Œsophageal Complications in Typhoid Fever (Studies II).

the end of the first and throughout the second week, but it may not occur until the third or even the fourth week. The number of discharges ranges from 3 to 8 or 10 in the twenty-four hours. They are usually abundant, thin, grayish-yellow, granular, of the consistency and appearance of pea-soup, and resemble very much, as Addison remarked, the normal contents of the small bowel. The reaction is alkaline and the odor offensive. On standing, the discharges separate into a thin serous layer, containing albumin and salts, and a lower stratum, consisting of epithelial *débris*, remnants of food, and numerous crystals of triple phosphates. Blood may be in small amount, and only recognized by the microscope. Sloughs of the Peyer's glands occur either as grayish-yellow fragments or occasionally as ovoid masses, an inch or more in length, in which portions of the bowel tissue may be found. The bacilli are not found in the stools until the end of the first or the middle of the second week. Constipation was present in 51 per cent of the cases.

Hæmorrhage from the bowels is a serious complication, occurring in from 3 to 5 per cent of all cases. It had occurred in 99 of the 2,000 fatal Munich cases. In 1,500 cases treated in my wards, hæmorrhage occurred in 118, and in 12 death occurred directly from the hæmorrhage. It was present in 3.77 per cent of Murchison's 1,564 cases. There may be only a slight trace of blood in the stools, but too often it is a profuse, free hæmorrhage, which rapidly proves fatal. It occurs most commonly between the end of the second and the beginning of the fourth week, the time of the separation of the sloughs. Occasionally it results simply from the intense hyperæmia. It usually comes on without warning. A sensation of sinking or collapse is experienced by the patient, the temperature falls, and may, as in the annexed chart, drop 6° or 7° in a few hours. Fatal collapse may supervene before the blood appears in the stool. Hæmorrhage usually occurs in cases of considerable severity. Graves and Trousseau held that it was not a very dangerous symptom, but statistics show that death follows in from 30 to 50 per cent of the cases.

It must not be forgotten that melæna may also be part of a general hæmorrhagic tendency (to be referred to later), in which case it is associated with petechiæ and hæmaturia. There may be a special family predisposition to intestinal hæmorrhages in typhoid fever.

Meteorism, a frequent symptom, is not serious if of moderate grade, but when excessive is usually of ill omen. Owing to defective tone in the walls, in severe cases to their infiltration with serum, gas accumulates in the small and large bowels, particularly in the latter. Pushing up the diaphragm, it interferes very much with the action of the heart and lungs, and may also favor perforation. Gurgling in the right iliac fossa exists in a large proportion of all the cases, and indicates simply the presence of gas and fluid fæces in the colon and cæcum.

Abdominal pain and tenderness were present in three-fifths of a series of 500 cases studied with special reference to the point by T. McCrae. In some it was only present at the onset. Pain occurred during the course in about one-third of the cases. This is due in some instances to conditions apart from the bowel lesions, such as pleurisy, distention of the bladder, and phlebitis. It may be associated with diarrhœa, severe constipation, a painful spleen, or acute abdominal complications. Pain occurs with some cases of hæmorrhage, but is most constantly present with perforation. In a large group no cause could be found for the pain, and if other symptoms be associated the condition may lead to error in diagnosis. Operation for appendicitis has been performed in the early stage of typhoid fever, owing to the combination of pain in the right iliac fossa, fever and constipation. This has happened twice at the Johns Hopkins Hospital.

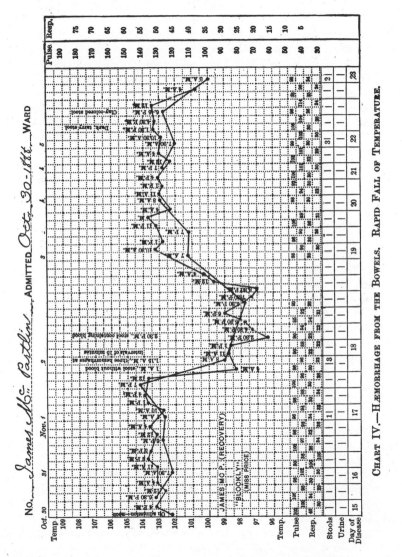

CHART IV.—HÆMORRHAGE FROM THE BOWELS. RAPID FALL OF TEMPERATURE.

PERFORATION.—From one-fourth to one-third of the deaths are due to perforation, and as there were 35,379 deaths from typhoid fever in the United States in the year 1900, this gives between 9,000 and 12,000 deaths from this cause. Watchful care on the part of the physician should result in a saving of at least one-third of the cases. While it may occur as early as the

7

first week, in the great majority it is at the height of the disease in the third week, and much more frequently in the severe cases, particularly those associated with tympanites and hæmorrhage. It may occur, however, in very mild cases and with great suddenness, when the patient is apparently progressing favorably.

Symptoms of Perforation.—By far the most important single indication is a sudden, sharp pain of increasing severity, often paroxysmal in character. It is rarely absent, except in the small group of cases with profound toxæmia. The situation is most frequent in the hypogastric region and to the right of the middle line. Tenderness on pressure is present in the great majority of cases, usually in the hypogastric and right iliac regions, sometimes diffuse; it may only be brought out on deep pressure. As LeConte points out, when the perforation happens to be in contact with the parietal peritonæum the local features on palpation are much more marked than when the perforated ulcer is next to a coil or to the mesentery. There may be early irritability of the bladder, with frequent micturition, and pain extending toward the penis. A third important sign is muscle rigidity, increased tension, and spasm on any attempt to palpate. With the onset of these features the patient may have signs of shock—a fall in temperature, an increase in the rapidity of the pulse and respirations, and slight sweating. Following these features in a few hours there is usually a reaction, and then the features of general peritonitis become manifest to a more or less marked degree. Among the general features, the facies of the patient shows changes; there is increased pallor, a pinched expression of the face, and as the symptoms progress and toward the end a marked Hippocratic facies, a dusky suffusion, and the forehead bathed in a clammy perspiration. The temperature, which often drops at the onset of a perforation, rises with the increase of the peritonitis. The pulse quickens, is running and thready, the heart's action becomes progressively more feeble, and there is an increase in the frequency of the respiration. Vomiting is a variable feature; it is present in a majority of the cases. Hiccough is common and may occur early, but more frequently late.

The local abdominal features are often more important than the general, as it is surprising to notice how excellent the condition of a patient may be with perforative peritonitis. Limitation of the respiratory movements is usually present, perhaps confined to the hypogastric area. Increasing distention is the rule, but perforation and peritonitis may occur, it is to be remembered, with an abdomen flat or even scaphoid. Increasing pain on pressure, increasing muscle spasm and tension of the wall are important signs. Percussion may reveal a flat note in the flanks, due to exudate. Auscultation may show absence of peristalsis, and auscultatory percussion may possibly show the presence of air free in the peritonæum. A friction may be present within a few hours of the onset of the perforation. Obliteration of the liver flatness in the nipple line may be caused by excessive tympany. Rapid obliteration of liver flatness in a flat, or a not much distended abdomen, is a valuable sign. Examination of the rectum may show fullness in the pelvis, or tenderness.

In a majority of all cases there is a rise in the leucocytes, and when present may be a valuable help, but it is not constant.

General peritonitis, without perforation of the bowel, may occur by extension from an ulcer, or by rupture of a softened mesenteric gland, or, as in one recent case in my series, from inflammation of the Fallopian tubes. It was present in 2.2 per cent of the Munich autopsies.

Perforation is almost invariably fatal. In a few cases healing takes place spontaneously, as is beautifully shown in one of the Pennsylvania Hospital specimens, or the orifice may be closed by a tag of omentum, as in a remarkable case reported by J. Milton Miller.

There is a group of cases in which hæmorrhage complicates the perforation and adds to the difficulty in diagnosis. In 7 of our 43 cases hæmorrhage accompanied the perforation; in 3 others the hæmorrhage had occurred some days before.

The diagnosis of perforation, easy enough at times, is not without serious difficulties. The conditions for which it has been mistaken in my wards have been: appendicitis, occurring during the course of the typhoid fever, phlebitis of the iliac vein with great pain, hæmorrhage, and in one case a local peritonitis without perforation, for which no cause was found. Recovery followed the exploratory operation, which was made in all but one (hæmorrhage case) of these cases.

The SPLEEN is usually enlarged, and the edge was felt below the costal margin in 71.6 per cent of my cases. Percussion is uncertain, as, owing to distention of the stomach and colon, even the normal area of dulness may not be obtainable. I have seen a very large spleen post mortem, when during life the increase in size was not observable.

LIVER.—Symptoms on the part of this organ are rare.

(*a*) *Jaundice* was present in only 8 cases of my series. Catarrh of the ducts, toxæmia, abscess, and occasionally gall-stones are the usual causes.

(*b*) *Abscess.*—Solitary abscess is exceedingly rare and occurred in but 3 cases in my series. It may follow the intestinal lesion or more commonly one of the complications, as parotitis or necrosis of bone. Suppurative pylephlebitis, which is more frequent than abscess, may follow perforation of the appendix. Suppurative cholangitis has been described.

(*c*) *Cholecystitis* occurred in 19 cases of the series. Camac * has collected 115 cases, in 21 of which perforation occurred. Pain in the region of the gall-bladder is the most constant symptom. Tenderness, muscle spasm with rigidity, and a gall-bladder tumor are present in a majority of the cases. Jaundice is inconstant. With perforation there may be a marked drop in the fever and the onset of signs of peritonitis. In simple cholecystitis the urgency of the symptoms may abate, and recovery may follow. Suppuration may occur with infection of the bile passages. Months or years after (eighteen years in Hunner's case) the bacilli may cause cholecystitis or gall-stones. Typhoid bacilli have been found by Cushing as a cause of cholecystitis in a patient who had never had typhoid fever.

(*d*) *Gall-Stones.*—Bernheim called attention to the frequency of cholelithiasis after typhoid fever. It is probably associated with the presence of typhoid bacilli in the gall-bladder (see under Gall-Stones).

---

* Studies in Typhoid Fever, Series III, Johns Hopkins Hospital Reports, vol. viii.

RESPIRATORY SYSTEM.—*Epistaxis*, an early symptom, precedes typhoid fever more commonly than any other febrile affection. It is occasionally profuse and serious.

Laryngitis is not very common. The ulcers and the perichondritis have already been described. Œdema, apart from ulceration, is rare. In the United States the laryngeal complications of typhoid fever seem much less frequent than on the Continent. I have twice seen severe perichondritis; both of the cases recovered, one after the expectoration of large portions of the thyroid cartilage.

Keen and Lüning have collected 221 cases of serious surgical complications of the larynx. General emphysema may follow the perforation of an ulcer. Stenosis is a very serious sequence.

From some recent studies it would appear that paralysis of the laryngeal muscles is much more common than we have supposed. Przedborski (Volkmann's Sammlung, No. 182) has systematically examined the larynx in 100 consecutive cases and found 25 with paralysis. The condition is nearly always due to neuritis, sometimes in connection with affections of other nerves.

Bronchitis is one of the most frequent initial symptoms. It is indicated by the presence of sibilant râles. The smaller tubes may be involved, producing urgent cough and even slight cyanosis. Collapse and lobular pneumonia may also occur.

Lobar pneumonia is met with under two conditions:

1. At the outset the *pneumo-typhus* of the Germans. This occurred in three of our cases. After an indisposition of a day or so, the patient is seized with a chill, has high fever, pain in the side, and within forty-eight hours there are signs of consolidation and the evidences of an ordinary lobar pneumonia. The intestinal symptoms may not occur until toward the end of the first week or later; the pulmonary symptoms persist, crisis does not occur; the aspect of the patient changes, and by the end of the second week the clinical picture is that of typhoid fever. Spots may then be present and doubts as to the nature of the case are solved. In other instances, in the absence of a characteristic eruption, the case remains doubtful, and it is impossible to say whether the disease has been pneumonia, in which the so-called typhoid symptoms have developed, or whether it was typhoid fever with early implication of the lungs. This condition may depend upon an early localization of the typhoid bacillus in the lung.

2. Lobar pneumonia forms a serious and by no means infrequent complication of the second or third week—in 19 of our cases. It was present in over 8 per cent of the Munich cases. The symptoms are usually not marked. There may be no rusty sputa, and, unless sought for, the condition is frequently overlooked. The etiological agent in these cases is still in dispute. Typhoid bacilli have been isolated from the sputum by Jehle, Rau, and others. They have also been isolated from the consolidated lungs at autopsy, but in such cases the pneumococci may have been originally present, and the typhoid bacilli secondary invaders. In all cases of pneumonia during typhoid fever occurring in the Johns Hopkins Hospital and coming to autopsy, the pneumococci could be demonstrated in the consolidated lung. Infarction, abscess, and gangrene are occasionally pulmonary complications.

Hypostatic congestion of the lungs and œdema, due to enfeebled circulation in the later periods of the disease, are very common. The physical signs are defective resonance at the bases, feeble breath-sounds, and, on deep inspiration, moist râles.

Hæmoptysis may occur. Creagh reports a case in which it caused death.

Pleurisy was present in about 8 per cent of the Munich autopsies. It may occur at the outset—pleuro-typhoid—or slowly during convalescence, in which case it is almost always purulent and due to the typhoid bacilli.

Pneumothorax is rare. Hale White has reported two cases, in both of which pleurisy existed. After death, no lesions of the lungs or bronchi were discovered. The condition may be due to straining, or to the rupture of a small pyæmic abscess. It may occur also during convalescence.

NERVOUS SYSTEM.—*Cerebro-spinal Form.*—As already noted, the disease may set in with intense and persisting headache, or an aggravated form of neuralgia. There are cases in which the effect of the poison is manifested on the nervous system early and with the greatest intensity. There are headache, photophobia, retraction of the neck, marked twitchings of the muscles, rigidity, and even convulsions. In such cases the diagnosis of meningitis is invariably made. The cases showing marked *meningeal features* during the course of the disease may be divided into three groups. First, those with symptoms suggestive of meningitis, but without localizing features and without at post mortem the anatomical lesions of meningitis. In every series of cases numerous such examples occur. Secondly, the cases of so-called serous meningitis. There is a localization of typhoid bacilli in the cerebro-spinal fluid and a mild inflammatory reaction, but without suppurative meningitis. Cole has collected thirteen such cases, five of them occurring in our series. Probably more frequent lumbar punctures will show that this occurs not infrequently. Thirdly, true typhoid suppurative meningitis due to B. typhosus. Only one such case occurred in our series, and Cole has collected thirteen from the literature. Meningitis in typhoid fever is occasionally due to other organisms, as tubercle bacilli, and the micrococcus intracellularis. Marked convulsive movements, local or general, with coma and delirium, are seen also in thrombosis of the cerebral veins and sinuses.

Delirium, usually present in very severe cases, is certainly less frequent under a rigid plan of hydrotherapy. It may exist from the outset, but usually does not occur until the second and sometimes not until the third week. It may be slight and only nocturnal. It is, as a rule, a quiet delirium, though there are cases in which the patient is very noisy and constantly tries to get out of bed, and, unless carefully watched, may escape. The patient does not often become maniacal. In heavy drinkers the delirium may have the character of delirium tremens. Even in cases which have no positive delirium, the mental processes are usually dulled and the aspect is listless and apathetic. In severe cases the patient passes into a condition of unconsciousness. The eyes may be open, but he is oblivious to all surrounding circumstances and neither knows nor can indicate his wants. The urine and fæces are passed involuntarily. In this pseudo-wakeful state, or coma vigil, as it is called, the eyes are open and the patient is constantly muttering. The lips and tongue are tremulous; there are twitchings of the fingers and wrists—subsultus tendinum and carphologia. He picks at the bedclothes or grasps at invisible objects. These are among the most serious symptoms of the disease and always indicate danger.

Convulsions in typhoid fever are rare. There were 8 instances in sixteen years among between fifteen and sixteen hundred cases. They occur: first, at the onset of the disease, particularly in children; secondly, as a manifestation of the toxæmia; and thirdly, as a result of severe cerebral complications—thrombosis, meningitis, or acute encephalitis. Occasionally in convalescence convulsions may occur from unknown causes. Of the 8 cases 3 died.

Neuritis, which is not uncommon—11 cases in the series—may be local, or a wide-spread affection of the nerves of the legs or of both arms and legs.

Local Neuritis.—This may occur during the height of the fever or after convalescence is established. It may set in with agonizing pain, and with sensitiveness of the affected nerve trunks. The local neuritis may affect the nerves of an arm or of a leg, and involve chiefly the extensors, so that there is wrist-drop or foot-drop. The arm or leg may be much swollen and the skin over it erythematous. *Painful muscles* are not uncommon, particularly in the calves. I have reported a series of cases (Studies III). Painful cramps may also occur. In some of the cases of painful legs the condition is a myositis; in others the swelling and pain may be due to thrombosis in the deeper veins.

A curious condition, probably a local neuritis, is that which was first described by Handford as *tender toes,* and which appears to be much more common after the cold-bath treatment. The tips and pads of the toes, rarely the pads at their bases, become exquisitely sensitive, so that the patient can not bear the weight of the bedclothes. There is no discoloration and no swelling, and it disappears usually within a week or ten days.

Multiple neuritis in typhoid fever comes on usually during convalescence. The legs may be affected, or the four extremities. The cases are often difficult to differentiate from those with subacute poliomyelitis. Recovery is the rule.

Poliomyelitis may occur with the symptoms of acute ascending paralysis and prove fatal in a few days. More frequently it is less acute, and causes either a paraplegia or a limited atrophic paralysis of one arm or leg.

Hemiplegia is a rare complication. Francis Hawkins has collected 17 cases from the literature; aphasia was present in 12. The lesion is usually thrombosis of the arteries, less often a meningo-encephalitis. The aphasia usually disappears.

True *tetany* occurs sometimes, and has been reported in connection with certain epidemics. It may set in during the full height of the disease.

Typhoid Psychoses.—There are three groups of cases: first, an initial delirium, which may be serious, and cause the patient to wander away from his home, or he may even become maniacal; secondly, the psychosis associated directly with the pyrexia and the toxæmia; in a few cases this outlasts the disappearance of the fever for months or even years; and, lastly, the asthenic psychosis of convalescence, more common after typhoid than after any other fever. The prognosis is usually good. Edsal has recently studied the condition in children, finding 69 cases in the literature, of which 43 recovered.

There is a distressing post-typhoid neurasthenia, in which for months or even for years the patient is unable to get into harmony with his surroundings.

SPECIAL SENSES.—*Eye.*—Conjunctivitis, simple or phlyctenular, sometimes with keratitis and iritis, may develop. Panophthalmitis has been reported in one case in association with hæmorrhage (Finlay). Loss of accommodation may occur, usually in the asthenia of convalescence. Oculo-motor paralysis has been seen, due probably to neuritis. Retinal hæmorrhages may occur alone or in association with other hæmorrhagic features. Double optic neuritis has been described in the course of the fever. It may be independent of meningitis. Atrophy may follow, but these complications are excessively rare. Cataract may follow inflammation of the uveal tract. Other rare complications are thrombosis of the orbital veins and orbital hæmorrhage. (See De Schweinitz in Keen's monograph for full consideration of the subject.)

Ear.—Otitis media is not infrequent, 2.5 per cent in Hengst's collected cases. We have never found the typhoid bacillus in the discharge. Serious results are rare; only one case of mastoid disease occurred in our series. The otitis may set in with a chill and an aggravation of the fever.

RENAL SYSTEM.—*Retention of urine* is an early symptom and may be the cause of abdominal pain. It may recur throughout the attack. *Suppression of urine* is rare. The urine is usually diminished at first, has the ordinary febrile characters, and the pigments are increased. Later in the disease it is more abundant and lighter in color.

Polyuria is not very uncommon. The amount of water depends very much on the fluid taken. In certain cases enormous quantities are passed, up to seven and eight quarts. While most common during convalescence, the increase may be sudden in the second week at the height of the fever, as in a case reported by Fussell. Patients treated by what is known as the washing-out method, in which large quantities of water are taken, may pass enormous amounts, 18 or 19 litres. One of my patients passed as much as 23 litres in one day!

The Diazo-reaction of Ehrlich.—Two solutions are employed, kept in separate bottles: one containing a saturated solution of sulphanilic acid in a solution of hydrochloric acid (50 cc. to 1,000 cc.); the other a half per cent solution of sodium nitrite. To make the test, a few cubic centimetres of urine are placed in a small test-tube with an equal quantity of a mixture of the solution of the sulphanilic acid (40 cc.) and the sodium nitrite (1 cc.), the whole being thoroughly shaken. One cubic centimetre of ammonia is then allowed to flow carefully down the side of the tube, forming a colorless zone above the yellow urine, and at the junction of the two a deep brownish-red ring will be seen if the reaction is present. With normal urine a lighter brownish ring is produced, without a shade of red. The color of the foam of the mixed urine and reagent, and the tint they produce when largely diluted with water, are characteristic, being in both cases of a delicate rose-red if the diazo-reaction be present; but if not, brownish-yellow. It was found in 894 of 1,467 cases. It may be present previous to the occurrence of the rash, and as late as the twenty-second day. The value of the test is lessened by its occurrence in cases of miliary tuberculosis, in malarial fever, and occasionally in the acute diseases associated with high fever. The urotoxic coefficient in typhoid fever is high and is said to be increased by the tubs. In cases passing large quantities of urine the diazo-reaction is very feeble or even absent.

Bacilluria occurs in about one-third of the cases, caused by the typhoid bacilli. The urine may be turbid from their presence and in the test-tube give a peculiar shimmer. There may be millions of bacilli to the cubic millimetre without pyuria or any symptoms of renal or bladder trouble. The bacilli may be present in the urine for years after the attack (see Gwyn, Studies III). Of 51 cases during the session of 1900–1901 in my clinic, Cole found typhoid bacilli in the urine in 16.

The renal complications in typhoid fever may be thus grouped:

(*a*) Febrile albuminuria is common and of no special significance. It was present in 999 of 1,500 cases, 66 per cent. Tube casts were present in 568 cases, 37.8 per cent. *Hæmoglobinuria* occurred in one case.

(*b*) Acute nephritis at the onset or during the height of the disease— the *nephro-typhus* of the Germans, the *fièvre typhoïde à forme rénale* of the French—may set in, with all the symptoms of acute Bright's disease, masking in many instances the true nature of the malady. After an indisposition of a few days there may be fever, pain in the back, and the passage of a small amount of bloody urine.

(*c*) Nephritis during convalescence is rare, and is usually associated with anæmia and œdema. Chronic nephritis is a most exceptional sequel of the disease.

(*d*) The lymphomatous nephritis, described by E. Wagner, and already referred to in the section on morbid anatomy, produces, as a rule, no symptoms.

(*e*) *Pyuria,* a not uncommon complication, may be associated with the typhoid or the colon bacillus, less often with staphylococci. It disappears during convalescence. It is usually due to a simple catarrh of the bladder, rarely to an intense cystitis.

(*f*) *Post-typhoid Pyelitis.*—One or both kidneys may be involved, either at the height of the disease or during convalescence. There may be blood and pus at first, later pus alone, varying in amount. A severe pyelonephritis may follow. *Perinephric abscess* is a rare sequel.

GENERATIVE SYSTEM.—*Orchitis* is occasionally met with. Kinnicutt has collected 53 cases in the literature. It is usually associated with a catarrhal urethritis. Induration or atrophy may occur, and more rarely suppuration. It was present in 4 cases in my series. In 1 case double hydrocele developed suddenly on the nineteenth day (Dunlap).

Acute mastitis, which may go on to suppuration, is a rare complication. It was present in 3 cases of my series, during the fever and in one late in convalescence.

OSSEOUS SYSTEM.—Among the most common and troublesome of the sequelæ of the disease are the *bone lesions.* In a few cases the bone lesions occur at the height of the disease or even earlier. A boy was admitted in the second week of an attack of typhoid fever with acute periostitis of the frontal bone and of one rib. Of 237 cases collected by Keen there were periostitis in 110, necrosis in 85, and caries in 13. They are, I am sure, much more frequent than the figures indicate. Six cases came under my notice in the course of a year, and formed the basis of Parsons' paper (Studies II). The legs are chiefly involved. In Keen's series the tibia was affected in 91 cases, the ribs in 40. The typhoid bone lesion is apt to form what the old writers called a cold abscess. Only a few of the cases are acute. Chronicity, indolence, and a remarkable tendency to recurrence are perhaps the three most striking features of the typhoid bone lesions. A bony node may be left by the typhoid periostitis.

Arthritis was present in 5 cases of my series. Rheumatic and septic forms are described, as well as a typhoid arthritis proper. The complication is exceedingly rare, and yet Keen has collected from the literature 84 cases. One of the most important points relating to it is the frequency with which spontaneous dislocations occur, particularly of the hip.

Typhoid Spine (Gibney).—During the disease in protracted cases, more often during convalescence, the patient complains of pain in the lumbar and sacral regions, perhaps after a slight jar or shock. Stiffness of the back, pain on movement, and tenderness on pressure are the chief features, but there are in addition marked nervous, sometimes hysterical manifestations. The diagnosis of spondylitis, Pott's disease, or perinephritic abscess, etc., may be made. The examination is negative. The patient is afebrile, as a rule. The outlook is good. In rare instances there may be perispondylitis, but usually the condition is a neurosis (Studies I).

The *muscles* may be the seat of the degeneration already referred to, but it rarely causes any symptoms. Hæmorrhage occasionally occurs into the muscles, and late in protracted cases abscesses may follow. Rupture of a muscle, usually the rectus abdominis, may occur, possibly associated with acute hæmorrhagic myositis.

Post-typhoid Septicæmia and Pyæmia.—In very protracted cases there may recur after defervescence a slight fever (100°–101°), with sweats, which is possibly septic. In other cases for two or three weeks there are recurring chills, often of great severity. They are usually of no moment in the absence of signs of complication. (See Studies II and III.)

Typhoid pyæmia is not very uncommon. (*a*) Extensive furunculosis may be associated with irregular fever and leucocytosis. (*b*) Following the fever there may be multiple subcutaneous " cold " abscesses, often with a dark, thin bloody pus. A score or more of these may appear in different parts. Pratt has isolated the bacillus in pure culture from the subcutaneous abscesses. (*c*) A crural thrombus may suppurate and cause a wide-spread pyæmia. (*d*) In rare instances suppuration of the mesenteric glands, of a splenic infarct, a sloughing parotid bubo, a perinephric or perirectal abscess, acute necrosis of the bones, or a multiple suppurative arthritis may cause pyæmia. In other cases following bed-sores or a furunculosis there occurs a general infection with pyogenic organisms, with fatal result. In three such cases in our series staphylococci were cultivated from the blood. In one case with many chills late in the disease, and the general condition excellent, typhoid bacilli were cultivated from the blood.

Association of other Diseases.—Erysipelas is a rare complication, most commonly met with during convalescence. In 1,420 cases at Basel it occurred 10 times. Griesinger states that it is met with in 2 per cent. Measles or scarlet fever may develop during the fever or in convalescence. Chicken-pox and noma have been reported in children. Pseudo-membranous inflammations may occur in the pharynx, larynx, or genitals.

Malarial and typhoid fevers may be associated, but a majority of the cases of so-called typho-malarial fever are either remittent malarial fever or true typhoid. It is interesting to note that among the 829 cases of typhoid fever plasmodia were found in the blood during the course of the disease in only 1 case. (See Lyon, Studies III.) Many of our typhoid-fever cases came from malarious regions.

The symptoms of influenza may precede the typhoid fever, or the two diseases may run concurrently. There are cases of chronic influenza which simulate typhoid fever very closely.

Typhoid Fever and Tuberculosis.—(*a*) The diseases may coexist. A person with chronic tuberculosis may contract the fever. Of 80 autopsies in typhoid fever, 4 presented marked tuberculous lesions. Miliary tuberculosis and typhoid fever may occur together. (*b*) Cases of typhoid fever with pulmonary and pleuritic symptoms may suggest tuberculosis at the onset. (*c*) There are five types of tuberculous infection which may simulate typhoid fever: the acute miliary form (page 298); tuberculous meningitis (page 301); tuberculous peritonitis (page 310); the acute toxæmia of certain local lesions (page 306); and forms of ordinary pulmonary tuberculosis. And, lastly, pulmonary tuberculosis may follow typhoid fever. In a large majority of such cases the disease has been tuberculosis from the onset, which has begun with a low fever and features suggestive of typhoid fever.

In epilepsy and in chronic chorea the fits and movements usually cease during an attack, and in typhoid fever in a diabetic subject the sugar may be absent during the height of the disease.

Varieties of Typhoid.—Typhoid fever presents an extremely complex symptomatology. Many forms have been described, some of which present exaggeration of common symptoms, others modification in the course, others again greater intensity of action of the poison on certain organs. As we have seen, when the nervous system is specially involved, it has been called the cerebrospinal form; when the kidneys are early and severely affected, nephro-typhoid; when the disease begins with pulmonary symptoms, pneumo-typhoid; with pleurisy, pleuro-typhoid; when the disease is characterized throughout by profuse sweats, the sudoral form of the disease. It is enough to remember that typhoid has no fixed and constant course, that it may set in occasionally with symptoms localized in certain organs, and that many of its symptoms are extremely variable—in one epidemic uniform and text-book-like, in another slight or not met with. This diversified symptomatology has led to many clinical errors, and in the absence of the salutary lessons of morbid anatomy it is not surprising that practitioners have so often been led astray. We may recognize with Murchison the following varieties:

1. The *mild* and *abortive* forms. Much attention has been paid of late to the milder varieties of typhoid fever—the typhus levissimus of Griesinger. Woodruff, of the United States Army, has called special attention to the great danger of neglecting these mild forms, which are often spoken of as mountain fever and malarial fever, " acclimation," " ground," and " miasmatic " fevers. During the prevalence of an epidemic there may be cases of fever so mild that the patient does not go to bed. The onset may be sudden, particularly in chil-

50

dren. The general symptoms are slight, the pulse rate not high, the fever rarely above 102°. Rose spots are usually present, with splenic enlargement. Diarrhœa is rare. The Widal reaction is present in a majority of the patients. There may be a marked tendency to relapse. While infrequent, characteristic complications and sequelæ may give the first positive clue to the nature of the trouble. J. B. Briggs has studied 44 of these mild cases from my clinic, in which the fever lasted 14 days or less. Rose spots were present in 24, and the Widal reaction in 26. There were three relapses. It can not be too forcibly impressed upon the profession that it is just by these mild cases, to which so little attention is paid, that the disease may be kept up in a community.

2. The *grave* form is usually characterized by high fever and pronounced nervous symptoms. In this category, too, come the very severe cases, setting in with pneumonia and Bright's disease, and with the very intense gastro-intestinal or cerebro-spinal symptoms.

3. The *latent* or *ambulatory* form of typhoid fever, which is particularly common in hospital practice. The symptoms are usually slight, and the patient scarcely feels ill enough to go to bed. He has languor, perhaps slight diarrhœa, but keeps about and may even attend to his work throughout the entire attack. In other instances delirium sets in. The worst cases of this form are seen in sailors, who keep up and about, though feeling ill and feverish. When brought to the hospital they often have symptoms of a most severe type of the disease. Hæmorrhage or perforation may be the first marked symptom of this ambulatory type. Sir W. Jenner has called attention to the dangers of this form, and particularly to the grave prognosis in the case of persons who have travelled far with the disease in progress.

Hæmorrhagic Typhoid Fever.—This is excessively rare. Among Ouskow's 6,513 cases there were 4 fatal cases with general hæmorrhagic features. Only three instances were present in our series. Hæmorrhages may be marked from the outset, but more commonly they come on during the course of the disease. The condition is not necessarily fatal. Several of those reported by Nicholls from the Royal Victoria Hospital, Montreal, recovered. (See Hamburger, Studies III.)

An *afebrile* typhoid fever is recognized by authors. Liebermeister says that the cases were not uncommon at Basel. The patients presented lassitude, depression, headache, furred tongue, loss of appetite, slow pulse, and even the spots and enlarged spleen. I have seen the temperature normal on the sixteenth day, while the spots did not come out until later.

TYPHOID FEVER IN CHILDREN.—Griffith collected a series of 325 cases in children under two and a half years; 111 of these were in the first year. Out of a total of 278 cases in which the result was recorded, 142 died. The cases are not very uncommon. The high mortality in Griffith's paper was probably due to the fact that only the more serious cases are reported. The abdominal symptoms are usually mild; fatal hæmorrhage and perforation are rare. Among sequelæ, aphasia, noma, and bone lesions are stated to be more common in children than in adults. Two of our cases were under one year of age.

TYPHOID FEVER IN THE AGED.—After the sixtieth year the disease runs a less favorable course, and the mortality is very high. The fever is not so high, but complications are more common, particularly pneumonia and heart-failure.

TYPHOID FEVER IN PREGNANCY.—Pregnancy affords no immunity against typhoid. In 1,500 of our cases to September 10, 1904, 438 of which were females, there were 6 cases. Goltdammer noted 26 pregnancies in 600 cases of typhoid fever in the female. It is more commonly seen in the first half of pregnancy. The pregnancy is interrupted in about 65 per cent of the cases, usually in the second week of the disease. In the obstetrical department of the Johns Hopkins Hospital (J. W. Williams) there have been (to January, 1905) three cases of puerperal infection with bacillus typhosus. One case showed a localized lesion of the chorion, from which cultures were obtained (Little).

TYPHOID FEVER IN THE FŒTUS.—From the recent studies of Fordyce, J. L. Morse, and F. W. Lynch, we may conclude that the typhoid bacillus may pass through the placenta to the child, causing a typhoid septicæmia, without intestinal lesions. Lynch has recently collected 16 such cases. Infection of the fœtus does not necessarily follow, but when infected the child dies, either in utero or shortly after birth. The Widal reaction has been obtained with fœtal blood. Its presence does not indicate that the child has survived infection in utero, as the agglutinating substances may filter through the placenta. They may also be transmitted to the nursling through the milk, and cause a transient reaction. The reaction could not be obtained with fœtal blood from which typhoid bacilli were cultivated (Lynch).

RELAPSE.—Relapses vary in frequency in different epidemics, and, it would appear, in different places. The percentages of different authors range from 3 per cent (Murchison), 11 per cent (Bäumler), to 15 or 18 per cent (Immermann). In 1,500 cases there were 172 relapses, 11.4 per cent.

We may recognize the ordinary, the intercurrent, and the spurious relapse.

The *ordinary relapse* sets in after complete defervescence. The average duration of the interval in Irvine's cases was a little over five days.

In one of my cases there was complete apyrexia for twenty-three days, followed by a relapse of forty-one days' duration; then apyrexia for forty-two days, followed by a second relapse of two weeks' duration. As a rule, two of the three important symptoms—step-like temperature at onset, roseola, an enlarged spleen—should be present to justify the diagnosis of a relapse. The intestinal symptoms are variable. The onset may be abrupt with a chill, or the temperature may have a typical ascent, as shown in Chart I. The number of relapses range from 1 to 5. In a case at the Pennsylvania Hospital in 1904 the disease lasted eleven months and four days, during which there were six relapses. The attack is usually less severe and of shorter duration. Of Murchison's 53 cases, the mean duration of the first attack was about twenty-six days; of the relapse, fifteen days. The mortality of relapse cases is not high.

The *intercurrent relapse* is common, often most severe, and is responsible for a great many of the most protracted cases. The temperature drops and the patient improves; but after remaining between 100° and 102° for a few days, the fever again rises and the patient enters upon another attack, which may be even more protracted, and of much greater intensity than the original one.

Spurious relapses are very common. They have already been referred to on page 72, under post-typhoid elevations of temperature. They are recrudescences of the fever due to a number of causes. It is not always easy to determine whether a relapse is present, particularly in cases in which the fever persists for only five or seven days without rose-spots and without enlargement of the spleen.

Undoubtedly a reinfection from within, yet of the conditions favoring the occurrence of relapse we as yet know little. Durham has advanced an interesting theory: Every typhoid infection is a complex phenomenon caused by groups of bacilli alike in species but not identical, as shown by their serum reactions. The antitoxin formed in the blood during the primary attack neutralizes only one (or several) groups, the remaining groups still preserving their pathogenic power. Following an error in diet, or some indiscretion, these latter groups may multiply sufficiently to cause a reinfection. Multiple relapses may be similarly explained. Bacteriological proof of this interesting theory has not yet been given.

Diagnosis.—There are several points to note. In the first place, typhoid fever is the most common of all continued fevers. Secondly, it is extraordinarily variable in its manifestations. Thirdly, there is no such hybrid malady as typho-malarial fever. Fourthly, errors in diagnosis are inevitable, even under the most favorable conditions.

DATA FOR DIAGNOSIS.—(*a*) *General.*—No single symptom or feature is characteristic. The onset is often suggestive, particularly the occurrence of epistaxis, and (if seen from the start) the ascending fever. The steadiness of the fever for a week or longer after reaching the fastigium is an important point. The irregular remittent character in the third week, and the intermittent features with chills, are common sources of error. While there is nothing characteristic in the pulse, dicrotism is so much more common early in typhoid fever that its presence is always suggestive. The rash is the most valuable single sign, and with the fever usually clinches the diagnosis. The enlarged spleen is of less importance, since it occurs in all febrile conditions, but with the fever and the rash it completes a diagnostic triad of the disease. The absence of leucocytosis and the presence of Ehrlich's reaction are valuable accessory signs.

(*b*) *Specific.*—(1) *Isolation of Typhoid Bacilli from the Blood.*—New methods have given better results in this procedure, which has been carried out extensively in my ward by Cole, and I can testify to its great value in doubtful cases and in the acute septic forms. The hypodermic puncture of a vein for the blood causes little or no pain.

(2) *Isolation of Typhoid Bacilli from the Stools.*—Cultures from the stools have proved of diagnostic value. A new and very satisfactory method is that of von Drigalski and Conradi (Zeit. f. Hygiene, Bd. 39), largely used in the campaign against typhoid in Germany, with which those familiar with bacteriologic methods are able to isolate the bacilli in a majority of the cases.

(3) *Isolation of Typhoid Bacilli from the Urine.*—Neumann, Horton-Smith, Richardson, and Gwyn have shown the great frequency of typhoid bacilli in the urine. In some cases they may be obtained before the Widal test is positive. Routine cultures do not offer great difficulties, and may frequently be of diagnostic value.

(4) *Isolation of Typhoid Bacilli from the Rose-spots.*—Neufeld, Curschmann, and Richardson have demonstrated the presence of the bacilli in rose-

spots in 32 of 40 cases examined. As the procedure causes considerable discomfort it can not be used as a routine method.

(5) *The Agglutination Test.*—In 1894 Pfeiffer showed that cholera spirilla, when introduced into the peritonæum of an immunized animal, or when mixed with the serum of immunized animals, lose their motion and break up. This "Pfeiffer's phenomenon" of agglutination and immobilization was thoroughly studied by Durham and also by A. S. Grünbaum, and the specificity of the reaction demonstrated. Widal took the method, and made it available in clinical work.

METHODS.—(*a*) *Macroscopic or Slow Method.*—This has not been largely used in clinical work, but on the whole the results are probably more satisfactory than with the microscopic method, and in hospitals, at least, the difficulties are no greater. Lately the use of cultures of dead bacilli has received quite wide application. This method is very satisfactory when the living, active bacilli can not be conveniently employed.

(*b*) *Microscopic or Rapid Method.*—The serum is mixed with a young bouillon culture of the typhoid bacillus, or with a suspension of a young agar culture, in such a manner as to dilute the serum to the required degree. A hanging-drop preparation of the mixture is made, and if the reaction is positive the bacilli will within a given time lose their motility and collect in clumps. Wyatt Johnston introduced the use of dried blood. It is convenient, but does not permit accurate dilutions. The use of glass bulbs to obtain the serum, and small glass pipettes to make accurate dilutions, is of value. As Cabot says, "the test is a quantitative, not a qualitative, one." Both the degree of dilution and the time limit are of importance. A safe standard, and the one in use at the Johns Hopkins Hospital, is a dilution of 1–50 and a time limit of one hour.

RESULTS.—Cabot's collection of 5,978 cases gives a positive reaction in 97.2 per cent. A positive reaction was obtained in 93 per cent of 849 cases tested before the eighth day. It may not appear until the relapse. In 4 of my cases it developed on the twenty-second, twenty-sixth, thirty-fifth, and forty-second days, respectively. It may be present even twenty or thirty years subsequent to the attack of fever.

While on the whole the serum reaction is of very great value, there are certain difficulties and objections which must be considered. A perfectly characteristic case with hæmorrhages, rose-spots, etc., may give no reaction throughout. In other cases the reaction is much delayed, becoming positive only during convalescence, or even during a relapse. It must be borne in mind that occasionally the reaction is not obtained with low dilutions, while with higher dilutions the reaction is characteristic.

COMMON SOURCES OF ERROR IN DIAGNOSIS.—An early and intense localization of the infection in certain organs may give rise to doubt at first.

Cases coming on with severe headache, photophobia, delirium, twitching of the muscles and retraction of the head are almost invariably regarded as *cerebrospinal meningitis.* Under such circumstances it may for a few days be impossible to make a satisfactory diagnosis. I have thrice performed autopsies on cases of this kind in which no suspicion of typhoid fever had been present, the intense cerebro-spinal manifestations having dominated the scene. Until the appearance of abdominal symptoms, or the rash, it may be quite impossible to

54

determine the nature of the case. Cerebro-spinal meningitis is, however, a rare disease; typhoid fever a very common one, and the onset with severe nervous symptoms is by no means infrequent. The lumbar puncture is now a great help.

I have already spoken of the misleading pulmonary symptoms, which occasionally occur at the very outset of the disease. The bronchitis rarely causes error, though it may be intense and attract the chief attention. More difficult are the cases setting in with chill and followed rapidly by *pneumonia*. I have brought such a case before the class one week as typical pneumonia, and a fortnight later shown the same case as undoubtedly one of typhoid fever. In another case, in which the onset was with definite pneumonia, no spots were present, and, though there were diarrhœa, meteorism, and the most pronounced nervous symptoms, the doubt still remains whether it was a case of typhoid fever or one of pneumonia in which severe secondary symptoms developed. There is less danger of mistaking the pneumonia which occurs at the height of the disease, and yet this is possible, as in a case admitted a few years ago to my wards—a man aged seventy, insensible, with a dry tongue, tremor, ecchymoses upon the wrists and ankles, no rose-spots, enlargement of the spleen, and consolidation of his right lower lobe. It was very natural, particularly since there was no history, to regard such a case as senile pneumonia with profound constitutional disturbance, but the autopsy showed the characteristic lesions of typhoid fever. Early involvement of the pleura or the kidneys may for a time obscure the diagnosis.

Of diseases with which typhoid fever may be confounded, malaria, certain forms of pyæmia, acute tuberculosis, and tuberculous peritonitis are the most important.

From *malarial fever*, typhoid is, as a rule, readily recognized. There is no such disease as typho-malarial fever—that is, a separate and distinct malady. Typhoid fever and malarial fever may coexist in the same patient. Of 1,500 cases of typhoid fever, in only three were the malarial parasites found in the blood during the fever. In patients returning from Cuba and Porto Rico during the late war the two conditions were often found together, but in this country it is excessively rare. The term typho-malarial fever should be abandoned. The autumnal type of malarial fever may present a striking similarity in its early days to typhoid fever. Differentiation may be made only by the blood examination. There may be no chills, the remissions may be extremely slight, there is a history perhaps of *malaise*, weakness, diarrhœa, and sometimes vomiting. The tongue is furred and white, the cheeks flushed, the spleen slightly enlarged, and the temperature continuous, or with very slight remissions. The æstivo-autumnal variety of the malarial parasite may not be present in the circulating blood for several days. Every year we had one or two cases in which the diagnosis was in doubt for a few days.

Pyæmia.—The long-continued fever of obscure, deep-seated suppuration, without chills or sweats, may simulate typhoid. The more chronic cases of ulcerative endocarditis are usually diagnosed enteric fever. The presence or absence of leucocytosis is an important aid. The Widal reaction and the blood cultures now offer additional and valuable help.

Acute miliary tuberculosis is not infrequently mistaken for typhoid fever. The points in differential diagnosis will be discussed under that disease. *Tuber-*

culous peritonitis in certain of its forms may closely simulate typhoid fever, and will be referred to in another section.

The early abdominal pain, etc., may lead to the diagnosis of appendicitis. (See Appendicitis.)

Prognosis.—(*a*) *Death-rate.*—The mortality is very variable, ranging in private practice from 5 to 12 and in hospital practice from 7 to 20 per cent. In some large epidemics the death-rate has been very low. In the Maidstone epidemic it was between 7 and 8 per cent. In recent years the mortality from typhoid fever has certainly diminished, and, under the influence of Brand, the reintroduction of hydrotherapy has reduced the death-rate in institutions in a remarkable manner, even as low as 5 or 6 per cent. Of the 1,500 cases treated in my wards, 9.1 per cent died. The mortality in the Spanish-American War was very low—7 per cent—and may be attributed to the picked set of men and to the care and attention which the patients received. In South Africa the mortality was 20.9 per cent to March 31, 1901.

(*b*) *Special Features in Prognosis.*—Unfavorable symptoms are high fever, toxic symptoms with delirium, meteorism, and hæmorrhage. Fat subjects stand typhoid fever badly. The mortality in women is greater than in men. The complications and dangers are more serious in the ambulatory form in which the patient has kept about for a week or ten days. Early involvement of the nervous system is a bad indication; and the low, muttering delirium with tremor means a close fight for life. Prognostic signs from the fever alone are deceptive. A temperature above 104° may be well borne for many days if the nervous system is not involved.

(*c*) *Sudden Death.*—It is difficult in many cases to explain this most lamentable of accidents in the disease. There are cases in which neither cerebral, renal, nor cardiac changes have been found; there are instances too in which it does not seem likely that there could have been a special localization of the toxins in the pneumogastric centres. McPhedran, in reporting a case of the kind, in which the post mortem showed no adequate cause of death, suggests that the experiments of McWilliam on sudden cardiac failure probably explain the occurrence of death in certain of the cases in which neither embolism nor uræmia is present. Under conditions of abnormal nutrition there is sometimes induced a state of *delirium cordis*, which may occur spontaneously, or, in the case of animals, on slight irritation of the heart, with the result of extreme irregularity and finally failure of action. Sudden death occurs more frequently in men than in women, according to Dewèvre's statistics, in a proportion of 114 to 26. It may occur at the height of the fever, and, as pointed out by Graves, may also happen during convalescence. There were four cases in my series.

Prophylaxis.—In cities the prevalence of typhoid fever is directly proportionate to the inefficiency of the drainage and the water-supply. With their improvement the mortality has been reduced one-half or even more. Fulton has shown that in the United States, at least, the disease exists to a proportionately greater extent in the country than it does in the city, and that the propagation of this disease is in general from the country to the town. In the water-supply of the latter the chances for dilution of the contaminating fluids are so much greater than in the country, where the privy vault is often in such close proximity to the well.

But it is not only through water that the disease is transmitted. Other methods play an important though not so frequent rôle. The bacilli may be carried by milk, oysters, uncooked vegetables, etc. Flies play an important rôle in the spread of the disease. Many cases undoubtedly arise by direct infection. But through whatever channel the infection occurs, for new cases to arise the virus must be obtained from another patient. It has been demonstrated by Jordan, Russell, Zeit and others that under ordinary circumstances the bacilli do not live and thrive long outside the body. To stamp out typhoid fever requires (1) *the recognition of all cases, including the typhoid carriers,* and (2) *the destruction of all typhoid bacilli as they leave the patient.* It is as much a part of the physician's duty to look after these points as to take care of the patient. Mild cases of fever are to be regarded with suspicion.

From the standpoint of prophylaxis, the question practically narrows down to disinfection of the urine, stools, sputum (in the few cases where bacilli are present), and of objects which may accidentally be contaminated by these excretions.

The nurse or attendant should be taught to regard every specimen of urine as a pure culture of typhoid bacilli, and to exercise the greatest care in preventing the scattering of drops of urine over the patient, bedding or floor, or over the hands of the attendant.

To disinfect the urine the best solutions are carbolic acid, 1–20, in an amount equal to that of the urine, or bichloride of mercury, 1–1,000, in an amount one-fifteenth that of the fluid to be sterilized. These mixtures with the urine should stand at least two hours.

Urotropin causes disappearance of the bacilli from the urine when bacilluria is present, but under no circumstances should its administration permit the disinfection of the urine to be neglected.

To disinfect stools carbolic acid is the most useful. It is cheap, and efficient when used in strong solutions. The stool should be mixed with at least twice its volume of 1–20 carbolic-acid solution and allowed to stand for several hours.

With hydrotherapy the disinfection of the bath water after use offers a serious and somewhat difficult problem.

E. Babucke has sought experimentally the best method for the disinfection of the bath water. He found chloride of lime the best substance to use, and found that even where the water contains coarse fecal matter, 250 gm. (one-half pound) of chloride of lime will render the ordinary bath of 200 litres sterile in one-half hour.

If there be any expectoration, the sputum should receive the same care as in tuberculosis. It is best to collect it in small cloths, which may be burned.

All the linen leaving the patient's bed or person should be soaked for two hours in 1–20 carbolic-acid solution, and then sent to the laundry, where it should be boiled. All dishes should be boiled before leaving the patient's room.

The nurse should wear a rubber apron when giving tubs or working over a typhoid patient, and this should be washed frequently with a carbolic acid or bichloride of mercury solution. The nurse should wear rubber gloves when giving tubs, or else soak her hands thoroughly in 1–1,000 bichloride solution after she has finished.

It is impossible here to deal with all the possible modes of spread of the infection. Keeping in mind that everything leaving the patient should be

57

sterilized whenever there is a chance of its having been contaminated by the discharges, a nurse of ordinary intelligence, even one of the family, can carry out very satisfactory prophylaxis.

Should the typhoid fever patient be isolated? To prevent direct infection of other members of the family a moderate degree of isolation should be carried out, though this need not be absolute as in the exanthemata. The windows should have fly screens in summer. After recovery the room should be disinfected.

An important question is as to the necessity for the isolation of typhoid patients in special wards in hospitals. At present this is not generally done in the United States. When, however, in a hospital with as good sanitary arrangements as the Johns Hopkins possesses, and in which all possible precautions are taken to prevent the infection spreading from patient to patient, 1.81 per cent of all the cases have been of hospital origin, the advisability of isolation of typhoid fever patients is certainly worth considering. On the other hand, in the general hospital, with students in the wards, the cases are more thoroughly studied, and in the graver complications, as perforation, it is of the greatest advantage to have the early co-operation of the house surgeon.

During the past few years an active campaign has been started in Germany, under the leadership of Professor Koch, with the object of ultimately stamping out this disease by means of early diagnosis and the institution of rigid measures for preventing the distribution of the infecting agent from the patients so diagnosed. With a corps of assistants he fitted up a laboratory in Trier, a locality where the disease had a firm hold. By bacteriological methods he was able to demonstrate that 72 persons were suffering from typhoid infection. So soon as the nature of a case was established, isolation and vigorous disinfection were practiced. The result was that within three months no more typhoid bacilli were discoverable, the patients were cured, no fresh cases arose, and, so far as that group of villages was concerned, typhoid was exterminated. Since, in other groups of villages situated under strictly comparable conditions, but where these methods of dealing with the disease were not practiced, typhoid continues to be prevalent, it may reasonably be inferred that the disappearance at Trier was not spontaneous, but due to the methods of identification and disinfection which were used.

When epidemics are prevalent the drinking-water and the milk used in families should be boiled. Travellers should drink light wines or mineral water rather than ordinary water or milk. Care should be taken to thoroughly cook oysters which have been fattened or freshened in streams contaminated with sewage.

While in camps it is easy to boil and filter the water; with troops on the march it is a very different matter, and it is impossible to restrain men from relieving their thirst the moment they reach water. Various chemical methods have been recommended—the use of bromine, hypochlorite of lime, permanganate of potassium, and the tablets of sodium bisulphate, none of which are probably very satisfactory.

VACCINATION.—A. E. Wright has introduced a method of vaccination against typhoid. A full description of the principles involved, as well as of the technique, is given in his work, A Short Treatise on Anti-Typhoid Inoculation, London, 1904. The material used is a bouillon culture of virulent bacilli

58

heated to 60° in order to kill them. By a somewhat complicated procedure the number of bacteria in this culture is estimated, and for the first inoculation a quantity of the vaccine containing 750 to 1,000 millions of bacteria is employed, and for the second inoculation a quantity containing 1,500 to 2,000 millions of bacilli is employed. Two inoculations are given at an interval of about two weeks. Following inoculation there is a mild local reaction and constitutional symptoms begin within two or three hours. As a sequence of the injection, there is an increase in both the bactericidal and agglutinating powers of the blood. Many thousand inoculations have now been made under Wright's direction, mainly on the British troops in India and South Africa. From the statistics so far available he concludes that the incidence of typhoid fever was diminished by at least one-half in the inoculated, while in the aggregate the proportion of deaths to cases among the inoculated has been rather less than half that among the uninoculated. The evidence so far points to a persistence of the protective effect for at least two years after inoculation. Wright's conclusions are supported by the evidence of a large number of English army officers. Wherever, therefore, large bodies of persons are likely to be exposed to unusual dangers of infection the procedure may be employed.

Treatment.—(*a*) GENERAL MANAGEMENT.—The profession was long in learning that typhoid fever is not a disease to be treated mainly with drugs. Careful nursing and a regulated diet are the essentials in a majority of the cases. The patient should be in a well-ventilated room (or in summer out of doors during the day), strictly confined to bed from the outset, and there remain until convalescence is well established. The bed should be single, not too high, and the mattress should not be too hard. The woven wire bed, with soft hair mattress, upon which are two folds of blanket, combines the two great qualities of a sick-bed, smoothness and elasticity. A rubber cloth should be placed under the sheet. An intelligent nurse should be in charge. When this is impossible, the attending physician should write out specific instructions regarding diet, treatment of the discharges, and the bed-linen.

(*b*) DIET.—Milk, eggs, and water are the essential foods during the febrile period. An adult receives four ounces of milk, diluted with two ounces of lime-water or soda-water, every four hours; and four ounces of albumen-water, made from the white of one or two eggs, every four hours. In this way he is fed every two hours. The juice of half a lemon or an ounce of fresh orange juice is added to the albumen-water, which may be sweetened with a little sugar. The great majority of our patients have this diet alone during the fever. Whey is substituted for the milk if there are curds in the stools or if there is much distention or if the plain milk disagrees in any way. If necessary, milk is cut off altogether and the albumen-water increased. Buttermilk, boiled milk, koumiss, or peptonized milk may be used. The beef extracts, meat juices, and artificially prepared foods are unnecessary, and in private practice among people in moderate circumstances add greatly to the expense of the illness. Such a diet is simple, reduces the work of feeding to a minimum, and agrees with a great majority of all patients. Water is given at fixed intervals. A good plan is to have a jug of water beside the patient and a tubing with a glass mouth-piece, so that he can drink as much as he wishes. A washing-out plan of treatment is advised by E. W. Cushing and T. W. Clarke, of the Lake-side Hospital, Cleveland. A gallon or more may be taken in the day. The water causes polyuria, and is a sort of internal hydrotherapy by which the toxins may be washed out. Barley water, lemonade, or iced-tea may be used. A small cup of coffee in the morning is very grateful. Bouillon or strained vegetable soup may serve as a change. Ice cream may be taken at any time, and is an agreeable variation, particularly for children.

It is possible that we give too much food. Of late years the disease has been treated by what has been called therapeutic fasting—little or no food, only water.

Alcohol is unnecessary in a great majority of the cases. Of late years I have used it much less freely; but when the heart is feeble and the toxic symptoms are severe, eight to twelve ounces of whisky may be given in the twenty-four hours.

(*c*) HYDROTHERAPY.—The use of water, inside and outside, was no new treatment in fevers at the end of the eighteenth century, when James Currie (a friend of Burns and the editor of his poems) wrote his Medical Reports on the Effects of Water, Cold and Warm, as a Remedy in Fevers and other Diseases. In this country it was used with great effect and recommended strongly by Nathan Smith, of Yale. Since 1861 the value of bathing in fevers has been specially emphasized by the late Dr. Brand, of Stettin.

Hydrotherapy may be carried out in several different ways, of which, in typhoid fever, the most satisfactory are sponging, the wet pack, and the full bath.

(*a*) *Cold Sponging.*—The water may be tepid, cold, or ice-cold, according to the height of the fever. A thorough sponge-bath should take from fifteen to twenty minutes. The ice-cold sponging is not quite as formidable as the full cold bath, for which, when there is an insuperable objection in private practice, it is an excellent alternative. But frequently it is difficult to get the friends to appreciate the advantages of the sponging. When such is the case, and in children and delicate persons, it can be made a little less formidable by sponging limb by limb and then the back and abdomen.

(*b*) The *cold pack* is not so generally useful in typhoid fever, but in cases with very pronounced nervous symptoms, if the tub is not available, the patient may be wrapped in a sheet wrung out of water at 60° or 65°, and then cold water sprinkled over him with an ordinary watering-pot.

(*c*) *The Bath.*—The tub should be long enough so that the patient can be completely covered except his head. Our rule for some years has been to give a bath at 70° every third hour when the temperature was above 102.5°. The patient remains in the tub for fifteen or twenty minutes, is taken out, wrapped in a dry sheet, and covered with a blanket. While in the tub the limbs and trunk are rubbed thoroughly, either with the hand or with a suitable rubber. It is well to give the first one or two baths at a temperature of 80° or 85°. There is no routine temperature. If the bath at 70° is not well taken, raise the temperature to 75° or 80°. It is important to see that the canvas supports are properly arranged, and that the rubber pillow is comfortable for the patient's head. The first bath should not be given at night, and it should be superintended by the house-physician. The amount of complaint made by the patient is largely dependent upon the skill and care with which the baths are given. Food is usually given, sometimes a stimulant, after the bath. The blueness and shivering, which often follow the bath, are not serious features. The rectal temperature is taken immediately after the bath, and again three-quarters of an hour later. Contra-indications are peritonitis, hæmorrhage, phlebitis, severe abdominal pain, and great prostration. The accompanying chart (Chart V) shows the number of baths

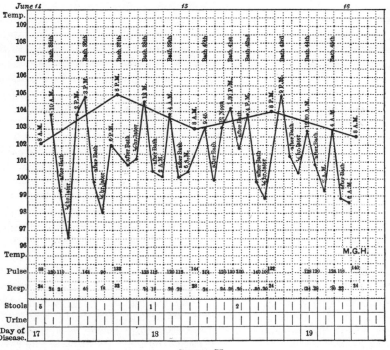

CHART V.

and the influence on the fever during two days of treatment. The good effects of the baths are: (1) The effect on the nervous system. The delirium lessens, the tremor diminishes, and the toxic features are less marked. The excretion of the toxins by the kidneys is stimulated. (2) The fever is reduced, though this is not the chief effect of the tubs; indeed at the height of the disease there may be very little reduction. (3) The heart rate usually falls, the pulse becomes smaller and harder, and the blood pressure rises 15 or 20 mm. of Hg. (4) With hydrotherapy the initial bronchitis is benefited, and there is less chance of passive congestion of the bases of the lungs. (5) The liability to bed-sores is diminished and the frequent cleansing of the skin is beneficial. Should boils occur, one bath-tub should be used for that patient alone. (6) The mortality is reduced. In general hospitals from six to eight patients in every hundred are saved by this plan of treatment. At the Brisbane Hospital, where F. E. Hare used it so thoroughly, the mortality was reduced from 14.8 per cent to 7.5. There is a remarkable uniformity in the death-rate of institutions using the method—usually from 6 to 8 per cent. At the Royal Victoria Hospital, Montreal, the rate for the six years was 5.4 per cent. At the Johns Hopkins Hospital the mortality among 1,500 cases was 137, or 9.1 per cent.

(*d*) MEDICINAL TREATMENT.—In hospital practice medicines are not often needed. A great majority of my cases do not receive a dose. In private practice it may be safer, for the young practitioner especially, to order a mild fever mixture. The question of medicinal antipyretics is important: they are used far too often and too rashly in typhoid fever. An occasional dose of antifebrin or antipyrin may do no harm, but the daily use of these drugs is most injurious. Quinine in moderate doses is still much employed. The local use of guaiacol on the skin, 3ss. painted on the flank, causes a prompt fall in the temperature.

In the various antiseptic drugs which have been advised I have no faith. Most of them do no harm, except that in private practice their use has too often diverted the practitioner from more rational and safer courses.

(*e*) SERUM THERAPY.—Numerous attempts have been made to obtain specific sera, which have been of two varieties, bactericidal and antitoxic. As Wasserman has shown, the probable reason why the former have failed is owing to the lack of sufficient complement in the patient's blood, and at present no available method has been found to increase this complement. As the isolation of a soluble typhoid toxin has presented insuperable difficulties so far, it is questionable whether an antitoxin of any value has yet been obtained. With the reported isolation of typhoid toxins of considerable strength by Conradi, and also by Macfadyen, it is possible that in the near future an antitoxin serum of great value may be produced. One of the most important problems in connection with this disease is the isolation of a strong soluble toxin, the results of which would probably be very far-reaching. Chantemesse (Presse Med., 1904, No. 86) has published the results obtained in several of the Paris hospitals with an antitoxic serum. The toxin is obtained in the filtered cultures of typhoid bacilli grown on a medium containing splenic pulp and human defibrinated blood. By injection of this into horses a serum has been produced, which, during a period of three and a half years, has been employed in the treatment of 765 cases, 545 by Chantemesse himself, and 220 cases in children by Josias and Brunon. Of these 765 cases only 30 died, a mortality of about 4 per cent, while in the other Paris hospitals during the same period there occurred a mortality of 18 per cent, in none of them under 12 per cent.

A third method is by means of the so-called extract of Jez, by the use of which good results have been reported by Eichhorst and others, though so far on a relatively small number of cases. This extract is obtained from the bone-marrow, spleen, thymus, brain, and spinal cord of animals highly immunized to typhoid bacilli. Large amounts must be used. Remembering the considerable period of time after the discovery of the diphtheria antitoxin before a serum of high value was obtained, it is not too much to hope that some of these experiments may lead to important results.

(*f*) TREATMENT OF THE SPECIAL SYMPTOMS.—The abdominal *pain* and *tympanites* are best treated with fomentations or turpentine stupes. The latter, if well applied, give great relief. Sir William Jenner used to lay great stress on the advantages of a well-applied turpentine stupe. He directed it to be applied as follows: A flannel roller was placed beneath the patient, and then a double layer of thin flannel, wrung out of very hot water, with a drachm of turpentine mixed with the water, was applied to the abdomen and covered with the ends of the roller. When the gas is in the large bowel, a tube may be passed or a turpentine enema given. For tympanites, with a dry tongue, turpentine may be given, or the oil of cinnamon, ℥ iii–v, every two hours (Caiger). If whey and albumen-water are substituted for milk, the distention lessens. Charcoal, bismuth, β-naphthol, and eserine, $\frac{1}{30}$ gr. hypodermically, may be tried. Opium should not be given.

For the *diarrhœa*, if severe—that is, if there are more than three or four stools daily—a starch and opium enema may be given; or, by the mouth, a combination of bismuth, in large doses, with Dover's powder; or the acid diarrhœa mixture, acetate of lead (gr. ii), dilute acetic acid (℥ xv–xx), and acetate of morphia (gr. $\frac{1}{6}$–$\frac{1}{8}$). The amount of food should be reduced, and whey and albumen-water in small amounts be substituted for the milk. An ice-bag or cold compresses relieve the soreness which sometimes accompanies the diarrhœa.

Constipation is present in many cases, and though I have never seen it do harm, yet it is well every third or fourth day to give an ordinary enema. If a laxative is needed during the course of the disease, the Hunyadi-janos or Friedrichshall water may be given.

Hæmorrhage.—As absolute rest is essential, the greatest care should be taken in the use of the bed-pan. It is perhaps better to allow the patient to pass the motions into the draw-sheet. Ice may be given, and a light ice-bag placed on the abdomen. The amount of food should be restricted for eight or ten hours. If there is a tendency to collapse, stimulants should be given, and, if necessary, hypodermic injections of ether. Injection of salt solution beneath the skin or directly into a vein may revive a failing heart. Turpentine is warmly recommended by certain authors. Should opium be given? One-fifth of the cases of perforation occur with hæmorrhage, and the opium may obscure the features upon which alone the diagnosis of perforation may be made. Of late we have abandoned the use of opium and have given the calcium chloride or lactate in doses of gr. xv every four hours. Gelatine we have also used a good deal, but it seems of doubtful value.

Perforation and Peritonitis.—Early diagnosis and early operation mean the saving of one-third of the cases of this heretofore uniformly fatal complication. The aim should be to operate for the perforation, and not to wait until a general peritonitis diminishes by one-half the chances of recovery. An incessant, intelligent watchfulness on the part of the medical attendant and the early co-operation of the surgeon are essentials. Every case of more than ordinary severity should be watched with special reference to this complication. Thorough preparation by early observation, careful notes, and knowledge of the conditions will help to prevent needless exploration. No case is too desperate; we have had one recovery after three operations. Twenty cases of perforation in my series were operated upon with seven recoveries; in an eighth case the patient died of the toxæmia on the eighth day after the laparotomy. The figures now published give from 25 to 33 per cent of recoveries. In doubtful cases it is best to operate, as experience shows that patients stand an exploration very well.

Cholecystitis.—A majority of the cases recover, but if the symptoms are very severe and progressive, operation should be advised.

Bone Lesions.—The typhoid periostitis of the ribs or of the tibia does not always go on to suppuration, though, as a rule, it requires operation. Unless the practitioner is accustomed to do very thorough surgical work, he should hand over the patient to a competent surgeon, who will clear out the diseased parts with the greatest thoroughness. Recurrence is inevitable unless the operation is complete.

For the progressive *heart-weakness*, alcohol, strychnine and ether hypodermically in full doses, digitalis, and the saline infusions may be tried.

The *nervous symptoms* of typhoid fever are best treated by hydrotherapy. Special advantages of this plan are that the restlessness is allayed, the delirium quieted, and sedatives are rarely needed. In the cases which set in early with severe headache, meningeal symptoms, and high fever, the cold bath, or in private practice the cold pack, should be employed. An ice-cap may be placed on the head, and if necessary morphia administered hypodermically. For the nocturnal restlessness, so distressing in some cases, Dover's powder should be given. As a rule, if a hypnotic is indicated, it is best to give opium in some form. Pulmonary complications should, if severe, receive appropriate treatment.

Bacilluria.—When bacilli are present, as demonstrated by cultures or shown by the microscope, urotropin may be given in ten-grain doses and kept up, if necessary, for several weeks. A patient should not be discharged with bacilli in his urine.

In protracted cases very special care should be taken to guard against *bedsores*. Absolute cleanliness and careful drying of the parts after an evacuation should be enjoined. The patient should be turned from side to side and propped with pillows, and the back can then be sponged with spirits. On the first appearance of a sore, the water- or air-bed should be used.

(*g*) THE MANAGEMENT OF CONVALESCENCE.—Convalescents from typhoid fever frequently cause greater anxiety than patients in the attack. The question of food has to be met at once, as the patient acquires a ravenous appetite and clamors for a fuller diet. My custom has been not to allow solid food until the temperature has been normal for ten days. This is, I think, a safe rule, leaning perhaps to the side of extreme caution; but, after all, with eggs, milk toast, milk puddings, and jellies, the patient can take a fairly varied diet. Many leading practitioners allow solid food to a patient so soon as he desires it. Peabody gives it on the disappearance of the fever; the late Austin Flint was also in favor of giving solid food early. I had a lesson in this matter which I have never forgotten. A young lad in the Montreal General Hospital, in whose case I was much interested, passed through a tolerably sharp attack of typhoid fever. Two weeks after the evening temperature had been normal, and only a day or two before his intended discharge, he ate several mutton chops, and within twenty-four hours was in a state of collapse from perforation. A small transverse rent was found at the bottom of an ulcer which was in process of healing. It is not easy to say why solid food, particularly meats, should disagree, but in so many instances an indiscretion in diet is followed by slight fever, the so-called *febris carnis*, that it is in the best interests of the patient to restrict the diet for some time after the fever has fallen. Whether an error in diet may cause relapse is doubtful. The patient may be allowed to sit up for a short time about the end of the first week of convalescence, and the period may be prolonged with a gradual return of strength. He should move about slowly, and when the weather is favorable should be in the open air as much as possible. He should be guarded at this period against all unnecessary excitement. Emotional disturbance not infrequently is the cause of recrudescence of the fever. Constipation is not uncommon in convalescence and is best treated by enemata. A protracted diarrhœa, which is usually due to ulceration in the colon, may retard recovery. In such cases the diet should be restricted to milk, and the patient should be confined to bed; large doses of bismuth and astringent injections will prove useful. The recrudescence of the fever does not require special measures. The treatment of the relapse is essentially that of the original attack.

Post-typhoid insanity requires the judicious care of an expert. The cases usually recover. The swollen leg after phlebitis is a source of great worry. A bandage should be worn during the day or a well-fitting elastic stocking. The outlook depends on the completeness with which the collateral circulation is established. In a good many cases there is permanent disability.

The *post-typhoid neuritis*, a cause of much alarm and distress, usually gets well, though it may take months, or even a couple of years, before the paralysis disappears. After the subsidence of the acute symptoms systematic massage of the paralyzed and atrophic muscles is the most satisfactory treatment.

The condition spoken of as the typhoid spine may drag on for months and prove very obstinate. The neurotic state has to be treated. Separation from solicitous and sympathetic friends, hydrotherapy in the form of the wet pack, and the Paquelin cautery are the most efficacious means of cure. An encouraging prognosis may be followed by rapid improvement.

II. TYPHUS FEVER.

Definition.—An acute infectious disease of unknown origin, highly contagious, characterized by sudden onset, maculated rash, marked nervous symptoms, and a cyclical course terminating by crisis, usually about the end of the second week. Post mortem there are no special lesions other than those associated with fever.

The disease is known by the names of hospital fever, spotted fever, jail fever, camp fever, and ship fever, and in Germany is called *exanthematic* typhus, in contradistinction to *abdominal* typhus.

Etiology.—Typhus fever has been one of the great epidemics of the world. Until the middle of the nineteenth century it prevailed extensively in all the larger cities of Europe, and at times extended to wide-spread outbreaks. As Hirsch has remarked, " The history of typhus is written in those dark pages of the world's story which tell of the grievous visitations of mankind by war, famine, and misery of every kind." Few countries have suffered more than Ireland, particularly between the years 1817 and 1819 and in 1846. In Eng-

typhoid fever

French clinicians of the early nineteenth century differentiated typhoid fever from other fevers. Nathan Smith's essay is the first significant American account of the disease, and the Philadelphian William Gerhard clearly distinguished it from typhus fever on clinical and anatomical grounds. Osler personally studied large numbers of typhoid patients in all of their clinical forms and correlated the pathological and clinical manifestations. To him belongs the credit for compiling the wealth of the then available knowledge and correlating it with his own views to provide the classic writings on typhoid fever. Osler's chapter in the 1909 edition fulfills every criterion for providing pertinent and essential details of an infectious disease. Remarkable for its clarity, his interpretation of epidemiology and pathogenesis coincides with current concepts and his description of the clinical features and complications reads as this great teacher spoke to his students.

Nothing is missing; the subject is given encyclopedic coverage and includes the clinical variations of typhoid fever from ambulatory to rapidly fatal forms. It is mainly in areas of specific treatment and management of complications that significant progress can be reported. Better understanding of epidemiology and methods of control have also accrued since 1909.

Etiology

Prevalence   Typhoid fever is now prevalent in those emerging countries where health standards have not reached levels enjoyed in America, European countries, and the Soviet Union. In the United States from 1900 to 1904, the death rate in registration areas was 33.8 per 100,000, with an annual toll of 40,000. From 1954 to 1963, there were 11,510 cases reported, with 317 deaths. Carriers are responsible for most cases in this country. The disease was of no importance to the military in World War II.

Immunity   Osler held that one attack conferred immunity, which is generally true, although second attacks do occur with infection by heterologous phage types. Osler observed that infection may occur without overt clinical illness, a fact which is observed repeatedly in sizeable outbreaks and in volunteer studies. Typhoid bacilli may be isolated from the blood or feces of these asymptomatic patients, who are a constant threat to the community and may become permanent carriers.

The Organism   Little more is known of the morphology of *Salmonella typhosa* and those factors which make it virulent. The bacillus has somatic and flagellar antigenic components, and the Phase I and II variations of the H antigen make it possible to classify salmonellae into subgroups. The virulence or surface antigen (Vi) is thought to account for pathogenicity, and strains without it are less virulent for primates and, probably, for man.

The prevalence of mixed infections was known to Osler, and it is not uncommon to isolate two salmonellae simultaneously from the blood or feces of a single patient. With better bacteriological and serological methods, it is now possible to relate various clinical syndromes to specific serotypes of salmonellae, e.g., gastroenteritis, *S. typhimurium*; bacteremia or focal infection, *S. choleraesuis*; enteric fever, *S. typhosa* and other salmonellae; and the carrier state, primarily *S. typhosa.*

Typhoid Carriers   About 3 percent of typhoid patients become permanent carriers, although the explanation for this is unknown. The only new data pertain to the propensity of the typhoid bacillus to persist in calculi. Combined cholecystectomy and antibiotics are necessary for clearance of typhoid carriers with cholelithiasis; in this condition, antibiotics given alone will fail. The paradox of the carrier state in cholecystectomized subjects may be explained on the basis of hepatic calcinosis. Typhoid carriers may shed bacilli continuously or intermittently. The spheroplast concept has been proposed but not proved to explain this unique example of microbial persistence.

Morbid anatomy and pathogenesis

The older morphological descriptions are very accurate. It is now known that *S. typhosa* localizes and propagates within the cytoplasm of cells. Studies in tissue culture have shown that typhoid bacilli may survive intracellularly for as long as two weeks of exposure to antibiotics. They form spheroplasts under similar experimental conditions. Biopsy specimens from the upper small intestine taken early in the illness show a reaction consisting of mononuclear and polymorphonuclear leukocytes, which indicates that inflammation occurs in the early stages. Repeated injections of endotoxin in tolerant animals produce hemorrhagic lesions of the intestine, liver, spleen, and marrow similar to the morphological lesion in typhoid patients.

Fewer of the classic complications, such as perforation or hemorrhage of the intestinal ulcer, occur today in previously healthy typhoid patients treated reasonably early in their illness. Debilitated, malnourished patients treated late in their illness develop complications of all types described so vividly by Osler.

Typhoid fever

Available evidence suggests that typhoid bacilli multiply in the intestine for several days, penetrate the intestinal mucosa, reach the systemic circulation via the lymphatics, and are distributed to Peyer's patches and lymphoid follicles of the intestine and elsewhere. Salmonellae are inhibited by an acid pH created by intestinal anaerobes such as *Bacteroides.* Prior treatment of animals with streptomycin, which inhibits these bacteria, increases susceptibility, presumably by elevation of pH. The relationship in humans is unknown but is under study.

The organism elaborates a lipid-polysaccharide-protein complex, or endotoxin, which in its purified form produces many of the clinical manifestations of typhoid fever when inoculated in small doses intravenously. The lipid component is regarded as the toxic fraction which causes headache, chills, malaise, fever of three to six hours, and leukopenia. Tolerance to this material develops in animals and man following repeated daily injections or continuous infusion. This pyrogenic tolerance develops both in normal subjects and in typhoid patients. Isotopically tagged macromolecules of endotoxin are avidly removed by the reticuloendothelial system during tolerance. Quantitative studies in volunteers suggest strongly that endotoxin is not primarily responsible for the clinical manifestation of typhoid fever.

Endotoxin of *S. typhosa* and other gram-negative bacilli, when given to animals or humans, provokes hyperreactivity of the vessels for catecholamines. In typhoid patients following injection of a small dose of norepinephrine, elevation of blood pressure, hypersensitivity of the nailfold capillaries, and hemorrhagic necrosis of the skin are observed. Conceivably endotoxin contributes to focal necrosis and hemorrhage in the intestinal tract and other organs during illness by altering vascular reactivity to the catecholamines.

Clinical manifestations

This section by Osler is one of the classic records of any disease and little comment is warranted. A few remarks may interest the contemporary reader. The initial medical diagnosis today might be "virus pneumonia" because of cough and diffuse bronchitic signs, infectious mononucleosis, lymphoma, or other virus infections. Osler's account is thorough, including descriptions of afebrile typhoid patients, hemorrhagic typhoid vesicular rose spots, and widespread sudamina which desquamate diffusely. He stressed the rarity of jaundice, herpes labialis, or profuse sweating in typhoid and noted the association of alopecia.

There is little newer knowledge about the hematological alterations. Although anemia is common, the development of hemolytic anemia was not described in 1909. In rare instances it accompanies typhoid fever and occurs independently of antibiotic treatment. It may be fatal.

Bradycardia, dicrotism, myocarditis, thrombophlebitis, diarrhea, intestinal hemorrhage and perforation, parotitis, superimposed pneumonia, cholecystitis, suppurative cholangitis and pylephlebitis, meningitis, neuritis, psychoses, acute nephritis, osteomyelitis, and chondritis now occur less frequently in patients adequately treated early. These sequelae of typhoid occur, however, in those areas of the world where nutritional standards are low and the disease is prevalent.

Management

Specific Treatment   Until 1948, the treatment of typhoid fever was symptomatic and supportive. Chloramphenicol was then shown to shorten the illness drastically and reduce the mortality. Osler reported a mortality of about 12 percent, with most deaths attributable to profound toxemia, to intestinal perforation with peritonitis, or to intestinal hemorrhage. Convalescence was prolonged and was frequently marked by secondary complications.

Chloramphenicol is bacteriostatic and is given to adults in an oral loading dose of 50 mg per kg, with similar doses daily in three divided doses for two weeks or two courses of five days each separated by eight days without antibiotic. The patient improves in two days and is afebrile in three and a half days, on the average, after initiating therapy. When the patient is afebrile, the antibiotic dosage may be reduced to 25 mg per kg per day. Smaller amounts of chloramphenicol are beneficial but not optimal. Lower dosage regimens present economic advantages when supplies are limited. The tetracycline antibiotics and the synthetic penicillins are moderately effective but do not compare with chloramphenicol in treatment (Figures 1 and 2).

Corticosteroids are antitoxemic and drastically shorten the toxic-febrile stage in typhoid fever. They are indicated only in those patients with severe toxic-febrile manifestations. If used, they should be administered along with chloramphenicol and not continued for longer than three days. Such regimens are not accompanied by a higher incidence of intestinal perforation or hemorrhage.

General Care   General management of the patient has been simplified by virtue of the specific control of the active infection. Adequate nutrition is maintained by administering liquids high in calories and proteins and later by low residue diets. Intensive replacement of fluids and electrolytes is indi-

Typhoid fever

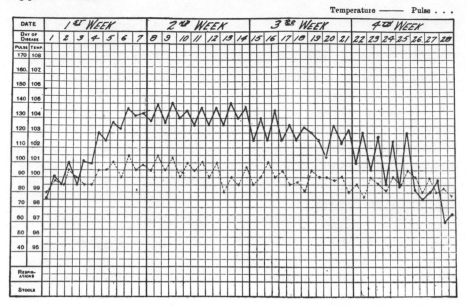

Figure 1. Typical temperature curve of moderately severe, uncomplicated typhoid fever.

Figure 2. Typhoid fever. Case T5, one of the first such patients to receive chloramphenicol, became afebrile after three days of treatment. From Woodward et al. *Ann. Intern. Med.*, 29:131, 1948.

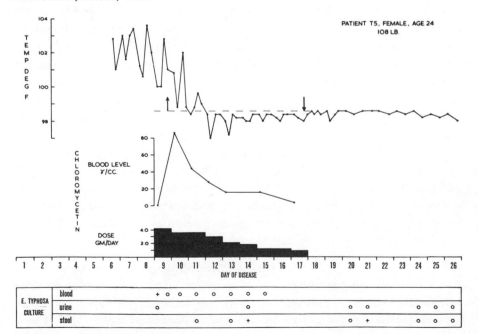

cated in severely dehydrated toxic patients. Transfusions of whole blood, given slowly, aid severely ill, anemic patients. Tepid sponging is indicated in the presence of hyperpyrexia.

Good nursing care is always essential and includes special attention to oral hygiene, adequate bathing, careful observation of the pulse, the onset of vomiting or severe abdominal pain, and the presence of bloody or tarry stools. Laxatives and the indiscreet use of enemas are ill-advised because of the danger of inciting intestinal perforation or hemorrhage.

Complications

Problem of Relapse
Osler found that relapse rates varied in different clinics from 3 to 18 percent; however, he reported a rate of 8.8 percent for an entire group of 28,051 cases. In spite of the application of various antibiotic regimens, including continuous or interrupted courses of chloramphenicol, with or without the supplemental administration of typhoid vaccine, relapses occur in about 20 percent of cases. One of the most important factors contributing to the frequency of relapse is the total dosage of chloramphenicol; as the dosage is decreased, the relapse rates increase.

The immunological reactions responsible for the patient's eventual recovery from typhoid fever are poorly understood. Presumably they require some weeks to become effective and are not fully developed in the individual who relapses whether he did or did not receive antibiotics. The height of the serological titer to the somatic (0), the flagellar (H), or Vi antigens cannot be equated with immunity; i.e., a patient may relapse in spite of a high typhoid 0 titer.

Problem of Intestinal Perforation
The management of a perforated intestine and peritonitis in the typhoid patient has changed radically since the introduction of chloramphenicol and the broad-spectrum antibiotics. Osler considered perforation without operation almost invariably fatal and even with surgical intervention, 13 of his 20 patients died. His overall incidence of intestinal perforation was 3.1 percent. The current incidence is now less, with adequate specific and general treatment of patients up to the tenth day or so of illness.

The debilitated toxic condition of the patient, the weakened circulation, the friability of the intestinal lesion, the stress of anesthesia and of the operative procedure have all contributed to make the typhoid patient with intestinal perforation and peritonitis a poor surgical risk. Medical treatment alone consisting of 1, control of the infection with antibiotics;

Typhoid fever

2, fluid and blood replacement to combat shock; and 3, the introduction of gastric suction to decompress the distended bowel has given surprisingly good results. The mortality from this complication is now about 30 percent, which is a significant improvement. Should it become obvious to the clinician and surgeon in attendance that the infectious process is failing to localize, as evidenced by the findings on examination, persistence of shock, continued leukocytosis, and other signs, it may be surmised that the ulcer is not healing and that surgical intervention is indicated. The medical approach appears to be the treatment of choice.

Diagnosis

Osler stressed the variable clinical pattern of typhoid fever from mild to grave forms and the importance of the febrile pattern. Initially the fever ascends stepwise for several days, stabilizes and maintains a high level for a week or more, and later becomes irregularly remittent and intermittent (see Fig. 1). He felt that the typhoid rash and the fever curve clinched the diagnosis.

The confirmatory laboratory tests are similar to those available in 1909, including specific bacteriological isolation of typhoid bacilli from the whole blood, blood clot, bone marrow, feces, urine, and pus. Bacteriological techniques have been changed and simplified.

Leukopenia remains a valuable laboratory finding in typhoid fever, and a moderate leukocytosis suggests a complication of the disease.

The Ehrlich diazo reaction of urine, introduced in 1883, is a red coloration given by the froth of urine of typhoid patients when mixed with diazo reagents. The test is performed simply and, if interpreted correctly, is useful particularly when laboratory facilities are limited.

The Widal reaction carries the same specificity as it did in 1909. Specific antibodies appear in the patient's serum to the H and O antigens, producing coarse and fine agglutination, respectively. The antibodies rise on about the seventh to the tenth day of illness, and the O titer is much more specific. A rising titer of the O agglutinin to 1:160 in a febrile patient with symptoms resembling typhoid fever is very suggestive but not absolutely diagnostic. In some instances, the agglutination titer does not rise or reach diagnostic levels. The agglutination titer is not an index of the state of immunity of the patient or susceptibility to relapse. The Vi antibody rises in typhoid patients but is not a reliable diagnostic test. It appears in carriers.

72

Mortality

Osler reported a variable mortality rate ranging in private practice from 5 to 12 percent and in hospital practice from 7 to 20 percent. Of 1,500 cases treated on his wards, 9.1 percent died. He regarded hydrotherapy as an effective measure responsible for lowering fatality. Chloramphenicol treatment combined with adequate supportive care under favorable conditions reduces the mortality to the order of a few percent at the most.

Prophylaxis

General Measures   Osler recognized the need to isolate typhoid patients in order to prevent patient spread. When the fecal-oral route of infection through contamination of water, milk or food became fully appreciated, sharper control measures were focused on elevating health standards, isolating the active patient, and restricting the carrier from handling food. The application of these health practices reduced the incidence of typhoid fever in the military, and only later was a reduction of incidence and mortality reflected in civilians. The decline is not attributable to the specific effect of vaccination.

Vaccination   Osler accepted the validity of the typhoid vaccine and cited the initial work of A.E. Wright published in 1904. Typhoid immunization was introduced in the U.S. Army by Russell in 1908. Initially, the vaccine was a heat-killed preparation of whole typhoid bacilli; later vaccines were prepared by phenol or alcohol inactivation which preserved somatic and Vi antigens respectively. Uncontrolled vaccine trials of many types were conducted until the midcentury, always with conflicting results. Under WHO auspices, controlled field trials were conducted in Yugoslavia from 1954 to 1956. The phenol vaccine gave protection for four years, but the alcohol vaccine was less effective. Additional appraisal was made by members of the Ministry of Health, Georgetown, British Guiana, from 1960 to 1963. Protection against infection by phenolized and acetone-inactivated vaccines was reported in primary school children aged 5 to 15 years. Studies in volunteers confirm that the phenol and acetone types of vaccine protect against a low infective challenge at an I.D.$_{25}$ dose, which is comparable to water-borne exposure. No protection is afforded at an I.D.$_{50}$ or higher dose, which is comparable to the degree of infection following the ingestion of contaminated food. Hence, the vaccine is effective but with limitations.

Theodore E. Woodward

Typhoid fever

REFERENCES

Ashcroft, M.T., Ritchie, J.M., and Nicholson, C.C. Controlled field trial in British Guiana school children of heat-killed phenolized and acetone-killed lyophilized typhoid vaccines. Amer. J. Hyg., 79:196, 1964.

Hornick, R.B., Woodward, T.E., McCrumb, F.R., Jr., Snyder, M.J., Dawkins, A.T., Jr., Buckeley, J.T., de la Macorra, F., and Carozza, F.A., Jr. Studies of induced typhoid fever. Evaluation of vaccine effectiveness. Trans. Ass. Amer. Physicians, Vol. 79, 1966.

Rowland, H.A.K. The treatment of typhoid fever. J. Trop. Med. Hyg., 64:101, 1961.

Woodward, T.E., and Smadel, J.E. Management of typhoid fever and its complications. Ann. Intern. Med., 60:144, 1964.

Should the fluid be sterile and tuberculosis suspected, a guinea-pig may be inoculated.

Prognosis.—Hirsch states that the mortality has ranged in various epidemics from 20 to 75 per cent. In children the death-rate is much higher than in adults.

Treatment.—The high rate of mortality which has existed in most epidemics indicates the futility of the various therapeutical agents which have been recommended. When we consider the nature of the local disease and the fact that, so far as we know, tuberculous and other secondary forms of cerebro-spinal meningitis are invariably fatal, we may wonder rather that recovery follows in any case.

In strong robust patients the local abstraction of blood by wet cups on the nape of the neck relieves the pain. General bloodletting is rarely indicated. Cold to the head and spine, which was used in the first epidemics by New England physicians, is of great service. A bladder of ice to the head, or an ice-cap, and the spinal ice-bag may be continuously employed. The latter is very beneficial. Hydrotherapy should be systematically used, in the form of the tub bath, at 98°, as recommended by Aufrecht. Netter speaks highly of its good effects, and we have also seen it do good. It may be given every third hour. If any counter-irritation is thought necessary, the skin of the back of the neck may be lightly touched with the Paquelin thermocautery. Blisters, which have been used so much, are of doubtful benefit. The lumbar puncture seems helpful in cases with coma or convulsions, and in any case it does no harm. Of internal remedies opium may be given freely, best as morphia hypodermically. Mercury has no special influence on meningeal inflammation. Iodide of potassium is warmly recommended by some writers. Quinine in large doses, ergot, belladonna and Calabar bean have had advocates. Bromide of potassium may be employed in the milder cases, but it is not so useful as morphia to control the spasms. Intraspinal injections have been tried, and in one of our cases Cushing opened and drained the spinal canal. Diphtheria antitoxin has been used with success in the recent New York epidemic.

A serum has been prepared and has been used with encouraging success. Flexner recommends doses of 30 cc. of his serum to be injected directly into the spinal meninges after the withdrawal of 50 cc. of cerebro-spinal fluid. Of 400 cases thus treated, collected by Flexner and Jobling, 295 recovered.

The diet should be nutritious, consisting of milk and strong broths while the fever persists. Many cases are very difficult to feed, and Heubner recommends forced alimentation with the stomach-tube. The cases seem to bear stimulants well, and whisky or brandy may be given freely when there are signs of a failing heart.

XV. LOBAR PNEUMONIA.

(Croupous or Fibrinous Pneumonia; Pneumonitis; Lung Fever.)

Definition.—An infectious disease characterized by inflammation of the lungs, toxæmia of varying intensity, and a fever that usually terminates by crisis. Secondary infective processes are common. The *Micrococcus lanceolatus* of Fraenkel is present in a large proportion of the cases.

History.—The disease was known to Hippocrates and the old Greek physicians, by whom it was confounded with pleurisy. Among the ancients, Aretæus gave a remarkable description. " Ruddy in countenance, but especially the cheeks; the white of the eyes very bright and fatty; the point of the nose flat; the veins in the temples and neck distended; loss of appetite; pulse, at first, large, empty, very frequent, as if forcibly accelerated; heat indeed, externally, feeble, and more humid than natural, but, internally, dry and very hot, by means of which the breath is hot; there is thirst, dryness of the tongue, desire of cold air, aberration of mind; cough mostly dry, but if anything be brought up it is a frothy phlegm, or slightly tinged with bile, or with a very florid tinge of blood. The blood-stained is of all others the worst." At the end of the seventeenth and the beginning of the eighteenth century Morgagni and Valsalva made many accurate clinical and anatomical observations on the disease. Our modern knowledge dates from Laennec (1819), whose masterly description of the physical signs and morbid anatomy left very little for subsequent observers to add or modify.

Incidence.—One of the most wide-spread and fatal of all acute diseases, pneumonia has become the " Captain of the Men of Death," to use the phrase applied by John Bunyan to consumption. In England and Wales in 1903 there were 40,725 deaths from this cause; 13,208 were attributed to lobar pneumonia, 17,425 to broncho-pneumonia, 10 to epidemic pneumonia, 216 to septic pneumonia, while 19,869 were registered as from pneumonia without further qualification. In 1902 there were 26,526 deaths from all forms of pneumonia, 21,623 in 1901, and 26,147 in 1900. The total number of deaths rose above 20,000 in 1890 and 1891 after the influenza, and fell again in 1894 to 18,000 (Tatham). The United States Census Report for 1900 gives 106.1 deaths from pneumonia per 1,000 deaths, against 90.6 in 1890 and 83.30 in 1880. An apparent increase is noted in the larger cities, particularly New York and Chicago. In Greater New York in 1904, out of a total of 42,700 deaths, there were 8,360 deaths from pneumonia, 19.5 per cent, against 16.5 per cent in 1903, 17 per cent in 1902, 16 per cent in 1901, and 14.7 per cent in 1898. In Chicago for the year 1903, out of a total of 28,914 deaths, 4,629, or 16 per cent, were from pneumonia, an increase of 18 per cent since the year 1900 (Reynolds).

Etiology.—Age.—To the sixth year the predisposition to pneumonia is marked; it diminishes to the fifteenth year, but then for each subsequent decade it increases. For children Holt's statistics of 500 cases give: First year, 15 per cent; from the second to the sixth year, 62 per cent; from the seventh to the eleventh year, 21 per cent; from the twelfth to the fourteenth year, 2 per cent. Lobar pneumonia has been met with in the new-born. The relation to age is well shown in the last U. S. Census Report for 1900. The death-rate in persons from fifteen to forty-five years was 100.05 per 100,000 of population; from forty-five to sixty-five years it was 263.12; and in persons sixty-five years of age and over it was 733.77. Pneumonia may well be called the friend of the aged. Taken off by it in an acute, short, not often painful illness, the old man escapes those " cold gradations of decay " so distressing to himself and to his friends.

Sex.—Males are more frequently affected than females.

Race.—In the United States pneumonia is more fatal in negroes than among the whites. Among the former, at the Johns Hopkins Hospital, the mortality was rarely under 30 per cent, against an average of about 25 per cent in the latter.

SOCIAL CONDITION.—The disease is more common in the cities. Individuals who are much exposed to hardship and cold are particularly liable to the disease. Newcomers and immigrants are stated to be less susceptible than native inhabitants.

PERSONAL CONDITION.—Debilitating causes of all sorts render individuals more susceptible. Alcoholism is perhaps the most potent predisposing factor. Robust, healthy men are, however, often attacked.

PREVIOUS ATTACK.—No other acute disease recurs in the same individual with such frequency. Instances are on record of individuals who have had ten or more attacks. The percentage of recurrences has been placed as high as 50. Netter gives it as 31, and he has collected the statistics of eleven observers who place the percentage at 26.8. Among the highest figures for recurrences are those of Benjamin Rush, 28, and Andral, 16.

TRAUMA—CONTUSION-PNEUMONIA.—Pneumonia may follow directly upon injury, particularly of the chest, without necessarily any lesion of the lung. Litten gives 4.4 per cent, Stern 2.8 per cent. There have been several well-marked cases at the Johns Hopkins Hospital. Stern describes three clinical varieties: first, the ordinary lobar pneumonia following a contusion of the chest wall; secondly, atypical cases, with slight fever and not very characteristic physical signs; thirdly, cases with the physical signs and features of bronchopneumonia. The last two varieties have a favorable prognosis. According to Ballard, workers in certain phosphate factories, where they breathe a very dusty atmosphere, are particularly prone to pneumonia.

COLD has been for years regarded as an important etiological factor. The frequent occurrence of an initial chill has been one reason for this wide-spread belief. As to the close association of pneumonia with exposure there can be no question. We see the disease occur either promptly after a wetting or a chilling due to some unusual exposure, or come on after an ordinary catarrh of one or two day's duration. Cold is now regarded simply as a factor in lowering the resistance of the bronchial and pulmonary tissues.

CLIMATE AND SEASON.—Climate does not appear to have very much influence, as pneumonia prevails equally in hot and cold countries. It is stated to be more prevalent in the Southern than in the Northern States, but an examination of the Census Reports shows that there is very little difference in the various state groups.

Much more important is the influence of *season*. Statistics are almost unanimous in placing the highest incidence of the disease in the winter and spring months. In Montreal, January, the coldest month of the year, but with steady temperature, has usually a comparatively low death-rate from pneumonia. The large statistics of Seitz from Munich and of Seibert of New York give the highest percentage in February and March.

Bacteriology of Acute Lobar Pneumonia.—(*a*) MICROCOCCUS LANCEOLATUS, PNEUMOCOCCUS OR DIPLOCOCCUS PNEUMONIÆ OF FRAENKEL AND WEICHSELBAUM.—In September, 1880, Sternberg inoculated rabbits with his own saliva and isolated a micrococcus. The publication was not made until April, 1881. Pasteur discovered the same organism in the saliva of a child dead of hydrophobia in December, 1880, and the priority of the discovery belongs to him, as his publication is dated January, 1881. There was, however, no suspicion that this organism was concerned in the etiology of lobar pneumonia, and it was not really until April, 1884, that Fraenkel determined that the organism found by Sternberg and Pasteur in the saliva, and known as the coccus of sputum septicæmia, was the most frequent germ in pneumonia.

The organism is a somewhat elliptical, lance-shaped coccus, usually occurring in pairs; hence the term diplococcus. It is readily demonstrated in cover-glass preparations with the usual dyes and by the Gram method. About the organism in the sputum a capsule can always be demonstrated. Its cultural and biological properties present many variations, for a consideration of which the student is referred to the text-books on bacteriology. Scarcely any peculiarity is constant. A large number of varieties have been cultivated. Its kinship to *Streptococcus pyogenes* is regarded by many as very close, but the alkaline serum-water medium, containing inulin, recommended by His, serves to distinguish the pneumococcus from the streptococcus.

Distribution in the Body.—In the bronchial secretions and in the affected lung the pneumococcus is readily demonstrated in smears, and in the latter in sections. By using large quantities of blood (3 to 6 cc.) diluted over twelve times with a liquid culture medium, preferably broth, Kinsey was able to isolate the pneumococcus from the blood during life in 19 of 25 cases.

(*b*) PNEUMOCOCCUS UNDER OTHER CONDITIONS.—(1) *In the Mouth.*— The studies of the New York Pneumonia Commission have shown that the pneumococcus is present in the mouths of a large proportion of healthy individuals, the various observers giving 80 to 90 per cent of positive results. The virulence is not always uniform, and Langcope and Fox were able to show that the saliva of the same individual increased in virulence during the winter months. Some persons always harbor a virulent variety. Buerger at the Mt. Sinai Hospital studied the communicability of the organism from one person to another, and it was found repeatedly that normal individuals—i. e., persons in whose mouths the pneumococcus was proved by repeated examinations to be absent—acquired the organisms by association with cases of pneumonia, or with healthy persons in whose saliva pneumococci were present.

(2) *Outside the Body.*—The viability of the pneumococcus is not great. It has been found occasionally in the dust and sweepings of rooms, but Wood has shown (New York Commission Report) that the germs exposed to sunlight die in a very short time—an hour and a half being the limit. In moist sputum kept in a dark room the germs lived ten days, and in a badly ventilated room in which a person with pneumonia coughed, the germs suspended in the air retained their vitality for several hours.

(3) *The Pneumococcus in Other Diseases.*—The organism is very widely distributed, and occurs in many conditions other than croupous pneumonia. An acute *septicæmia* without local lesion may occur, resembling the typhoid septicæmia, already described. In a case reported by Townsend, a girl, aged six, had pain in the abdomen, vomiting, and a temperature of 104.2°. There was no exudate in the throat. She died thirty hours after the onset of the symptoms. There was found a general infection with the pneumococcus in blood, lungs, spleen, and kidneys. As Rosenau has shown, a bacteriæmia may precede the development of the local lesion in the lungs. In *terminal infec-*

tions the pneumococcus plays an important rôle. Flexner found it four times in acute peritonitis, eleven times in acute pericarditis, five times in acute endocarditis, and three times both in pleurisy and in acute meningitis.

The germ has been associated with wide-spread epidemics of catarrh of the upper air passages, *pneumococcus catarrh,* almost like influenza, and sometimes with gastro-intestinal disturbances.

An extraordinary number of local affections are due to the pneumococcus. It is a common cause of the primary and secondary *broncho-pneumonias.* Infection of the *accessory nasal sinuses* is most important. Darling found them involved in 92 per cent of all pneumococcus infections coming to autopsy at Panama. *Meningitis* may be associated with pneumonia or endocarditis, but the so-called primary pneumococcus meningitis is almost always secondary to sinus infection, 90 per cent in 25 cases (Darling). *Pericarditis, endocarditis, empyema, peritonitis, arthritis, conjunctivitis, otitis* may be primary infections with this ubiquitous germ.

(*c*) BACILLUS PNEUMONIÆ OF FRIEDLÄNDER.—This is a larger organism than the pneumococcus, and appears in the form of plump, short rods. It also shows a capsule, but presents marked biological and cultural differences from Fraenkel's pneumococcus. It occurred in 9 of Weichselbaum's 129 cases. It may cause broncho-pneumonia and other affections, but probably is not a cause of genuine lobar pneumonia. The exudate in pneumonias caused by this bacillus is usually more viscid and poorer in fibrin than that in diplococcus pneumonias.

(*d*) OTHER ORGANISMS.—Various bacteria may be associated with the pneumococcus in lobar pneumonia, the most common of these being *Streptococcus pyogenes,* the pyogenic staphylococci, and Friedländer's pneumobacillus; but while these latter may cause broncho-pneumonias, they have not been satisfactorily demonstrated to be other than secondary invaders in lobar pneumonia. Likewise the pneumonias caused by *Bacillus typhosus, Bacillus diphtheriæ,* and the influenza bacillus are not to be identified with true lobar pneumonia.

Clinically, the *infectious nature* of pneumonia was recognized long before we knew anything of the pneumococcus. Among the features which favored this view were the following: First, the disease is similar to other infections in its mode of outbreak. It may occur in endemic form, localized in certain houses, in barracks, jails, and schools. As many as ten occupants of one house have been attacked. I have seen three members of a family consecutively attacked with a most malignant type of pneumonia. Among the more remarkable endemic outbreaks is that reported by W. B. Rodman, of Frankfort, Ky. In a prison with a population of 735 there occurred in one year 118 cases of pneumonia with 25 deaths. The disease may assume epidemic proportions. In the Middlesborough epidemic, so carefully studied by Ballard, there were 682 persons attacked, with a mortality of 21 per cent. During some years pneumonia is so prevalent that it is practically pandemic. Direct contagion is suggested by the fact that a patient in the next bed to a pneumonia case may take the disease, or 2 or 3 cases may follow in rapid succession in a ward. It is very exceptional, however, for nurses or doctors to be attacked.

Secondly, as in other acute infections, the constitutional symptoms may bear no proportion whatever to the severity of the local lesion. As is well

79

known, a patient may have a very small apex pneumonia which does not seriously impair the breathing capacity, but which may be accompanied with the most intense toxic features.

Thirdly, the clinical course of the disease is that of an acute infection. It is the very type of a self-limited disease, running a definite cycle in a way seen only in infectious disorders.

Conditions Favoring Infection.—Some have already been referred to, but of many we are still ignorant. The one all-important fact, emphasized by the work of the New York Commission, is that a majority of us harbor the germ in mouth or nose or throat. It has been shown that the virulence varies at different periods, and with this may be associated the well-known seasonal prevalence of the disease. Some individuals are less resistant, and in no other acute disease may so many successive attacks occur in the same person. It is notorious that the negro race in the United States, in Panama, and in South Africa shows an extreme susceptibility; on the other hand, the Chinese in the South African compounds show an extraordinary resistance to the disease (Porter). Probably for each one of us it is a battle between the degree of resistance and the virulence of the organism which we harbor. A catarrh of the upper air passages, exposure, alcoholism, etc., weaken the defences, and give the ever-present enemy a chance, either for a frontal attack in the lungs, in an acute pneumonia, or to make a flanking assault on some unprotected region, causing a peritonitis, otitis, sinusitis, etc.

Immunity and Serum Therapy.—The pneumococcus does not produce in artificial cultures any strong, soluble toxin analogous to the diphtheria toxin or the tetanus toxin, but its poison is contained within the bacterial cells, from which it may be extracted in various ways, or it may be set free from the dead or degenerated cocci. The possibility that the pneumococcus may secrete a soluble toxin in the infected human or animal body may be admitted, but of this there is no conclusive demonstration. By the use of living or dead pneumococci or their extracts, animals may be vaccinated against this organism, so that their blood-serum is capable of protecting susceptible animals against many times the minimal fatal dose of the virulent pneumococcus. Strong protective serum has thus been obtained from rabbits, horses, asses, cows, and other animals subjected to repeated inoculations with dead and living cultures of the pneumococcus. This specific serum is neither antitoxic nor bactericidal. Metchnikoff believes that it acts by stimulating the leucocytes to ingest and destroy the pneumococci, but A. E. Wright and Douglas have shown that the protective constituent, which they call an opsonin, enters into chemical combination with the cocci, rendering them thereby more readily engulfed and digested by the phagocytes. Neufeld and Rimpau have reached a similar conclusion as to the mode of action of this immune serum. M. Wassermann finds that the specific protective substances are formed in the bone-marrow, and thence distributed to the blood. There is evidence that similar specific substances are produced in human beings infected with this organism, and the crisis of pneumonia is explained by the formation and accumulation of these substances in the body.

Many trials have been made of the curative value of antipneumococcic serum in the treatment of pneumonia, the serum made by Pane having been most extensively employed. Thus far it has not been shown that this serum influences in any marked degree the course of the disease in man. Pässler claims to have observed favorable results from the use of a polyvalent serum prepared according to a method devised by Römer, and he advocates its employment especially in patients with symptoms of severe infection.

Morbid Anatomy.—Since the time of Laennec, pathologists have recognized three stages in the inflamed lung: engorgement, red hepatization, and gray hepatization.

In the stage of *engorgement* the lung tissue is deep red in color, firmer to the touch, and more solid, and on section the surface is bathed with blood and serum. It still crepitates, though not so distinctly as healthy lung, and excised portions float. The air-cells can be dilated by insufflation from the bronchus. The capillary vessels are greatly distended, the alveolar epithelium swollen, and the air-cells occupied by a variable number of blood-corpuscles and detached alveolar cells. In the stage of *red hepatization* the lung tissue is solid, firm, and airless. If the entire lobe is involved it looks voluminous, and shows indentations of the ribs. On section, the surface is dry, reddish-brown in color, and has lost the deeply congested appearance of the first stage. One of the most remarkable features is the friability; in striking contrast to the healthy lung, which is torn with difficulty. The surface has a granular appearance due to the fibrinous plugs filling the air-cells. The distinctness of this appearance varies greatly with the size of the alveoli, which are about 0.10 mm. in diameter in the infant, 0.15 or 0.16 in the adult, and from 0.20 to 0.25 in old age. On scraping the surface with a knife a reddish viscid serum is removed, containing small granular masses. The smaller bronchi often contain fibrinous plugs. If the lung has been removed before the heart, it is not uncommon to find solid moulds of clot filling the blood-vessels. Microscopically, the air-cells are seen to be occupied by coagulated fibrin in the meshes of which are red blood-corpuscles, mononuclear and polynuclear leucocytes, and alveolar epithelium. The alveolar walls are infiltrated and leucocytes are seen in the interlobular tissues. Cover-glass preparations from the exudate, and thin sections show, as a rule, the diplococci already referred to, many of which are contained within cells. Staphylococci and streptococci may also be seen in some cases. In the stage of *gray hepatization* the tissue has changed from a reddish-brown to a grayish-white color. The surface is moister, the exudate obtained on scraping is more turbid, the granules in the acini are less distinct, and the lung tissue is still more friable. The air-cells are densely filled with leucocytes, the fibrin network and the red blood-corpuscles have largely disappeared. A more advanced condition of gray hepatization is that known as *purulent infiltration*, in which the lung tissue is softer and bathed with a purulent fluid. Small abscess cavities may form, and by their fusion larger ones, though this is a rare event in ordinary pneumonia.

Resolution.—The changes in the exudate which lead to its resolution are due to an autolytic digestion by proteolytic enzymes which are present much more abundantly in gray hepatization than in the preceding stage. The dissolved exudate is for the most part excreted by the kidneys. By following the nitrogen excess in the urine the progress of resolution may be followed and even an estimate formed of the amount of the exudate thus eliminated. In a study from my clinic H. W. Cook found in cases of delayed resolution that the nitrogen excess in the urine (which persisted until the lung was clear) was very large, and he suggests that delayed resolution may really be a matter of continued exudation.

General Details of the Morbid Anatomy.—In 100 autopsies, made by me at the General Hospital, Montreal, in 51 cases the right lung was affected, in 32 the left, in 17 both organs. In 27 cases the entire lung, with the exception, perhaps, of a narrow margin at the apex and anterior border, was consolidated. In 34 cases, the lower lobe alone was involved; in 13 cases, the upper lobe alone. When double, the lower lobes were usually affected together, but in three instances the lower lobe of one and the upper lobe of the other were attacked. In 3 cases, also, both upper lobes were affected. Occasionally the disease involves the greater part of both lungs; thus, in one instance the left organ with the exception of the anterior border was uniformly hepatized, while the right was in the stage of gray hepatization, except a still smaller portion in the corresponding region. In a third of the cases, red and gray hepatization existed together. In 22 instances there was gray hepatization. As a rule the unaffected portion of the lung is congested or œdematous. When the greater portion of a lobe is attacked, the uninvolved part may be in a state of almost gelatinous œdema. The unaffected lung is usually congested, particularly at the posterior part. This, it must be remembered, may be largely due to post-mortem subsidence. The uninflamed portions are not always congested and œdematous. The upper lobe may be dry and bloodless when the lower lobe is uniformly consolidated. The average weight of a normal lung is about 600 grammes, while that of an inflamed organ may be 1,500, 2,000, or even 2,500 grammes.

The bronchi contain, as a rule, at the time of death a frothy serous fluid, rarely the tenacious mucus so characteristic of pneumonic sputum. The mucous membrane is usually reddened, rarely swollen. In the affected areas the smaller bronchi often contain fibrinous plugs, which may extend into the larger tubes, forming perfect casts. The bronchial glands are swollen and may even be soft and pulpy. The pleural surface of the inflamed lung is invariably involved when the process becomes superficial. Commonly, there is only a thin sheeting of exudate, producing slight turbidity of the membrane. In only two of the hundred instances the pleura was not involved. In some cases the fibrinous exudate may form a creamy layer an inch in thickness. A serous exudation of variable amount is not uncommon.

Lesions in Other Organs.—The heart, particularly its right chamber, is distended with firm, tenacious coagula, which can be withdrawn from the vessels as dendritic moulds. In no other acute disease do we meet with coagula of such solidity. The spleen is often enlarged, though in only 35 of the 100 cases was the weight above 200 grammes. The kidneys show parenchymatous swelling, turbidity of the cortex, and, in a very considerable proportion of the cases—25 per cent—chronic interstitial changes.

Pericarditis is not infrequent, and occurs more particularly with pneumonia of the left side and with double pneumonia. In 5 of the 100 autopsies it was present, and in 4 of them the lappet of lung overlying the pericardium with its pleura was involved. *Endocarditis* is more frequent and occurred in 16 of the 100 cases. In 5 of these the endocarditis was of the simple character; in 11 the lesions were ulcerative. Of 209 cases of malignant endocarditis which I collected from the literature, 54 occurred in pneumonia. Kanthack found an antecedent pneumonia in 14.2 per cent of cases of infective endocarditis. In the recent figures collected by E. F. Wells, of 517 fatal cases of acute endocarditis, 22.3 per cent were in pneumonia. It is more common on the left than on the right side of the heart. Of 61 of a series of 107 cases of endocarditis in Professor Welch's laboratory in which cultures were made, pneumococci were found in 21. In 7 of the cases there was a general pneumococcic infection. *Myocarditis* and fatty degeneration of the heart may be present in protracted cases.

Meningitis, which is not infrequent, may be associated with malignant endocarditis. It was present in 8 of the 100 autopsies. Of 20 cases of meningitis in ulcerative endocarditis 15 occurred in pneumonia. The meningitis is usually of the convex.

Croupous or diphtheritic inflammation may occur in other parts. A *croupous colitis,* as pointed out by Bristowe, is not very uncommon. It occurred in 5 of my 100 post mortems. It is usually a thin, flaky exudation, most marked on the tops of the folds of the mucous membrane. In one case there was a patch of *croupous gastritis,* covering an area 2 by 8 cm., situated to the left of the cardiac orifice.

The liver shows parenchymatous changes, and often extreme engorgement of the hepatic veins.

Symptoms.—Course of the Disease in Typical Cases.—We know but little of the incubation period in lobar pneumonia. It is probably very short. There are sometimes slight catarrhal symptoms for a day or two. As a rule, the disease sets in abruptly with a severe chill, which lasts from fifteen to thirty minutes or longer. In no acute disease is an initial chill so constant or so severe. The patient may be taken abruptly in the midst of his work, or may awaken out of a sound sleep in a rigor. The temperature taken during the chill shows that the fever has already begun. If seen shortly after the onset, the patient has usually features of an acute fever, and complains of headache and general pains. Within a few hours there is pain in the side, often of an agonizing character; a short, dry, painful cough begins, and the respirations are increased in frequency. When seen on the second or third day, the picture in typical pneumonia is more distinctive than that presented by any other acute disease. The patient lies flat in bed, often on the affected side; the face is flushed, particularly one or both cheeks; the breathing is hurried, accompanied often with a short expiratory grunt; the alæ nasi dilate with each inspiration; herpes is usually present on the lips or nose; the eyes are bright, the expression is anxious, and there is a frequent short cough which makes the patient wince and hold his side. The expectoration is blood-tinged and extremely tenacious. The temperature may be 104° or 105°. The pulse is full and bounding and the pulse-respiration ratio much disturbed. Examination of the lungs shows the physical signs of consolidation—blowing breathing and fine râles. After persisting for from seven to ten days the crisis occurs, and with a fall in the temperature the patient passes from the condition of extreme distress and anxiety to one of comparative comfort.

Special Features.—*The fever* rises rapidly, and the height may be 104° or 105° within twelve hours. Having reached the fastigium, it is remarkably constant. Often the two-hour temperature chart will not show for two days more than a degree of variation. In children and in cases without chill the

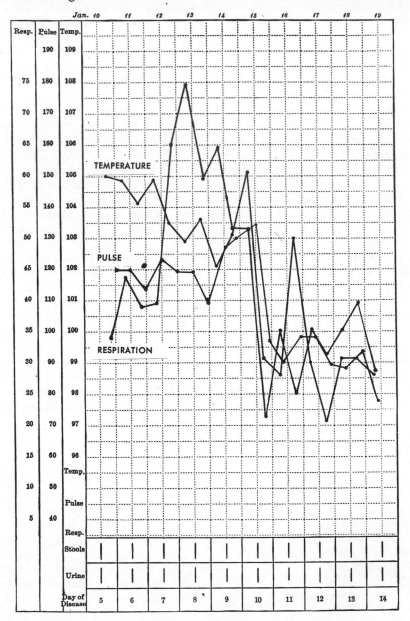

CHART X.—FEVER, PULSE, AND RESPIRATION IN LOBAR PNEUMONIA.

rise is more gradual. In old persons and in drunkards the temperature range is lower than in children and in healthy individuals; indeed, one occasionally meets with an afebrile pneumonia.

84

THE CRISIS.—After the fever has persisted for from five to nine or ten days there is an abrupt drop, known as the crisis, which is one of the most characteristic features of the disease. The day of the crisis is variable. It is very uncommon before the third day, and rare after the twelfth. I have seen it as early as the third day. From the time of Hippocrates it has been thought to be more frequent on the uneven days, particularly the fifth and seventh. A *precritical rise* of a degree or two may occur. In one case the temperature rose from 105° to nearly 107°, and then in a few hours fell to normal. Not even after the chill in malarial fever do we see such a prompt and rapid drop in the temperature. The usual time is from five to twelve hours, but often in an hour there may occur a fall of six or eight degrees (S. West). The temperature may be subnormal after the crisis, as low as 96° or 97°. Usually there is an abundant sweat, and the patient sinks into a comfortable sleep. The day after the crisis there may be a slight post-critical rise. A *pseudo-crisis* is not very uncommon, in which on the fifth or sixth day the temperature drops from 104° or 105° to 102°, and then rises again. When the fall takes place gradually within twenty-four hours it is called a protracted crisis. If the fever persists beyond the twelfth day, the fall is likely to be by lysis. In children this mode of termination is common, and occurred in one-third of a series of 183 cases reported by Morrill. Occasionally in debilitated individuals the temperature drops rapidly just before death; more frequently there is an ante-mortem elevation. In cases of delayed resolution the fever may persist for six or eight weeks. The crisis is the most remarkable single phenomenon of pneumonia. With the fall in the fever the respirations become reduced almost to normal, the pulse slows, and the patient passes from perhaps a state of extreme hazard and distress to one of safety and comfort, and yet, so far as the physical examination indicates, there is with the crisis no special change in the local condition in the lung.

PAIN.—There is early a sharp, agonizing pain, generally referred to the region of the nipple or lower axilla of the affected side, and much aggravated on deep inspiration and on coughing. It is associated, as Aretæus remarks, with involvement of the pleura. It is absent in central pneumonia, and much less frequent in apex pneumonia. The pain may be severe enough to require a hypodermic injection of morphia. As has been recognized for many years, the pain may be altogether abdominal, either central or in the right iliac fossa, suggesting appendicitis. Crozer Griffith, calling attention to the frequency of the simulation in children, reports 8 cases, and has collected 34 cases from the literature, many in adults. The operation for appendicitis has been performed.

DYSPNŒA is an almost constant feature. Even early in the disease the respirations may be 30 in the minute, and on the second or third day between 40 and 50. The movements are shallow, evidently restrained, and if the patient is asked to draw a deep breath he cries out with the pain. Expiration is frequently interrupted by an audible grunt. At first with the increased respiration there may be no sensation of distress. Later this may be present in a marked degree. In children the respirations may be 80 or even 100. Many factors combine to produce the shortness of breath—the pain in the side, the toxæmia, the fever, and the loss of function in a considerable area of the lung tissue. Sometimes there appear to be nervous factors at work.

85

That it does not depend upon the consolidation is shown by the fact that after the crisis, without any change in the local condition of the lung, the number of respirations may drop to normal. The ratio between the respirations and the pulse may be 1 to 2 or even 1 to 1.5, a disturbance rarely so marked in any other disease.

COUGH.—This usually comes on with the pain in the side, and at first is dry, hard, and without any expectoration. Later it becomes very characteristic—frequent, short, restrained, and associated with great pain in the side. In old persons, in drunkards, in the terminal pneumonias, and sometimes in young children, there may be no cough. After the crisis the cough usually becomes much easier and the expectoration more easily expelled. The cough is sometimes persistent, continuous, and by far the most aggravated and distressing symptom of the disease. Paroxysms of coughing of great intensity after the crisis suggest a pleural exudate.

SPUTUM.—A brisk hæmoptysis may be the initial symptom. At first the sputum may be mucoid, but usually after twenty-four hours it becomes blood-tinged, viscid, and very tenacious. At first quite red from the unchanged blood, it gradually becomes rusty or of an orange yellow. The tenacious viscidity of the sputum is remarkable; it often has to be wiped from the lips of the patient. When jaundice is present it may be green or yellow. In low types of the disease the sputum may be fluid and of a dark brown color, resembling prune juice. The amount is very variable, ranging from 100 to 300 cc. in the twenty-four hours. In 100 cases in my clinic studied by Emerson, in 16 there was little or no sputum; in 32 it was typically rusty; in 33 blood-streaked; in 3 cases the sputum was very bloody. In children and very old people there may be no sputum whatever. After the crisis the quantity is variable, abundant in some cases, absent in others.

Microscopically, the sputum consists of leucocytes, mucus corpuscles, red blood-corpuscles in all stages of degeneration, and bronchial and alveolar epithelium. Hæmatoidin crystals are occasionally met with. Of micro-organisms the pneumococcus is usually present, and sometimes Friedländer's bacillus and the influenza bacillus. Very interesting constituents are small cell moulds of the alveoli and the fibrinous casts of the bronchioles; the latter may be very plainly visible to the naked eye, and sometimes may form good-sized dendritic casts. Chemically, the expectoration is particularly rich in calcium chloride.

Physical Signs.—INSPECTION.—The position of the patient is not constant. He usually rests more comfortably on the affected side, or he is propped up with the spine curved toward it. Orthopnœa is rare.

In a small lesion no differences may be noted between the sides; as a rule, movement is much less on the affected side, which may look larger. With involvement of a lower lobe, the apex on the same side may show greater movement. The compensatory increased movement on the sound side is sometimes very noticeable even before the patient's chest is bared. The intercostal spaces are not usually obliterated. When the cardiac lappet of the left upper lobe is involved there may be a marked increase in the area of visible cardiac pulsation. Pulsation of the affected lung may cause a marked movement of the chest wall (Graves). Other points to be noticed in the inspection are the frequency of the respiration, the action of the accessory muscles, such as the sterno-cleido-mastoids and scaleni, and the dilatation of the nostrils with each inspiration.

MENSURATION may show a definite increase in the volume of the side affected, rarely more, however, than 1 or 1½ cm.

PALPATION.—The lack of expansion on the affected side is sometimes more readily perceived by touch than by sight. The pleural friction may be felt. On asking the patient to count, the voice fremitus is greatly increased in comparison with the corresponding point on the healthy side. It is to be remembered that if the bronchi are filled with thick secretion, or if, in what is known as massive pneumonia, they are filled with fibrinous exudate, the tactile fremitus may be diminished. It is always well to ask the patient to cough before testing the fremitus.

PERCUSSION.—In the stage of engorgement the note is higher pitched and may have a somewhat tympanitic quality, the so-called Skoda's resonance. This can often be obtained over the lung tissue just above a consolidated area. L. A. Conner calls attention to a point which all observers must have noticed, that, when the patient is lying on his side, the percussion at the dependent base is " deeper and more resonant than that of the upper side," which by contrast may seem abnormal, and there may even be a faint tubular element added to the vesicular breathing on the compressed side. When the lung is hepatized, the percussion note is dull, the quality varying a good deal from a note which has in it a certain tympanitic quality to one of absolute flatness. There is not the wooden flatness of effusion and the sense of resistance is not so great. During resolution the tympanitic quality of the percussion note usually returns. For weeks or months after convalescence there may be a higher-pitched note on the affected side. Wintrich's change in the percussion note when the mouth is open may be very well marked in pneumonia of the upper lobe. Occasionally there is an almost metallic quality over the consolidated area, and when this exists with a very pronounced amphoric quality in the breathing the presence of a cavity may be suggested. In deep-seated pneumonias there may be for several days no change in the percussion note.

AUSCULTATION.—Quiet, suppressed breathing in the affected part is often a marked feature in the early stage, and is always suggestive. Only in a few cases is the breathing harsh or puerile. Very early there is heard at the end of inspiration the fine crepitant râle, a series of minute cracklings heard close to the ear, and perhaps not audible until a full breath is drawn. This is probably a fine pleural crepitus, as J. B. Leaming maintained; it is usually believed to be produced in the air-cells and finer bronchi by the separation of the sticky exudate. In the stage of red hepatization and when dulness is well defined, the respiration is tubular, similar to that heard in health over the larger bronchi. It is heard first with expiration (a point noted by James Jackson, Jr.), and is soft and of low pitch. Gradually it becomes more intense, and finally presents an intensity unknown in any other pulmonary affection—of high pitch, perfectly dry, and of equal length with inspiration and expiration. It is simply the propagation of the laryngeal and tracheal sounds through the bronchi and the consolidated lung tissue. The permeability of the bronchi is essential to its production. Tubular breathing is absent in the excessively rare cases of massive pneumonia in which the larger bronchi are completely filled with exudation. When resolution begins mucous râles of all sizes can be heard. At first they are small and have been called the *redux-crepitus*. The voice-sounds and the expiratory grunt are transmitted through the consolidated lung with great intensity. This bronchophony may have a curious nasal quality, to which the term ægophony has been given. There are cases in which the consolidation is deeply seated—so-called central pneumonia, in which the physical signs are slight or even absent, yet the cough, the rusty expectoration, and general features make the diagnosis certain.

Circulatory Symptoms.—During the chill the *pulse* is small, but in the succeeding fever it becomes full and bounding. In cases of moderate severity it ranges from 100 to 116. It is not often dicrotic. In strong, healthy individuals and in children there may be no sign of failing pulse throughout the attack. With extensive consolidation the left ventricle may receive a very much diminished amount of blood and the pulse in consequence may be small. In the old and feeble it may be small and rapid from the outset. The pulse may be full, soft, very deceptive, and of no value whatever in prognosis.

BLOOD PRESSURE.—During the first few days there is no change. The extent of involvement seems to have no effect upon the peripheral blood pressure. In the toxic cases the pressure may begin to fall early; a drop of 15–20 mm. Hg. is perfectly safe, but a progressive fall indicates the need of stimulation. A sudden drop is rarely seen except just before death. A slow, gradual fall of more than 20 mm. Hg. means cardio-vascular asthenia, and calls for an increase in the stimulation. The crisis has no effect on the blood pressure. The *heart-sounds* are usually loud and clear. During the intensity of the fever, particularly in children, *bruits* are not uncommon both in the mitral and in the pulmonic areas. The second sound over the pulmonary artery is accentuated. Attention to this sign gives a valuable indication as to the condition of the lesser circulation. With distention of the right chambers and failure of the right ventricle to empty itself completely the pulmonary second sound becomes much less distinct. When the right heart is engorged there may be an increase in the dulness to the right of the sternum. With gradual heart weakness and signs of dilatation the long pause is greatly shortened, the sounds approach each other in tone and have a fœtal character (embryocardia).

There may be a sudden early collapse of the heart with very feeble, rapid pulse and increasing cyanosis. I have known this to occur on the third day. Even when these symptoms are very serious recovery may take place. In other instances without any special warning death may occur even in robust, previously healthy men. The heart weakness may be due to paralysis of the vaso-motor centre and consequent lowering of the general arterial pressure. The soft, easily compressed pulse, with the gray, ashy facies, cold hands and feet, the clammy perspiration, and the progressive prostration tell of a toxic action on the vaso-motor centres. Endocarditis and pericarditis will be considered under complications.

BLOOD.—Anæmia is rarely seen. Bollinger has called attention to an oligæmia due to the large amount of exudate. A decrease in the red cells may occur at the time of the crisis. There is in most cases a leucocytosis, which appears early, persists, and disappears with the crisis. The leucocytes may

13

number from 12,000 to 40,000 or even 100,000 per cubic millimetre.   The fall in the leucocytes is often slower than the drop in the fever, particularly when resolution is delayed.   The annexed chart shows well the coincident drop in the fever and in the number of the leucocytes.   The leucocytosis bears relation to the extent of the exudate.   In malignant pneumonia the leucocy-

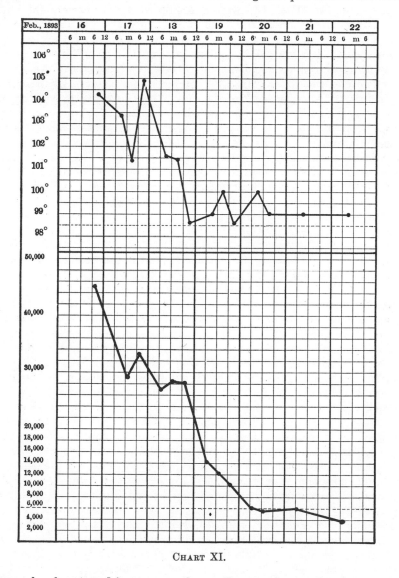

CHART XI.

tosis may be absent, and in any case the continuous absence may be regarded as an unfavorable sign.   A striking feature in the blood-slide is the richness and density of the fibrin network.   This corresponds to the great increase in the fibrin elements, the proportion rising from 4 to 10 parts per thousand.   The blood-plates are greatly increased.

Digestive Organs.—The tongue is white and furred, and in severe toxic cases rapidly becomes dry. Vomiting is not uncommon at the onset in children. The appetite is lost. Constipation is more common than diarrhœa. A distressing and sometimes dangerous symptom is meteorism. Fibrinous, pneumococcic exudates may occur in the conjunctivæ, nose, mouth, prepuce, and anus (Cary). The liver may be depressed by the large right lung, or enlarged from the engorged right heart, or as a result of the infection. The spleen is usually enlarged, and the edge can be felt during a deep inspiration.

Skin.—Among *cutaneous* symptoms one of the most interesting is the association of herpes with pneumonia. Not excepting malaria, we see labial herpes more frequently in this than in any other disease, occurring, as it does, in from 12 to 40 per cent of the cases. It is supposed to be of favorable prognosis, and figures have been quoted in proof of this assertion. It may also occur on the nose, genitals, and anus. Its significance and relation to the disease are unknown. At the height of the disease sweats are not common, but at the crisis they may be profuse. Redness of one cheek is a phenomenon long recognized in connection with pneumonia, and is usually on the same side as the disease. A diffuse erythema is occasionally seen, and in rare cases purpura. Jaundice is referred to among the complications.

Urine.—Early in the disease it presents the usual febrile characters of high color, high specific gravity, and increased acidity. A trace of albumin is very common. There may be tube-casts, and in a few instances the existence of albumin, tube-casts, and blood indicates the presence of an acute nephritis. The urea and uric acid are usually increased at first, but may be much diminished before the crisis, to increase greatly with its onset. Robert Hutchison's researches show that a true retention of chlorides within the body takes place, the average amount being about 2 grams daily. It is a more constant feature of pneumonia than of any other febrile disease, and this being the case, a diminution of the chlorides in the urine may be of value in the diagnosis from pleurisy with effusion or empyema. It is to be remembered that in dilatation of the stomach chlorides may be absent. Hæmaturia is a rare complication.

Cerebral Symptoms.—Headache is common. In children convulsions occur frequently at the outset. Apart from meningitis, which will be considered separately, one may group the cases with marked cerebral features into—

First, the so-called cerebral pneumonias of children, in which the disease sets in with a convulsion, and there are high fever, headache, delirium, great irritability, muscular tremor, and perhaps retraction of the head and neck. The diagnosis of meningitis is usually made, and the local affection may be overlooked.

Secondly, the cases with maniacal symptoms. These may occur at the very outset, and I once performed an autopsy on a case in which there was no suspicion whatever that the disease was other than acute mania. The house physician should give instructions to the nurses to watch such cases very carefully. On March 22, 1894, a patient who had been doing very well, with the exception of slight delirium, while the orderly was out of the room for a few moments, got up, raised the window, and jumped out, sustaining a fracture of the leg and of the upper lumbar vertebræ, of which he died.

Thirdly, alcoholic cases with the features of delirium tremens. It should be an invariable rule, even if fever be not present, to examine the lungs in a case of *mania a potu.*

Fourthly, cases with toxic features, resembling rather those of uræmia. Without a chill and without cough or pain in the side, a patient may have fever, a little shortness of breath, and then gradually grow dull mentally, and within three days be in a condition of profound toxæmia with low, muttering delirium.

It is stated that apex pneumonia is more often accompanied with severe delirium. Occasionally the cerebral symptoms occur immediately after the crisis. Mental disturbance may persist during and after convalescence, and in a few instances delusional insanity follows, the outlook in which is favorable.

Complications.—Compared with typhoid fever, pneumonia has but few complications and still fewer sequelæ. The most important are the following:

Pleurisy is an inevitable event when the inflammation reaches the surface of the lung, and thus can scarcely be termed a complication. But there are cases in which the pleuritic features take the first place—cases to which the term pleuro-pneumonia is applicable. The exudation may be sero-fibrinous with copious effusion, differing from that of an ordinary acute pleurisy in the greater richness of the fibrin, which may form thick, tenacious, curdy layers. Pneumonia on one side with extensive pleurisy on the other is sometimes a puzzling complication to diagnose, and an aspirator needle may be required to settle the question. *Empyema* is one of the most common complications, and has of late increased in frequency. During the eight years, 1883–'90, there were at Guy's Hospital 7 cases of empyema among 445 cases of pneumonia, while in the eight years, 1891–'98, there were 38 cases among 896 cases of pneumonia (Hale White). Influenza may be responsible for the increase. The pneumococcus is usually present; in a few the streptococcus, in which case the prognosis is not so good. Recurrence of the fever after the crisis or persistence of it after the tenth day, with sweats, leucocytosis, and perhaps an aggravation of the cough, are suspicious symptoms. The dulness persists at the base, or may extend. The breathing is feeble and there are no râles. Such a condition may be closely simulated, of course, by the thickened pleura. Exploratory aspiration may settle the question at once. There are obscure cases in which the pus has been found only after operation, as the collection may be very small.

Pericarditis was present in 31 of 665 patients in my wards at the Johns Hopkins Hospital (Chatard). It is often a terminal affair and overlooked. The mortality is very high; 29 of the 31 cases died. Pleurisy is an almost constant accompaniment, being present in 28 of the 29 autopsies in our series. In only 3 cases was the effusion purulent and in large amount.

Endocarditis.—The valves on the left side are more commonly attacked, and particularly if the seat of arterio-sclerosis. It is particularly liable to attack persons with old valvular disease. There may be no symptoms indicative of this complication even in very severe cases. It may, however, be suspected in cases (1) in which the fever is protracted and irregular; (2) when signs of septic mischief arise, such as chills and sweats; (3) when embolic phenomena appear. The frequent complication of meningitis with the endocarditis of pneumonia, which has already been mentioned, gives prominence to the cerebral symptoms in these cases. The physical signs may be very deceptive. There are instances in which no cardiac murmurs have been heard. In others the occurrence under observation of a loud, rough murmur, particularly if diastolic, is extremely suggestive.

Thrombosis.—Ante-mortem clotting in the heart, upon which the old writers laid great stress, is very rare. Thrombosis in the peripheral veins is also uncommon. Two cases occurred at my clinic, which have been reported by Steiner, who was able to collect only 41 cases from the literature. In 27 out of 32 cases which were fully reported, the thrombosis occurred during convalescence. It is almost always in the femoral veins. A rare complication is *embolism* of one of the larger arteries. I saw in Montreal an instance of embolism of the femoral artery at the height of pneumonia, which necessitated amputation at the thigh. The patient recovered. *Aphasia* has been met with in a few instances, setting in abruptly with or without hemiplegia.

Meningitis is perhaps the most serious complication of pneumonia. It varies very much at different times and in different regions. My Montreal experience is rather exceptional, as 8 per cent of the fatal cases had this complication. It usually comes on at the height of the fever, and in the majority of the cases is not recognized unless, as before mentioned, the base is involved, which is not common. Occurring later in the disease, it is more easily diagnosed. In some cases it is associated with infective endocarditis. The pneumococcus has been found in the exudate.

Peripheral neuritis is a rare complication, of which several cases have been described.

Gastric complications are rare. A croupous gastritis has already been mentioned. The *croupous colitis* may induce severe diarrhœa.

Abdominal Pain.—It is by no means uncommon to have early pain, either in the region of the umbilicus or in the right iliac fossa, and a suspicion of appendicitis is aroused; indeed, a catarrhal form of this disease may occur coincidently with the pneumonia. In other instances so localized may the pain be in the region of the pancreas, associated with meteorism and high fever, that the diagnosis of acute hæmorrhagic pancreatitis is made. Such a case occurred in February, 1905, in the wards of my colleague Dr. Halsted. The patient was admitted in a desperate condition, all the symptoms were abdominal, and the apex pneumonia was not discovered. *Peritonitis* is a rare complication, of which we have had only two or three instances. It is sometimes in the upper peritonæum, and a direct extension through the diaphragm. It is usually in the severer cases and not easy to recognize. In one case, indeed, in which there was a friction along the costal border, which we thought indicated a peritonitis, it was communicated from the diaphragmatic pleura. Meteorism is not infrequent, and is sometimes serious. In some cases it may be due to a defect in the mechanical action of the diaphragm, in others to an acute septic catarrh of the bowels, or to a toxic paresis of the walls, occasionally to peritonitis. *Jaundice* occurs with curious irregularity in different outbreaks of the disease. In Baltimore it was more common among the negro patients. It sets in early, is rarely very intense, and has not the characters of obstructive jaundice. There are cases in which it assumes a very serious form. The mode of production is not well ascertained. It does not appear to bear any definite relation to the degree of hepatic engorgement, and it is not always due to catarrh of the ducts. Possibly it may be, in great part, hæmatogenous.

Parotitis occasionally occurs, commonly in association with endocarditis. In children, middle-ear disease is not an infrequent complication.

Bright's disease does not often follow pneumonia.

The relations of arthritis and pneumonia are very interesting. It may precede the onset, and the pneumonia, possibly with endocarditis and pleurisy, may occur as complications. In other instances at the height of an ordinary pneumonia one or two joints may become red and sore. On the other hand, after the crisis has occurred pains and swelling may come on in the joints.

Relapse.—There are cases in which from the ninth to the eleventh day the fever subsides, and after the temperature has been normal for a day or two a rise occurs and fever may persist for another ten days or even two weeks. Though this might be termed a relapse, it is more correct to regard it as an instance of an anomalous course of delayed resolution. Wagner, who has studied the subject carefully, says that in his large experience of 1,100 cases he met with only 3 doubtful cases. When it does occur, the attack is usually abortive and mild. In the case of Z. R. (Medical No. J. H. H., 4223), with pneumonia of the right lower lobe, crisis occurred on the seventh day, and after a normal temperature for thirteen days he was discharged. That night he had a shaking chill, followed by fever, and he had recurring chills with reappearance of the pneumonia. In a second case (Medical No. J. H. H., 4538) crisis occurred on the third day, and there was recurrence of pneumonia on the thirteenth day.

Recurrence is more common in pneumonia than in any other acute disease. Rush gives an instance in which there were 28 attacks. Other authorities narrate cases of 8, 10, and even more attacks.

Convalescence in pneumonia is usually rapid, and sequelæ are rare. After the crisis, sudden death has occurred when the patient has got up too soon. With the onset of fever and persistence of the leucocytosis the affected side should be very carefully examined for pleurisy. With a persistence of the dulness the physical signs may be obscure, but the use of a small exploratory needle will help to clear the diagnosis.

Clinical Varieties.—Local variations are responsible for some of the most marked deviations from the usual type.

Apex pneumonia is said to be more often associated with adynamic features and with marked cerebral symptoms. The expectoration and cough may be slight.

Migratory or *creeping pneumonia,* a form which successively involves one lobe after the other.

Double pneumonia has no peculiarities other than the greater danger connected with it.

Massive pneumonia is a rare form, in which not alone the air-cells but the bronchi of an entire lobe or even of a lung are filled with the fibrinous exudate. The auscultatory signs are absent; there is neither fremitus nor tubular breathing, and on percussion the lung is absolutely flat. It closely resembles pleurisy with effusion. The moulds of the bronchi may be expectorated in violent fits of coughing.

Central Pneumonia.—The inflammation may be deep-seated at the root of the lung or centrally placed in a lobe, and for several days the diagnosis may be in doubt. It may not be until the third or fourth day that a pleural friction is detected, or that dulness or blowing breathing and râles are recognized. I saw in 1898 with Drs. H. Adler and Chew a young, thin-chested girl in whom at the end of the fourth day all the usual symptoms of pneumonia were present without any physical signs other than a few clicking râles at the left apex behind. The thinness of the patient greatly facilitated the examination. The general features of pneumonia continued, and the crisis occurred on the seventh day.

PNEUMONIA IN INFANTS.—It is sometimes seen in the new-born. In infants it very often sets in with a convulsion. The apex of the lung seems more frequently involved than in adults, and the cerebral symptoms are more marked. The torpor and coma, particularly if they follow convulsions, and the preliminary stage of excitement, may lead to the diagnosis of meningitis. Pneumonic sputum is rarely seen in children.

PNEUMONIA IN THE AGED.—The disease may be latent and set in without a chill; the cough and expectoration are slight, the physical signs ill-defined and changeable, and the constitutional symptoms out of all proportion to the extent of the local lesion.

PNEUMONIA IN ALCOHOLIC SUBJECTS.—The onset is insidious, the symptoms masked, the fever slight, and the clinical picture usually that of delirium tremens. The thermometer alone may indicate the presence of an acute disease. Often the local condition is overlooked, as the patient makes no complaint of pain, and there may be very little shortness of breath, no cough, and no sputum.

TERMINAL PNEUMONIA.—The wards and the post-mortem room show a very striking contrast in their pneumonia statistics, owing to the occurrence of what may be called terminal pneumonia. During the winter months patients with chronic pulmonary tuberculosis, arterio-sclerosis, heart disease, Bright's disease, and diabetes are not infrequently carried off by a pneumonia which may give few or no signs of its presence. There may be a slight elevation of temperature, with increase in the respirations, but the patient is near the end and perhaps not in a condition in which a thorough physical examination can be made. The autopsy may show pneumonia of the greater part of one lower lobe or of the apex, which had entirely escaped notice. In diabetic patients the disease often runs a rapid and severe course, and may end in abscess or gangrene.

Some of the most remarkable variations in the clinical course of pneumonia depend probably upon the severity, possibly upon the nature of the infection. Further investigation may enable us to say how far the associated organisms, so often present, may be responsible for the differences in the clinical course.

SECONDARY PNEUMONIAS.—These are met with chiefly in the specific fevers, particularly diphtheria, typhoid fever, typhus, influenza, and the plague. Anatomically, they rarely present the typical form of red or gray hepatization. The surface is smoother, not so dry, and it is often a pseudo-lobar condition, a consolidation caused by closely set areas of lobular involvement. Histologically, they are characterized in many instances by a more

94

cellular, less fibrinous exudate, which may also infiltrate the alveolar walls. Bacteriologically, a large number of different organisms have been found, the specific microbe of the primary disease, usually in association with the streptococcus pyogenes or the staphylococcus; in some instances the colon bacillus has been present.

The symptoms of the secondary pneumonias often lack the striking definiteness of the primary croupous pneumonia. The pulmonary features may be latent or masked altogether. There may be no cough and only a slight increase in the number of respirations. The lower lobe of one lung is most commonly involved, and the physical signs are obscure and rarely amount to more than impaired resonance, feeble breathing, and a few crackling râles.

EPIDEMIC PNEUMONIA has already been referred to. It is, as a rule, more fatal, and often displays minor complications which differ in different outbreaks. In some the cerebral manifestations are very marked; in others, the cardiac; in others again, the gastro-intestinal.

LARVAL PNEUMONIA.—Mild, abortive types are seen, particularly in institutions when pneumonia is prevailing extensively. A patient may have the initial symptoms of the disease, a slight chill, moderate fever, a few indefinite local signs, and herpes. The whole process may only last for two or three days; some authors recognize even a one-day pneumonia.

ASTHENIC, TOXIC, OR TYPHOID PNEUMONIA.—The toxæmic features dominate the scene throughout. The local lesions may be slight in extent and the subjective phenomena of the disease absent. The nervous symptoms usually predominate. There are delirium, prostration, and early weakness. Very frequently there is jaundice. Gastro-intestinal symptoms may be present, particularly diarrhœa and meteorism. In such a case, seen about the end of the first week, it may be difficult to say whether the condition is one of asthenic pneumonia or one of typhoid fever which has set in with early localization in the lung. Here the Widal reaction and cultures from the blood are important aids. In these cases there is really a pneumococcus septicæmia, and the organisms may sometimes be isolated from the blood. Possibly, too, there is a mixed infection, and the streptococcus pyogenes may be in large part responsible for the toxic features of the disease.

ASSOCIATION OF PNEUMONIA WITH OTHER DISEASES.—(a) With Malaria. —A malarial pneumonia is described by many observers and thought to be particularly prevalent in some parts of the United States. One hears of it, indeed, even where true malaria is rarely seen. With our large experience in malaria, amounting now to between two and three thousand cases, and a considerable number of pneumonia patients every year, we have only had a few cases in which the latter disease has set in during malarial fever, or vice versa. In either case the malaria yields promptly to the action of quinine. A special form of pneumonia due to the malarial parasite is unknown. Yet there are cases reported by Craig and others in which in an acute malarial infection the features suggest pneumonia at the onset, but the parasites are found in the blood, and under the use of quinine the fever drops rapidly and the pneumonia symptoms clear up. Such a case as the following we see occasionally: A patient was admitted, March 16, 1894, with tertian malarial fever. The lungs were clear. A pneumonia began thirty-six hours after admission. Quinine was given that evening, and the malarial organisms rapidly disappeared from the blood. There was successive involvement of the right lower, the middle, and the left lower lobe. The temperature fell by crisis on the 24th, and there were no features in the disease whatever suggestive of malaria. In other instances we have found a chill in the course of an ordinary pneumonia to be associated with a malarial infection, and quinine has rapidly and promptly caused the disappearance of the parasites from the blood.

(*b*) *Pneumonia and Acute Arthritis.*—We have already spoken under complications of this association, which is more frequently seen in children.

(*c*) *Pneumonia and Tuberculosis.*—Many subjects of chronic pulmonary tuberculosis die of an acute croupous pneumonia. A point to be specially borne in mind is the fact that acute tuberculous pneumonia may set in with all the features and physical signs of fibrinous pneumonia (**see page 175**).

For the consideration of the association of pneumonia with typhoid fever and influenza, the reader is referred to the sections on those diseases.

POST-OPERATION PNEUMONIA.—Before the days of anæsthesia, lobar pneumonia was a well-recognized cause of death after surgical injuries and operations. Norman Cheevers, in an early number of the Guy's Hospital Reports, calls attention to it as one of the most frequent causes of death after surgical procedures, and Erichsen states that of 41 deaths after surgical injuries 23 cases showed signs of pneumonia. The lobular form is the most frequent. I have already referred to the contusion-pneumonia described by Litten.

ETHER PNEUMONIA.—The question of a direct relation between ether narcosis and pneumonia has been much discussed of late years, having been raised by Mr. Lucas, of Guy's Hospital. The statistics are by no means unanimous. The London anæsthetists, particularly Hewitt and Silk, seem to have had a fortunate experience, Silk having found among 5,000 cases 13 of pneumonia; 8 of these were tongue or jaw cases. The German experience is very different. Von Beck states that, owing to the injurious after-effects upon the respiratory tract, the use of ether has been largely restricted in Czerny's clinic. Gurlt reports 52,177 cases, with 30 cases of pneumonia and 15 deaths. We usually had three or four cases each year at the Johns Hopkins Hospital. Czerny suggests that the relation of these ether pneumonias to abdominal operations is associated with the pain on coughing, which leads to an accumulation of secretion, and through this to retention or aspiration pneumonia. Among the various views brought forward to account for it are the rapid evaporation of the ether, causing chilling of the pulmonary tissues, chilling of the patient at the time of operation, infection from the inhaler, and direct action of the ether.

The probability is that the prolonged etherization lowers the vitality of the tissues of the finer bronchi and permits the pathogenic organisms (which are almost always present) to do their work. The pneumonia is more frequently lobular than lobar. Neuwerck, and subsequently Whitney, have suggested thorough disinfection of the mouth and throat before operation.

DELAYED RESOLUTION IN PNEUMONIA.—The lung is restored to its normal state by the liquefaction and absorption of the exudate. There are cases in which resolution takes place rapidly without any increase in (or, indeed, without any) expectoration; on the other hand, during resolution it is not uncommon to find in the sputa the little plugs of fibrin and leucocytes which have been loosened from the air-cells and expelled by coughing. A variable time is taken in the restoration of the lung. Sometimes within a week or ten days the dulness is greatly diminished, the breath-sounds become clear, and, so far as physical signs are any guide, the lung seems perfectly restored. It is to be remembered that in any case of pneumonia with extensive pleurisy a certain amount of dulness will persist for months, owing to thickening of the pleura.

Delayed resolution is a condition which causes much anxiety to the physician. While it is perhaps more frequent in debilitated persons, yet it is met with in robust, previously healthy individuals, and in cases which have had a very typical onset and course. The condition is stated to be most frequent in apex pneumonia. Venesection has been assigned as a cause. The solid exudate may persist for weeks and yet the integrity of the lung may ultimately be restored. Grissole describes the lung from a patient who died on the sixtieth day, in which the affected part showed a condition not unlike that of the acute stage.

Clinically, there are several groups of cases: First, those in which the crisis occurs naturally, the temperature falls and remains normal, but the local features persist—well-marked flatness with tubular breathing and râles. Resolution may occur very slowly and gradually, taking from two to three weeks. In a second group of cases the temperature falls by lysis, and with the persistence of the local signs there is slight fever, sometimes sweats and rapid pulse. The condition may persist for three or four weeks, or, as in one of my cases, for eleven weeks, and ultimately perfect resolution occur. During all this time there may be little or no sputum. The practitioner is naturally much exercised, and he dreads lest tuberculosis should supervene. In a third group the crisis occurs or the fever falls by lysis, but the consolidation persists and there may be intense bronchial breathing, with few or no râles, or the fever may recur and the patient may die exhausted. In 1 of my 100 autopsies a patient, aged fifty-eight, had died on the thirty-second day from the initial chill. The right lung was solid, grayish in color, firm, and presented in places a translucent, semi-homogeneous aspect. In these areas the alveolar walls were thickened, and the plugs filling the air-cells were undergoing transformation into new connective tissue. This fibroid induration may proceed gradually and be associated with shrinkage of the affected side, and the gradual production of a cirrhosis or chronic interstitial pneumonia.

Ordinary fibrinous pneumonia never terminates in tuberculosis. The instances of caseous pneumonia and softening which have followed an acute pneumonic process have been from the outset tuberculous.

TERMINATION IN ABSCESS.—This occurred in 4 of my 100 autopsies. Usually the lung breaks down in limited areas and the abscesses are not large, but they may fuse and involve a considerable proportion of a lobe. The condition is recognized by the sputum, which is usually abundant and contains pus and elastic tissue, sometimes cholesterin crystals and hæmatoidin crystals. The cough is often paroxysmal and of great severity; usually the fever is remittent, or in protracted cases intermittent in character, and there may be pronounced hectic symptoms. When a case is seen for the first time it may be difficult to determine whether it is one of abscess of the lung or a local empyæma which has perforated the lung.

97

GANGRENE.—This is most commonly seen in old debilitated persons. It was present in 3 of my 100 autopsies. It very often occurs with abscess. The gangrene is associated with the growth of the saprophytic bacteria on a soil made favorable by the presence of the pneumococcus or the streptococcus. Clinically, the gangrene is rendered very evident by the horribly fetid odor of the expectoration and its characteristic features. In some instances the gangrene may be found post mortem when clinically there has not been any evidence of its existence.

Prognosis.—Pneumonia is the most fatal of all acute diseases, killing more than diphtheria, and outranking even consumption as a cause of death.

Hospital statistics show that the mortality ranges from 20 to 40 per cent. Of 1,012 cases at the Montreal General Hospital, the mortality was 20.4 per cent. It appears to be somewhat more fatal in southern climates. Of 3,969 cases treated at the Charity Hospital, New Orleans, the death-rate was 38.01 per cent. The mortality at the Johns Hopkins Hospital has been about 25 per cent in the whites and 30 per cent in the colored. In 704 cases at the Pennsylvania Hospital the mortality was 29 per cent. At the Boston City Hospital, in 1,443 cases the mortality was 29.1 per cent. It has been urged that the mortality in this disease has been steadily increasing, and attempts have been made to connect this increase with the expectant plan of treatment at present in vogue. But the careful and thorough analysis by C. N. Townsend and A. Coolidge, Jr., of 1,000 cases at the Massachusetts General Hospital indicates clearly that, when all circumstances are taken into consideration, this conclusion is not justified.

According to the analysis of 708 cases at St. Thomas's Hospital by Hadden, H. W. G. McKenzie, and W. W. Ord, the mortality progressively increases from the twentieth year, rising from 3.7 per cent under that age to 22 per cent in the third decade, 30.8 per cent in the fourth, 47 per cent in the fifth, 51 per cent in the sixth, 65 per cent in the seventh decade. Of 465,400 cases collected by E. F. Wells from various sources, 94,826 died, a mortality of 20.4 per cent.

The mortality in private practice varies greatly. R. P. Howard treated 170 cases with only 6 per cent of deaths. Fussell has recently reported 134 cases with a mortality of 17.9 per cent. The mortality in children is sometimes very low. Morrill has recently reported 6 deaths in 123 cases of frank pneumonia. On the other hand, Goodhart had 25 deaths in 120 cases.

The following are among the circumstances which influence the prognosis:

Age.—As Sturges remarks, the old are likely to die, the young to recover. Under one year it is more fatal than between two and five. Fussell lost 5 out of 8 cases in sucklings. At about sixty the death-rate is very high, amounting to 60 or 80 per cent. From the reports of its fatality in some places, one may say that to die of pneumonia is almost the natural end of old people.

As already stated, the disease is more fatal in the negro than in the white race.

Previous habits of life and the condition of bodily health at the time of the attack form the most important factors in the prognosis of pneumonia. In analyzing a series of fatal cases one is very much impressed with the number of cases in which the organs shown signs of degeneration. In 25 of my

100 autopsies at the Montreal General Hospital the kidneys showed extensive interstitial changes. Individuals debilitated from sickness or poor food, hard drinkers, and that large class of hospital patients, composed of robust-looking laborers between the ages of forty-five and sixty, whose organs show signs of wear and tear, and who have by excesses in alcohol weakened the reserve power, fall an easy prey to the disease. Very few fatal cases occur in robust, healthy adults. Some of the statistics given by army surgeons show better than any others the low mortality from pneumonia in healthy picked men. The death-rate in the German army in over 40,000 cases was only 3.6 per cent.

Certain *complications* and terminations are particularly serious. The meningitis of pneumonia is probably always fatal. Endocarditis is extremely grave, much more so than pericarditis. Apart from these serious complications, the fatal event in pneumonia is due either to a gradual toxæmia or to mechanical interference with the respiration and circulation.

Much stress has been laid of late upon the factor of *leucocytosis* as an element in the prognosis. A very slight or complete absence of a leucocytosis is rightly regarded as very unfavorable.

Toxæmia is the important prognostic feature in the disease, to which in a majority of the cases the degree of pyrexia and the extent of consolidation are entirely subsidiary. It is not at all proportionate to the degree of lung involved. A severe and fatal toxæmia may occur with the consolidation of only a small part of one lobe. On the other hand, a patient with complete solidification of one lung may have no signs of a general infection. The question of individual resistance seems to be the most important one, and one sees even most robust-looking individuals fatally stricken within a few days.

Death is rarely due to direct interference with the function of respiration, even in double pneumonia. Sometimes it seems to be caused by the extensive involvement with œdema of the other parts of the lungs, an engorgement with progressive weakness of the right heart. But death is most frequently due to the action of the poisons on the vaso-motor centres, with progressive lowering of the blood pressure. This is a much more serious factor than direct weakness of the heart muscle itself.

Diagnosis.—No disease is more readily recognized in a large majority of the cases. The external characters, the sputa, and the physical signs combine to make one of the clearest of clinical pictures. After a study in the post-mortem room of my own and others' mistakes, I think that the ordinary lobar pneumonia of adults is rarely overlooked. Errors are particularly liable to occur in the intercurrent pneumonias, in those complicating chronic affections, and in the disease as met with in children, the aged, and drunkards. Tuberculo-pneumonic phthisis is frequently confounded with pneumonia. Pleurisy with effusion is, I believe, not often mistaken except in children. The diagnostic points will be referred to under pleurisy.

In diabetes, Bright's disease, chronic heart-disease, pulmonary phthisis, and cancer, an acute pneumonia often ends the scene, and is frequently overlooked. In these cases the temperature is perhaps the best index, and should, more particularly if cough occurs, lead to a careful examination of the lungs. The absence of expectoration and of pulmonary symptoms may make the diagnosis very difficult.

In children there are two special sources of error; the disease may be entirely masked by the cerebral symptoms and the case mistaken for one of meningitis. It is remarkable in these cases how few indications there are of pulmonary trouble. The other condition is pleurisy with effusion, which in children often has deceptive physical signs. The breathing may be intensely tubular and tactile fremitus may be present. The exploratory needle is sometimes required to decide the question. In the old and debilitated a knowledge that the onset of pneumonia is insidious, and that the symptoms are ill-defined and latent, should put the practitioner on his guard and make him very careful in the examination of the lungs in doubtful cases. In chronic alcoholism the cerebral symptoms may completely mask the local process. As mentioned, the disease may assume the form of violent mania, but more commonly the symptoms are those of delirium tremens. In any case, rapid pulse, rapid respiration, and fever are symptoms which should invariably excite suspicion of inflammation of the lungs. Under cerebro-spinal meningitis will be found the points of differential diagnosis between pneumonia and that disease.

Pneumonia is rarely confounded with ordinary consumption, but to differentiate acute tuberculo-pneumonic phthisis is often difficult. The case may set in with a chill. It may be impossible to determine which condition is present until softening occurs and elastic tissue and tubercle bacilli appear in the sputum. A similar mistake is sometimes made in children. With typhoid fever, pneumonia is not infrequently confounded. There are instances of pneumonia with the local signs well marked in which the patient rapidly sinks into what is known as the typhoid state, with dry tongue, rapid pulse, and diarrhœa. Unless the case is seen from the outset it may be very difficult to determine the true nature of the malady. On the other hand, there are cases of typhoid fever which set in with symptoms of lobar pneumonia—the so-called pneumo-typhus. It may be impossible to make a differential diagnosis in such a case unless the characteristic eruption occurs or the Widal reaction be given.

Prophylaxis.—We do not know the percentage of individuals who harbor the pneumococcus normally in the secretions of the mouth and throat. In a great majority of cases it is an auto-infection, and the lowered resistance due to exposure or to alcohol, or a trauma or anæsthetization, simply furnishes conditions which favor the spread and growth of a parasite already present. Individuals who have already had pneumonia should be careful to keep the teeth in good condition, and the mouth and throat in as healthy a state as possible. Antiseptic mouth washes may be used.

We know practically nothing of the conditions under which the pneumococcus lives outside the body, or how it gains entrance in healthy individuals. The sputum of each case should be very carefully disinfected. In institutions the cases should be isolated.

Treatment.—Pneumonia is a self-limited disease, which can neither be aborted nor cut short by any known means at our command. Even under the most unfavorable circumstances it may terminate abruptly and naturally. A patient was admitted to the Philadelphia Hospital on the evening of the seventh day after the chill, in which he had been seen by one of my assistants, who had ordered him to go to a hospital. He remained, however, in his house alone, without assistance, taking nothing but a little milk and bread and whisky, and was brought into the hospital by the police in a condition of active delirium. That night his temperature was 105° and his pulse above 120. In his delirium he tried to escape through the window of the ward. The following morning—the eighth day—the crisis occurred, and the temperature was below 98°. The entire lower lobe of the right side was found involved, and he entered upon a rapid convalescence. So also, under the favoring circumstances of good nursing and careful diet, the experience of many physicians in different lands has shown that pneumonia runs its course in a definite time, terminating sometimes spontaneously on the third, or the fifth day, or continuing until the tenth or twelfth.

There is no specific treatment for pneumonia. The young practitioner should bear in mind that patients are more often damaged than helped by the promiscuous drugging, which is still only too prevalent.

1. GENERAL MANAGEMENT OF A CASE.—The same careful hygiene of the bed and of the sick-room should be carried out as in typhoid fever. When conditions are favorable the bed may be wheeled into the open air. The patient should not be too much bundled up with clothing. For the heavy flannel undershirts should be substituted a thin, light flannel jacket, open in front, which enables the physician to make his examinations without unnecessarily disturbing the patient. The room should be bright and light, letting in the sunshine if possible, and thoroughly well ventilated. Only one or two persons should be allowed in the room at a time. Even when not called for on account of the high fever, the patient should be carefully sponged each day with tepid water. This should be done with as little disturbance as possible. Special care should be taken to keep the mouth and gums cleansed.

2. DIET.—Plain water, a pleasant table water, or lemonade should be given freely. When the patient is delirious the water should be given at fixed intervals. The food should be liquid, consisting chiefly of milk, either alone or, better, mixed with food prepared from some one of the cereals, and eggs, either soft boiled or raw.

3. SPECIAL TREATMENT.—Certain measures are believed to have an influence in arresting, controlling, or cutting short the disease. It is very difficult for the practitioner to arrive at satisfactory conclusions on this question in a disease so singularly variable in its course. How natural, when on the third or fourth day the crisis occurs and convalescence sets in, to attribute the happy result to the effect of some special medication! How easy to forget that the same unexpected early recoveries occur under other conditions! The following are among the measures which may be helpful:

(a) *Bleeding.*—The reproach of Van Helmont, that "a bloody Moloch presides in the chairs of medicine," can not be brought against this generation of physicians. Before Louis' iconoclastic paper on bleeding in pneumonia it would have been regarded as almost criminal to treat a case without venesection. We employ it nowadays much more than we did a few years ago, but more often late in the disease than early. To bleed at the very onset in robust, healthy individuals in whom the disease sets in with great intensity and high fever is, I believe, a good practice. I have seen instances in which it was very beneficial in relieving the pain and the dyspnœa, reducing the temperature, and allaying the cerebral symptoms.

(*b*) *Drugs.*—Certain drugs are credited with the power of reducing the intensity and shortening the duration of the attack. Among them veratrum viride still holds a place, doses of ℥ ij–v of the tincture given every two hours. Tartar emetic—a remedy which had great vogue some years ago—is now very rarely employed. To a third drug, digitalis, has been attributed of late great power in controlling the course of the disease. Petresco gives at one time as much as from 4 to 12 grammes of the powdered leaves, and claims that these colossal doses are specially efficacious in shortening the course of the disease and diminishing the mortality.

(*c*) *Antipneumococcic Serum.*—Anders' recent analyses of the reported cases do not give a very favorable impression of the value of the sera at present in use. More perhaps may be expected from the polyvalent serum of Römer, but even with it 4 of the 24 cases treated in Curschmann's clinic died (Pässler).

4. SYMPTOMATIC TREATMENT.—(*a*) *To relieve the Pain.*—The stitch in the side at onset, which is sometimes so agonizing, is best relieved by a hypodermic injection of a quarter of a grain of morphia. When the pain is less intense and diffuse over one side, the Paquelin cautery applied lightly is very efficacious, or hot or cold applications may be tried. When the disease is fairly established the pain is not, as a rule, distressing, except when the patient coughs, and for this the Dover's powder may be used in 5-grain doses, according to the patient's needs. Hot poultices, formerly so much in use, relieve the pain, though not more than the cold applications. For children they are often preferable.

(*b*) *To combat the Toxæmia.*—Until we have a specific, either drug or the product of the bacteriological laboratory, which will safely and surely neutralize the toxins of the disease, we must be content with measures which promote the elimination of the poisons. Unfortunately, we know very little of the channels by which they are got rid of, but on general principles we may suppose them to be the skin, the kidneys, and the bowels. By the tepid or the cold bath not only is the action of the skin promoted, but the vaso-motor centres are stimulated. Abundance of water should be given to promote the flow of urine, and the saline infusion seems to act helpfully in this way. The bowels should be kept freely open by saline laxatives.

(*c*) The third and all-important indication in the treatment of pneumonia is *to support the circulation.* We can not at present separate the effects of the fever from those of the toxins. It is possible, indeed, as some suppose, that the fever itself may be beneficial. Undoubtedly, however, high and prolonged pyrexia is dangerous to the heart, and should be combated. For this our most trusty weapon is *hydrotherapy*, which in pneumonia is used in several different ways. The ice-bag to the affected side is one of the most convenient and serviceable. It allays the pain, reduces the fever slightly, and, as a rule, the patient says he feels very much more comfortable. Broad, flat ice-bags are now easily obtained for the purpose, and if these are not available an ice poultice can be readily made, and by the use of oil-silk the clothing and bedding of the patient can be protected from the water. Cold sponging is the best form of hydrotherapy to employ as a routine measure. When done limb by limb the patient is but little disturbed, and it is refreshing and beneficial. With very pronounced nervous symptoms and persistent high temperature, or with hyperpyrexia, a cold bath of ten minutes' duration may be given. Probably the very best effect of the hydrotherapy is in the stimulating effect on the vaso-motor centres. The dusky skin, increasing cyanosis, increasing shortness of breath, with signs of œdema of the lungs, and the rapid, small, soft pulse, tell of a progressive lowering of the blood tension. Digitalin given hypodermically in full doses, $\frac{1}{20} - \frac{1}{40}$ gr., and strychnine, $\frac{1}{30} - \frac{1}{60}$ gr., are the most satisfactory drugs to support the blood pressure. Camphor and caffein and musk are also of value. The effect of adrenalin, even in intravenous injection, is too transitory to be of any value. Alcohol does not seem to raise the blood pressure in fever, and the studies of Briggs and Cook in my wards would indicate that it is not of much value in progressive vaso-motor collapse. This does not mean, however, that it may not have a value in the fever, and I should be sorry to give up its use in the severer forms of enteric and of pneumonia. Saline infusions promote elimination and may help in tiding over a period of vascular depression. A litre may be allowed to run by gravity beneath the skin, and if necessary may be repeated two or three times in the twenty-four hours.

Oxygen Gas.—It is doubtful whether the inhalation of oxygen in pneumonia is really beneficial. The work of Lorrain-Smith suggests, indeed, that it may under certain circumstances be positively harmful. He has shown experimentally that oxygen may be a serious irritant, actually producing inflammation of the lungs. If we are justified in applying his results to man, there can be but little doubt that the administration of oxygen may not be entirely " harmless," as stated in previous editions of this work. If the tension of the oxygen breathed rises to 80 per cent of an atmosphere, which it might easily do in certain methods of administration, it may be injurious. When used it should be allowed to flow gently from the nozzle held at a little distance, in which way it is freely diluted with air.

Treatment of Complications.—If the fever persists it is important to look out for pleurisy, particularly for the meta-pneumonic empyema. The exploratory needle should be used if necessary. A sero-fibrinous effusion should be aspirated, a purulent opened and drained. In a complicating pericarditis with a large effusion aspiration may be necessary. Delayed resolution is a difficult condition to treat. Fibrotysin, 2.5 cc. every other day, has been used successfully in a few cases (Crofton).

XVI. DIPHTHERIA.

Definition.—A specific infectious disease, characterized by a local fibrinous exudate, usually upon a mucous membrane, and by constitutional symptoms due to toxins produced at the site of the lesion. The presence of the Klebs-Loeffler bacillus is the etiological criterion by which true diphtheria is distinguished from other forms of membranous inflammation.

The clinical and bacteriological conceptions of diphtheria are at present not in full accord. On the one hand, there are cases of simple sore throat which the bacteriologists, finding the Klebs-Loeffler bacillus, call true diphtheria. On the other hand, cases of membranous, sloughing angina, diagnosed by the physician as diphtheria, are called by the bacteriologists, in

pneumonia

Osler's manifest interest in pneumonia stemmed from his days at the Montreal General Hospital at a time when the disease was the leading cause of death and is evidenced by his more than 15 publications on this and related topics (dating from 1878). His description of the association of meningitis and endocarditis with pneumonia, which appeared in 1881, the year in which Sternberg and Pasteur independently reported the first isolation of the pneumococcus, was perhaps his most original contribution to the subject of pneumococcal infection. At the time, however, Osler was uncertain of the significance of the "micrococci" which he observed in histological preparations of heart valves. In May of 1884, Osler attended the Congress of German Physicians, at which both Friedländer and Fraenkel presented their polemic observations on the bacterial etiology of pneumonia. The following year, he published his "Notes on the Morbid Anatomy of Pneumonia" based on autopsies of 105 cases. His continuing interest in the disease is shown by his institution of an annual review of the cases of pneumonia studied on the wards of the Johns Hopkins Hospital, one of which was reported in *The National Medical Review* in 1897. It was his stated aim to "make the cases teach the lesson of the disease." In this fashion, an enduring tradition was established at the Johns Hopkins Medical Institutions, and the developing knowledge of pneumonia is reflected in the continuing series of reports on this subject resulting from such studies.

It is clear from the foregoing facts that Osler was well grounded when he set forth to write the chapter on pneumonia in the first edition. The author's evolving views on this topic are apparent from his treatment of it in subsequent editions of the text. In the third edition, published in 1898, the chapter was revised extensively, expanded from 21 to 30 pages, and moved from Section IV entitled "Diseases of the Respiratory System" to Section I devoted to "Specific Infectious Diseases" where it was to remain, eventually to achieve the status of Chapter I in an edition edited by Christian. Osler's description of the symptoms, physical findings, and course of lobar pneumonia remain to this day an entirely adequate account of the natural history of the untreated disease. Among the more penetrating observations was his recognition that it was the toxemia accompanying infection rather than the involvement of the lungs that posed a threat to life. His comments thereon are relevant today, and despite the great strides that have been made in antimicrobial therapy, the toxemia of pneumococcal infection and the means specifically to combat it are as little understood now as they were in Osler's lifetime.

Knowledge of the pneumococcus and the other agents responsible for bacterial pneumonia was in a developing state when Osler wrote. His description of the pneumoccocus was largely morphological. He mentioned no other attribute of the organism than its ability to ferment inulin, described by Hiss in 1902, although its solubility in bile had been reported two years earlier by Neufeld. Immunological classification of pneumococcus was then just in its beginnings. That experimental infection conferred immunity to the same strain and could be transferred passively in experimental animals had been recognized before the turn of the century. Attempts to translate these observations to the treatment of pneumonia in man, however, had yielded uncertain results at best because of unawareness of the diversity of pneumococcal capsular types. By 1913, three well-defined types of pneumococcus had been described, and treatment of the disease by passive immunization was undergoing intensive investigation. In the revised reprinting of the eighth edition, which appeared in 1917, the first reference to the beneficial effects of serum therapy in Type I pneumococcal infection was made. This statement was to remain essentially unchanged until the publication of the twelfth edition in 1935 when a qualified endorsement of Type II antipneumococcal serum was given. Although therapeutic rabbit antipneumococcal serums were just being introduced at this time, the era of serotherapy was almost at its end. The attempt to develop satisfactory therapeutic serums had been, nonetheless, the stimulus to intensive examination of the pneumococcus and gave rise to some of the most important biological discoveries of the twentieth century. The recognition that the capsules of the pneumococcus, of which 82 distinct types are now known, are polysaccharides capable of stimulating the formation of antibodies marked a milestone in immunology. Of even greater impact on all of biology was the observation by Griffith of the transformation of pneumococcal capsular types and the subsequent elucidation of this phenomenon by Avery and his co-workers. The demonstration of the genetic activity of deoxyribonucleic acids in the pneumococcus was to provide the basis for the contemporary development of biochemical genetics.

Domag's discovery of the antibacterial activity of the sulfonamides in 1935 opened a new era in the treatment of infectious disease. Sulfapyridine was reported to be effective in pneumococcal pneumonia in 1938 and was followed in rapid succession by congeners of lesser toxicity. The status of the sulfonamides as drugs of choice for the treatment of pneumococcal pneumonia was, however, to be short-lived. The discovery of penicillin and the extraordinary potency of this bactericidal antibiotic in pneumococcal disease, reported in 1944, established it as the most suitable agent. Virtually devoid of toxicity, penicillin is nonetheless allergenic and not tolerated by some. For such patients, a number of alternative antimicrobial agents are now available, including the cephalosporins, tetracyclines, and macrolides. The utility of penicillin is described in the sixteenth edition of the textbook.

Pneumonia

Despite the absence of highly effective measures during the early decades of this century, the annual mortality from pneumonia fell from approximately 200 per 100,000 population in 1900 to 80 per 100,000 in 1938, the year in which sulfapyridine was introduced. Mortality fell even more sharply after the introduction of potent antimicrobial drugs and reached its nadir at 28.2 per 100,000 in 1956, since which time it has been rising slowly. Concomitant with the introduction of effective therapy, there has been a decline in interest in pneumococcal disease despite the fact that the incidence of pneumococcal infections seems to have undergone little change in recent years. Although no longer "Captain of the Men of Death," pneumonia remains the only infectious disease among the 10 leading causes of death in the United States in the 1960s, and in the country's greatly expanded population, there are today almost half as many deaths from pneumonia per annum as there were in 1900. The demonstration in 1945 that vaccines of purified pneumococcal capsular polysaccharides are effective prophylactic agents against infection with organisms of homologous capsular types provides today the potentially most effective, though unused, means to protect those at high risk of death from the toxemia of pneumococcal disease so well described by Osler.

Osler's changing philosophic outlook on pneumonia is reflected in succeeding editions of *The Principles and Practice of Medicine*. In the first two editions, he writes of pneumonia as "The special enemy of old age." In the third edition, his altered and widely quoted view of pneumonia as "the friend of the aged" appeared for the first time and was to be repeated in all subsequent versions of the text. Osler himself was to succumb to the complications of what he had styled "Captain of the Men of Death." His terminal illness is described by Cushing. Afflicted apparently by chronic bronchial disease, Osler was subject to recurring bouts of bronchopneumonia during his last six months of life. On November 1, 1919, he wrote: "No fever since the 16th but the cough persists & an occasional paroxysm — bouts as bad as senile whooping-cough. One night they nearly blew my candle out! No. 3 pneumococcus and *M. catarrhalis* — the organisms. Practically no physical signs — a little impairment of resonance at bases but no rales or tubular breathing." He was to live another eight weeks, his illness complicated by empyema yielding *H. influenzae* and by hemorrhage from his surgical wound. He died on December 29,1919, having been spared, at least in part, "those 'cold gradations of decay' so distressing to himself and to his friends."

Robert Austrian

106

REFERENCES

Avery, O.T., MacLeod, C.M., and McCarty, M. Studies on the chemical nature of the substance inducing transformation of pneumococcal types. J. Exp. Med., 79:137, 1944.

Dochez, A.R., and Gillespie, L.J. A biological classification of pneumococci by means of immunity reactions. J.A.M.A., 61:727, 1913.

Griffith, F. The significance of pneumococcal types. J. Hyg., 27:113, 1928.

Heidelberger, M., and Avery, O.T. The soluble specific substance of pneumococcus. J. Exp. Med., 38:73, 1923.

Tillett, W.S., McCormack, J.E., and Cambier, M.J. Treatment of lobar pneumonia with penicillin. J. Clin. Invest., 25:589, 1945.

(*c*) CUTANEOUS ACTINOMYCOSIS.—In several instances in connection with chronic ulcerative diseases of the skin the ray-fungus has been found. It is a very chronic affection resembling tuberculosis of the skin, associated with the growth of tumors which suppurate and leave open sores, which may remain for years.

(*d*) CEREBRAL ACTINOMYCOSIS.—Bollinger has reported an instance of primary disease of the brain. The symptoms were those of tumor. A second remarkable case has been reported by Gamgee and Delepine. The patient was admitted to St. George's Hospital with left-sided pleural effusion. At the post mortem three pints of purulent fluid were found in the left pleura; there was an actinomycotic abscess of the liver, and in the brain there were abscesses in the frontal, parietal, and temporo-sphenoidal lobes which contained the mycelium, but no clubs. A third case, reported by O. B. Keller, had *empyema necessitatis*, which was opened and actinomycetes were found in the pus. Subsequently she had Jacksonian epilepsy, for which she was trephined twice and abscesses opened, which contained actinomyces grains. Death occurred after the second operation.

Symptoms.—The fever is of an irregular type and depends largely on the existence of suppuration. The cough is an important symptom, and the diagnosis in 18 of the cases was made during life by the discovery of the actinomyces. Death results usually with septic symptoms. Occasionally there is a condition simulating typhoid fever. The average duration of the disease was ten months. Recovery is very rare. Clinically the disease closely resembles certain forms of pulmonary tuberculosis and of fœtid bronchitis. It is not to be forgotten in the examination of the sputum that, as Bizzozero mentions, certain degenerated epithelial cells may be mistaken for the organism. The radiating leptothrix threads about the epithelium of the mouth sometimes present a striking resemblance.

Diagnosis.—The disease is in reality a chronic pyæmia. The only test is the presence of the actinomyces in the pus. Metastases may occur as in pyæmia and in tumors. The tendency, however, is rather to the production of a local purulent affection which erodes the bones and is very destructive.

Treatment.—This is largely surgical and is practically that of pyæmia. Incision of the abscess, removal of the dead bone, and thorough irrigation are appropriate measures. Thomassen has recommended iodide of potassium, which, in doses of from 40 to 60 grains daily, has proved curative in a number of recent cases.

XXXI. SYPHILIS.

Definition.—A specific disease of slow evolution, caused by the *Spirochæta pallida*, propagated by inoculation (acquired syphilis) or by hereditary transmission (congenital syphilis).

I. GENERAL ETIOLOGY AND MORBID ANATOMY.

Since the sixth edition of this work appeared there have been three remarkable advances in our knowledge of syphilis—the discovery of the germ, the transmission of the disease to apes, and the serum diagnosis of the disease.

19

The *Spirochæta pallida,* discovered by Schaudinn, a spirally curved organism from 10 to 15 μ in length, is found in primary, secondary and tertiary lesions, and may be inoculated successfully into apes, monkeys, and rabbits. It is believed to be a protozoan, but it has not yet been cultivated. In the congenital lesions it is present in extraordinary numbers.

Modes of Infection.—(1) In a large majority of all cases the disease is transmitted by *sexual congress,* but the designation *venereal* disease (*lues venerea*) is not always correct, as there are many other modes of inoculation. In the St. Louis collection there are illustrations of 26 varieties of extra-genital chancres.

(2) *Accidental Infection.*—In surgical and in midwifery practice physicians are not infrequently inoculated. General infection may occur without a characteristic local sore. Midwifery chancres are usually on the fingers, but they may be on the back of the hand. The lip chancre is the most common of these erratic or extra-genital forms, and may be acquired in many ways apart from direct infection. Mouth and tonsillar sores result as a rule from improper practices. Wet-nurses are sometimes infected on the nipple, and it occasionally happens that relatives of a syphilitic child are accidentally contaminated.

(3) *Hereditary Transmission.*—This is most common from (*a*) the father, the mother being healthy (sperm inheritance). *S. pallida* has not yet been found in the sperm cell, but we do not know its life phases, and from what we do know of the history of syphilis, it seems probable that all the sperms cells are infective. A syphilitic father may beget an apparently healthy child, even when the disease is fresh and full-blown. On the other hand, in very rare instances, a man may have had syphilis when young, undergo treatment, and for years present no signs of disease, and yet his first-born may show very characteristic lesions. The closer the begetting to the primary sore, the greater the chance of infection. A man with tertiary lesions may beget healthy children. As a general rule it may be said that with judicious treatment the transmissive power rarely exceeds three or four years.

(*b*) Maternal transmission (germ inheritance). While the father may not be affected, in a large number of instances both parents are diseased, the one having infected the other, in which case the chances of fœtal infection are greatly increased. Heredity through the mother alone is much more fatal to the offspring than paternal heredity. It is a remarkable and interesting fact that a woman who has borne a syphilitic child is herself immune, and can not be infected, though she may present no signs of the disease. This is known as Beaumès' or Colles' law, and was thus stated by the distinguished Dublin surgeon: " That a child born of a mother who is without obvious venereal symptoms, and which, without being exposed to any infection subsequent to its birth, shows this disease when a few weeks old, this child will infect the most healthy nurse, whether she suckle it, or merely handle and dress it; and yet this child is never known to infect its own mother, even though she suckle it while it has venereal ulcers of the lips and tongue." In a majority of these cases the mother has received a sort of protective inoculation, without having had actual manifestations of the disease. A child showing no taint, but born of a woman suffering with syphilis may with impunity be suckled by its mother (Profeta's law).

(*c*) Placental transmission. The mother may be infected after conception, in which case the child may be, but is not necessarily, born syphilitic. If the infection is late in pregnancy, after the seventh month, the child usually escapes.

Morbid Anatomy.—The *primary lesion,* or chancre, shows: (*a*) A diffuse infiltration of the connective tissue with small, round cells. (*b*) Larger epithelioid cells. (*c*) Giant cells. (*d*) Changes in the small arteries and veins, chiefly thickening of the intima, and alterations in the nerve-fibres going to the part. The sclerosis is due in part to this acute obliterative endarteritis. Associated with the initial lesions are changes in the adjacent lymph-glands, which undergo hyperplasia, and finally become indurated.

The *secondary lesions* of syphilis are too varied for description here. They consist of condylomata, skin eruptions, affections of the eye, etc.

The *tertiary lesions* consist of circumscribed tumors known as gummata, various skin lesions, and a special type of arteritis.

Gummata.—Syphilomata occur in the bones or periosteum—here they are called nodes—in the muscles, skin, brain, lung, liver, kidneys, heart, testes, and adrenals. They vary in size from small, almost microscopic bodies to large solid tumors from 3 to 5 cm. in diameter. They are usually firm and hard, but in the skin and on the mucous membranes they tend to break down rapidly and ulcerate. On cross-section a medium-sized gumma has a grayish-white, homogeneous appearance, presenting in the centre a firm, caseous substance, and at the periphery a translucent, fibrous tissue. Often there are groups of three or more surrounded by dense sclerotic tissue.

The arteritis will be considered in a separate section.

II. Acquired Syphilis.

Primary Stage.—This extends from the appearance of the initial sore until the onset of the constitutional symptoms, and has a variable duration of from six to twelve weeks. The initial sore appears within a month after inoculation, and it first shows itself as a small red papule, which gradually enlarges and breaks in the centre, leaving a small ulcer. The tissue about this becomes indurated so that it ultimately has a gristly, cartilaginous consistence—hence the name, hard or indurated chancre. The size attained is variable, and when small the sore may be overlooked, particularly if it is just within the urethra. The glands in the lymph-district of the chancre enlarge and become hard. Suppuration both in the initial lesion and in the glands may occur as a secondary change. The general condition of the patient in this stage is good. There may be no fever and no impairment of health.

Secondary Stage.—The first constitutional symptoms are usually manifested within three months of the appearance of the primary sore. They rarely occur earlier than the sixth or later than the twelfth week:

(*a*) *Fever,* slight or intense, and very variable in character, may occur early before the skin rash; more frequently it is the " fever of invasion " with the secondary symptoms, or the fever may occur at any period. It may be a mild continuous pyrexia, in other instances, with marked remissions, but the most remarkable form is the intermittent, often mistaken for malaria. Such cases have been reported by Yeo and by Sidney Phillips. The fever may reach

110

105° and the paroxysms persist for months. We have had several cases in which typhoid fever was suspected (T. B. Futcher, New York Medical Journal, 1901), and in others tuberculosis.

(*b*) *Anæmia.*—In many cases the syphilitic poison causes a pronounced anæmia which gives to the face a muddy pallor, and there may even be a light-yellow tinging of the conjunctivæ or of the skin, a hæmatogenous icterus. This syphilitic cachexia may in some instances be extreme. The red blood-corpuscles do not show any special alterations. The blood-count may fall to three millions per cubic millimetre, or even lower. The anæmia may come on suddenly. In a case of syphilitic arthritis in a young girl, following three or four inunctions of mercury, the blood-count fell below two millions per cubic millimetre in a few days.

(*c*) *Cutaneous Lesions.*—The earliest and most common is a *macular syphilide* or *syphilitic roseola*, which occurs on the trunk, and on the front of the arms. The face is often exempt. The spots, which are reddish-brown and symmetrically arranged, persist for a week or two. There may be multiple relapses of roseola, sometimes at long intervals, even eleven years (Fournier). The *papular syphilide*, which forms acne-like indurations about the face and trunk, is often arranged in groups. Other forms are the *pustular rash*, which may so closely simulate variola that the patient may be sent to a small-pox hospital. A *squamous syphilide* occurs, not unlike ordinary psoriasis, except that the scales are less abundant. The rash is more copper-colored and not specially confined to the extensor surfaces.

In the moist regions of the skin, such as the perinæum and groins, the axillæ, between the toes, and at the angles of the mouth, the so-called *mucous patches* occur, which are flat, warty outgrowths, with well-defined margins and surfaces covered with a grayish secretion. They are among the most distinctive lesions of syphilis.

Frequently the hair falls out (alopecia), either in patches or by a general thinning. Occasionally the nails become affected (syphilitic onychia).

(*d*) *Mucous Lesions.*—With the fever and the roseolous rash the throat and mouth become sore. The pharyngeal mucosa is hyperæmic, the tonsils are swollen and often present small, kidney-shaped ulcers with grayish-white borders. Mucous patches are seen on the inner surfaces of the cheeks and on the tongue and lips. Hypertrophy of the papillæ in various portions of the mucous membrane produces the syphilitic warts or condylomata which are most frequent about the vulva and anus.

(*e*) *Arthritis* and pains in the limbs are common secondary symptoms. Occasionally the joint affection is severe and rheumatic fever is suspected.

(*f*) *Other Lesions.*—*Iritis* is common, and usually affects one eye before the other. It comes on from three to six months after the chancre. There may be only slight ciliary congestion in mild cases, but in severer forms there is great pain, and the condition is serious and demands careful management. *Choroiditis* and *retinitis* are rare secondary symptoms. Ear affections are not common in the secondary stage, but instances are found in which sudden deafness occurs, which may be due to labyrinthine disease; more commonly the impaired hearing is due to the extension of inflammation from the throat to the middle ear. Epididymitis and parotitis are rare. Jaundice may occur, the *icterus syphiliticus precox*. The acute nephritis will be referred to later.

Tertiary Stage.—No hard and fast line can be drawn between the lesions of the secondary and those of the tertiary period; and, indeed, in exceptional cases, manifestations which usually appear late may set in even before the primary sore has properly healed. The special affections of this stage are certain skin eruptions, gummatous growths in the viscera, and amyloid degenerations.

(a) The late *syphilides* show a greater tendency to ulceration and destruction of the deeper layers of the skin, so that in healing scars are left. They are also more scattered and seldom symmetrical. One of the most characteristic of the syphilides is rupia, the dry stratified crusts of which cover an ulcer which involves the deeper layers of the skin and in healing leaves a scar. It may be a secondary lesion.

(b) *Gummata.*—These may occur in the skin, subcutaneous tissue, muscles, or internal organs. The general character has been already described. In the skin they tend to break down and ulcerate, leaving ugly sores which heal with difficulty. In the solid organs they undergo fibroid transformation and produce puckering and deformity. On the mucous membranes these tertiary lesions lead to ulceration, in the healing of which cicatrices are formed; thus, in the larynx great narrowing may result, and in the rectum ulceration with fibroid thickening and retraction may lead to stricture. Gummatous ulcers may be infective.

(c) *Amyloid Degeneration.*—Syphilis plays a most important *rôle* in the production of this affection. Of 244 instances analyzed by Fagge, 76 had syphilis, and of these 42 had no bone lesions. It follows the acquired form and is very common in association with rectal syphilis in women. In congenital lues amyloid degeneration is rare.

Quaternary Stage.—Long years it may be from the primary sore and from any active manifestations, certain diseases may follow, not directly syphilitic, but dependent in some way upon its poison, and hence termed meta- or parasyphilitic affections, the chief of which are locomotor ataxia and dementia paralytica and aneurism.

III. Congenital Syphilis.

With the exception of the primary sore, every feature of the acquired disease may be seen in the congenital form.

The intra-uterine conditions leading to the death of the fœtus do not here concern us. The child may be born healthy-looking, or with well-marked evidences of the disease. In the majority of instances the former is the case, and within the first month or two the signs of the disease appear.

Symptoms.—(a) *At Birth.*—When the disease exists at birth the child is feebly developed and wasted, and a skin eruption is usually present, commonly in the form of bullæ about the hands and feet (pemphigus neonatorum syphiliticus). The child snuffles, the lips are ulcerated, the angles of the mouth fissured, and there is enlargement of the liver and spleen. The bone symptoms may be marked, and the epiphyses may even be separated. In such cases the children rarely survive long.

(b) *Early Manifestations.*—When born healthy the child thrives, is fat and plump, and shows no abnormity whatever; then from the fourth to the eighth week, rarely later, a nasal catarrh occurs, *syphilitic rhinitis*, which impedes respiration, and produces the characteristic symptom which has given the name *snuffles* to the disease. The discharge may be sero-purulent or bloody. The child nurses with great difficulty. In severe cases ulceration takes place with necrosis of the bone, leading to a depression at the root of the nose and a deformity characteristic of congenital syphilis. This coryza may be mistaken at first for an ordinary catarrh, but the coexistence of other manifestations usually makes the diagnosis clear. The disease may extend into the Eustachian tubes and middle ears and lead to deafness.

The *cutaneous lesions* arise with or shortly after the onset of the snuffles. The skin often has a sallow, earthy hue. The eruptions are first noticed about the nates. There may be an erythema or an eczematous condition, but more commonly there are irregular reddish-brown patches with well-defined edges. A papular syphilide in this region is by no means uncommon. Fissures occur about the lips, either at the angles of the mouth or in the median line. These *rhagades*, as they are called, are very characteristic. There may be marked ulceration of the muco-cutaneous surfaces. The secretions from these mouth lesions are very virulent, and it is from this source that the wet-nurse is usually infected. Not only the nurse, but members of the family, may be contaminated. There are instances in which other children have been accidentally inoculated from a syphilitic infant. The hair of the head or of the eyebrows may fall out. The syphilitic *onychia* is not uncommon. Enlargement of the glands is not so frequent in the congenital as in the acquired disease. When the cutaneous lesions are marked, the contiguous glands can usually be felt. As pointed out by Gee, the spleen is enlarged in many cases. The condition may persist for a long time. Enlargement of the liver, though often present, is less significant, since in infants it may be due to various causes. These are among the most constant symptoms of congenital syphilis, and usually arise between the third and twelfth weeks. Frequently they are preceded by a period of restlessness and wakefulness, particularly at night. Some authors have described a peculiar syphilitic cry, high-pitched and harsh. Among rarer manifestations are hæmorrhages—the *syphilis hæmorrhagica neonatorum*. The bleeding may be subcutaneous, from the mucous surfaces, or, when early, from the umbilicus. All of such cases, however, are not syphilitic, and the disease must not be confounded with the acute hæmoglobinuria of new-born infants. E. Fournier has described a remarkable enlargement of the subcutaneous veins.

(*c*) *Late Manifestations.*—Children with congenital syphilis rarely thrive. Usually they present a wizened, wasted appearance, and a prematurely aged face. In the cases which recover, the general nutrition may remain good and the child may show no further manifestations of the disease; commonly, however, at the period of second dentition or at puberty the disease reappears. Although the child may have recovered from the early lesions, it does not develop like other children. Growth is slow, development tardy, and there are facial and cranial characteristics which often render the disease recognizable at a glance. A young man of nineteen or twenty may neither look older nor be more developed than a boy of ten or twelve. Fournier describes this condition as *infantilism*. The forehead is prominent, the frontal eminences are marked, and the skull may be very asymmetrical. The bridge of the nose is depressed, the tip *retroussé*. The lips are often prominent, and there are striated lines running from the corners of the mouth. The *teeth* are deformed and may present appearances which Jonathan Hutchinson claims are specific and peculiar. The upper central incisors of the permanent set are the teeth which give information. The specific alterations are—the teeth are peg-shaped, stunted in length and breadth, and narrower at the cutting edge than at the root. On the anterior surface the enamel is well formed, and not eroded or honeycombed. At the cutting edge there is a single notch, usually shallow, sometimes deep, in which the dentine is exposed.

Among late manifestations, particularly apt to appear about puberty, is the interstitial *keratitis*, which usually begins as a slight steaminess of the corneæ, which present a ground-glass appearance. It affects both eyes, though one is attacked before the other. It may persist for months, and usually clears completely, though it may leave opacities, which prevent clear vision. *Iritis* may also occur. Of *ear affections*, apart from those which follow the pharyngeal disease, a form occurs about the time of puberty or earlier, in which deafness comes on rapidly and persists in spite of all treatment. It is unassociated with obvious lesions, and is probably labyrinthine in character. *Bone lesions*, occurring oftenest after the sixth year, are not rare among the late manifestations of hereditary syphilis. The tibiæ are most frequently attacked. It is really a chronic gummatous periostitis, which gradually leads to great thickening of the bone. The nodes of congenital syphilis, which are often mistaken for rickets, are more commonly diffuse and affect the bones of the upper and lower extremities. They are generally symmetrical and rarely painful. They may occur late, even after the twenty-first year.

Joint lesions are rare. Clutton has described a symmetrical synovitis of the knee in hereditary syphilis. Enlargement of the spleen, sometimes with the lymph-glands, may be one of the late manifestations, and may occur either alone or in connection with disease of the liver.

Gummata of the liver, brain, and kidneys have been found in late hereditary syphilis. General paresis may follow.

Is syphilis transmitted to the third generation? Opinion on this subject has been divided. Occasionally cases of pronounced congenital syphilis are met with in the children of parents who are perfectly healthy, and who have not, so far as is known, had syphilis; and yet, as remarked by Coutts in reporting such a group of cases, they do not always bear careful scrutiny. E. Fournier, in his *L'Hérédo-Syphilis Tardive* (1907), cites interesting examples which appear to prove the transmission to the third generation, and this appears to be the view of the French syphilographers. Mr. Hutchinson is still opposed to this view.

IV. VISCERAL SYPHILIS.

1. *Syphilis of the Brain and Cord.*

There are three anatomical changes in the central nervous system—new growths, arteritis, and chronic degenerative (sclerotic) processes.

(1) The new formations or *gummata* form definite tumors, ranging in size from a pea to a walnut, usually multiple and attached to the pia mater, sometimes to the dura. Very rarely they are found unassociated with the meninges. When small they present a uniform, translucent appearance, but when large the centre undergoes a fibro-caseous change, while at the periphery

there is a firm, translucent, grayish tissue. They may resemble large tuberculous tumors. The growths are most common in the cerebrum. They may be multiple and may even attain a considerable size without becoming caseous. Occasionally gummata undergo cystic degeneration. In the cord large growths are not so common.

In the neighborhood of the growths gummous meningitis occurs, in which all the membranes are involved. This is more common at the base, about the chiasma and the interpeduncular space, and along the Sylvian fissures.

(2) *Arteritis,* in the form of nodular tumors on the vessels, which may break down or lead to rupture, or there is a progressive obliterative endarteritis. Heubner's view of the specific character of these changes is disputed.

(3) *Degenerative fibroid changes,* not distinctive anatomically, but clinically directly connected with the disease, are known as post- or meta-syphilitic.

Secondary Changes.—In the brain gummatous arteritis is one of the common causes of softening, which may be extensive, as when the middle cerebral artery is involved, or when there is a large patch of meningitis. In such instances the process is really a meningo-encephalitis, and the symptoms are due to the secondary changes, not directly to the gumma. In the neighborhood of a gumma intense encephalitis or myelitis may occur, and within a few days change the clinical picture.

Syphilitic disease of the nerve-centres occurs usually in the acquired form. In the congenital cases the tumors usually occur early, but may be as late as the twenty-first year. Of late years it has been recognized that the nervous lesions may occur very early in the disease, even before the induration of the primary sore has gone. In a majority of the cases brain symptoms come on within three or four years after infection.

Symptoms.—The chief features of cerebral syphilis are those of tumor cerebri, which will be considered later. They may be classified here as follows:

(1) Psychical features. A sudden and violent onset of delirium may be the first symptom. In other instances prior to the occurrence of delirium there have been headache, alteration of character, and loss of memory. The condition may be accompanied by convulsions. There may be no neuritis, no palsy, and no localizing symptoms.

(2) More commonly following headache, giddiness, or an excited state which may amount to delirium, the patient has an epileptic seizure or a hemiplegic attack, or there is involvement of the nerves of the base. Some of these cases display a prolonged torpor, a special feature of brain syphilis to which both Buzzard and Heubner have referred, which may persist for as long as a month.

(3) In some cases the clinical picture is that of general paralysis—dementia paralytica.

(4) Many cases of cerebral syphilis display the symptoms of brain tumor —headache, optic neuritis, vomiting, and convulsions. Of these symptoms convulsions are the most important, and both Fournier and Wood have laid great stress on the value of this symptom in persons over thirty. The first symptoms may, however, rather resemble those of embolism or thrombosis; thus there may be sudden hemiplegia, with or without loss of consciousness.

The symptoms of *spinal syphilis* are extremely varied and may be caused by large gummatous growths attached to the meninges, in which case the

115

features are those of tumor, by gummatous arteritis with secondary softening, by meningitis with secondary cord changes, or by scleroses occurring late in the disease. Syphilitic myelitis will be considered under affections of the spinal cord.

Diagnosis.—The history is of the first importance, but it may be extremely difficult to get a trustworthy account. Careful examination should be made for traces of the primary sore, for the cicatrices of bubo, for scars of the skin eruption or throat ulcers, and for bone lesions. The character of the symptoms is often of great assistance. They are multiform, variable, and often such as could not be explained by a single lesion; thus there may be anomalous spinal symptoms or involvement of the nerves of the brain on both sides. And lastly the result of treatment has a definite bearing on the diagnosis, as the symptoms may clear up and disappear with the use of antisyphilitic remedies.

2. *Syphilis of the Respiratory Organs.*

1. *Syphilis of the Trachea and Bronchi.*—L. A. Conner (Am. Jour. of Med. Sci., July, 1903) has analyzed 128 recorded cases of syphilis of the trachea and bronchi. In 56 per cent of the cases the trachea was alone involved. In only 10 per cent were characteristic lesions of syphilis found in the lungs. Bronchial dilatation below the lesion was found in 15 per cent of the cases. In ten of the cases the lesion occurred in congenital syphilis.

2. *Syphilis of the Lung.*—This is a very rare disease. In the 2,800 post mortems at the Johns Hopkins Hospital there were 12 cases with syphilitic disease in the lungs; in 8 of these the lesions were in congenital syphilis. In 11 cases there were definite gummata. Clinically the presence of syphilis of the lung was suspected in three cases. Some years ago Fowler visited the museums of the London hospitals and the Royal College of Surgeons, and could find only twelve specimens illustrating syphilitic lesions of the lungs, two of which are doubtful. For the most full and satisfactory consideration of pulmonary syphilis, the reader is referred to chapter xxxvii of Fowler and Godlee's work on Diseases of the Lungs.

It occurs under the following forms:

(1) *The white pneumonia of the fœtus.* This may affect large areas or an entire lung, which then is firm, heavy, and airless, even though the child may have been born alive. On section it has a grayish-white appearance— the so-called white hepatization of Virchow. The chief change is in the alveolar walls, which are greatly thickened and infiltrated, and the section is like one of the pancreas—" pancreatization " of the lung. In the early stages, for example, in a seven or eight months' fœtus, there may be scattered miliary foci of this induration chiefly about the arteries. The air-cells are filled with desquamated and swollen epithelium.

(2) In the form of definite *gummata*, which vary in size from a pea to a goose-egg. They occur irregularly scattered through the lung, but, as a rule, are more numerous toward the root. They present a grayish-yellow caseous appearance, are dry and usually imbedded in a translucent, more or less firm, connective tissue. In a case from my wards described by Councilman, there was extensive involvement of the root of the lungs. Bands of connective tissue passed inward from the thickened pleura, and between these strands and surrounding the gummata there was in places a mottled red

pneumonic consolidation. In the caseous nodules there is typical hyaline degeneration. In a few rare instances there are most extensive caseous gummata with softening and formation of bronchiectatic cavities, and clinically a picture of pulmonary tuberculosis without the presence of tubercle bacilli. In one case, a man aged twenty-seven, admitted in April, 1902, had had for a year cough and bloody expectoration and died of severe hæmoptysis. Bacilli were never found in the sputum. There were extensive caseous gummata throughout both lungs, with much fibrous thickening, and in the lower lobe of the right lung a cavity 3 × 5 cm. in diameter, on the wall of which a branch of the pulmonary artery was eroded. This is the only instance among my cases in which there was an extensive destruction of the lung tissue with the clinical picture simulating pulmonary phthisis.

(3) A majority of authors follow Virchow in recognizing the fibrous interstitial pneumonia at the root of the lung and passing along the bronchi and vessels as probably syphilitic. This much may be said, that in certain cases gummata are associated with these fibroid changes. Again; this condition alone is found in persons with well-marked syphilitic history or with other visceral lesions. It seems in many instances to be a purely sclerotic process, advancing sometimes from the pleura, more commonly from the root of the lung, and invading the interlobular tissue, gradually producing a more or less extensive fibroid change. It rarely involves more than a portion of a lobe or portions of the lobes at the root of the lung. The bronchi are often dilated.

Diagnosis.—It is to be borne in mind, in the first place, that hospital physicians and pathologists the world over bear witness to the extreme rarity of lung syphilis. In the second place, the therapeutic test upon which so much reliance is placed is by no means conclusive. With pulmonary tuberculosis there should now be no confusion, owing to the readiness with which the presence of bacilli is determined. Bronchiectasis in the lower lobe of a lung, dependent upon an interstitial pneumonia of syphilitic origin, could not be distinguished from any other form of the disease. In persons with well-marked syphilitic lesions elsewhere, when obscure pulmonary symptoms occur, or if there are signs of chronic interstitial pneumonia with dilated bronchi, and no tubercle bacilli are present, the condition may possibly be due to syphilis. So far as my experience goes, tuberculous phthisis occurring in a syphilitic subject has no special peculiarities. The lesions of syphilis and tuberculosis could of course coexist in a lung.

3. *Syphilis of the Liver.*

1. INHERITED.—(*a*) *Congenital.*—Gubler in 1852 first described the diffuse hepatitis, which occurs in a large percentage of all deaths in congenital lues. While there may be little or no macroscopical change, the liver preserves its form and is usually enlarged, hard and resistant, and has a yellowish color, compared by Trousseau to sole-leather, or by Gubler to that of flint. Small grayish nodules may be seen on the section. In other cases there are definite gummata with extensive sclerosis.

The child may be still-born or die shortly after birth, or it may be healthy when born and the liver enlarges within a few weeks. The organ is firm; the edge may be readily felt, usually far below the navel. The spleen is also enlarged. The general features are those of a hypertrophic cirrhosis, but jaundice and ascites are not common. Hochsinger (whose exhaustive work on hereditary syphilis has just been completed, 1904) states that of 45 cases recovery took place in 30.

(*b*) *Delayed Congenital Syphilis.*—The condition is by no means rare. Of 132 cases of syphilis hereditaria tarda collected by Forbes, in 34 the liver was involved. The children are nearly always ill-developed, sometimes with marked clubbing of the fingers and showing signs of infantilism. Jaundice is rare. The liver is usually enlarged, or it may show nodular masses.

2. ACQUIRED SYPHILIS.—(*a*) In the *secondary stages* of the disease the liver is not often involved. Jaundice may occur coincident with the rash and with the enlargement of the superficial glands. Rolleston thinks it is probably due to a catarrhal condition of the smaller ducts, part of a general syphilitic hepatitis. There are cases in which it has passed on to a state of acute yellow atrophy. The liver is slightly enlarged. The prognosis is generally good. (*b*) *Tertiary lesions.* The frequency with which the liver is involved in syphilis in adults is very variously estimated. J. L. Allen, quoted by Rolleston, found 37 cases of hepatic gummata among 11,629 autopsies at St. George's Hospital, 27 cases in which cicatrices alone were present. Flexner at the Philadelphia Hospital found 88 cases of hepatic syphilis among 5,088 autopsies. Among 2,300 autopsies at the Johns Hopkins Hospital (Professor Welch) there have been 47 cases of syphilis of the liver, gummata in 19, scars in 16, cirrhosis in 21 cases; 6 of the cases were congenital. My experience coincides with that of Einhorn and of Stockton, who hold that in the United States the disease is by no means uncommon. In 21 cases the diagnosis of syphilis of the liver was made clinically.

Anatomically the lesions may be either gummata or scars or a syphilitic sclerosis. The gummata range in size from a pea to an orange. When small they are pale and gray; the larger ones present yellowish centres; but later there is a " pale, yellowish, cheese-like nodule of irregular outline, surrounded by a fibrous zone, the outer edge of which loses itself in the lobular tissue, the lobules dwindling gradually in its grasp. This fibrous zone is never very broad; the cheesy centre varies in consistence from a gristle-like toughness to a pulpy softness; it is sometimes mortar-like, from cretaceous change " (Wilks). They may form enormous tumors, as in the remarkable one figured on page 351 in Rolleston's work on Diseases of the Liver. They may be felt as large as an orange beneath the skin in the epigastrium and they may disappear with the same extraordinary rapidity as the subcutaneous or periosteal gumma. Macroscopically they may indeed at first look like massive cancer. Extensive caseation, softening and calcification may occur. The syphilitic scars are usually linear or star-shaped. They may be very numerous and divide the liver into small sections—the so-called botyroid organ, of which a remarkable example is figured in my *Lectures on Abdominal Tumors.* The syphilitic cirrhosis is usually combined with gummata, or with marked scarring in the portal canal, leading to lobulation of the organ, but the ordinary multilobular cirrhosis is not common.

Symptoms.—In the first place the clinical picture may be that of cirrhosis —slight jaundice, fever, portal obstruction, ascites. There may not be the slightest suspicion of the syphilitic nature of the case. One of my patients had been tapped thirteen times before admission to the hospital. The diagnosis was made by finding the gummata on the shins. She recovered promptly.

In a second group of cases the patient is anæmic, passes large quantities of pale urine containing albumin and tube-casts; the liver is enlarged, perhaps irregular, and the spleen also is enlarged. Dropsical symptoms may supervene, or the patient may be carried off by some intercurrent disease. Extensive amyloid degeneration of the spleen, the intestinal mucosa, and of the liver, with gummata, are found.

Thirdly, in a very important group the symptoms are those of tumor of the liver, causing pain and distress, and on examination an irregular mass is discovered. The tumor may be large, causing a prominent bulging in the epigastrium. Naturally carcinoma is thought of, as there may be nothing to suggest syphilis. In other cases the history or the presence of gummata elsewhere should aid in the diagnosis. In other instances the rapid disappearance under treatment even of a large visible tumor makes the syphilitic nature quite positive. Lastly, in a few cases the irregular fever with enlargement and irregularity of the liver may suggest suppuration, or the uniform great enlargement of the organ hypertrophic biliary cirrhosis, while there are some cases in which the spleen is so greatly enlarged, the anæmia so pronounced, and the liver small and contracted that the diagnosis of splenic anæmia is made.

4. *Syphilis of the Digestive Tract.*

The *œsophagus* is very rarely affected. Stenosis is the usual result. Syphilis of the *stomach* is excessively rare. Flexner has reported a remarkable case in association with gummata of the liver. He has collected 14 cases in the literature. Syphilitic ulceration has been found in the small intestine and in the cæcum.

The most common seat in this tract is the *rectum*. The affection is found most commonly in women, and results from the growth of gummata in the submucosa above the internal sphincter. The process is slow and tedious, and may last for years before it finally induces stricture. The symptoms are usually those of narrowing of the lower bowel. The condition is readily recognized by rectal examination. The history of gradual on-coming stricture, the state of the patient, and the fact that there is a hard, fibrous narrowing, not an elevated crater-like ulcer, usually render easy the diagnosis from malignant disease. In medical practice these cases come under observation for other symptoms, particularly amyloid degeneration; and the rectal disease may be entirely overlooked, and only discovered post mortem.

5. *Circulatory System.*

Syphilis of the Heart.—A fresh, warty endocarditis due to syphilis is not recognized, though occasionally in persons dead of the disease this form is present, as is not uncommon in conditions of debility. Outgrowths on the valves in connection with gummata have been reported by Janeway and others. Loomis groups the lesions into: (1) Gummata, recent or old; (2) fibroid induration, localized or diffuse; (3) amyloid degeneration; and (4) endarteritis obliterans. I. Adler claims that changes in the blood-vessels of the walls of the heart are common both in congenital and acquired syphilis, even in cases without clinical symptoms or gross lesions.

Rupture may take place, as in the cases reported by Dandridge and Nalty, or sudden death, as in the cases of Cayley and Pearce Gould; indeed, sudden death is frequent, occurring in 21 of 63 cases (Mracek).

Syphilis of the Arteries.—Syphilis plays an important *rôle* in arterio-sclerosis and aneurism. Its connection with these processes will be considered later; here we shall refer only to the syphilitic affection of the smaller vessels, which occurs in two forms:

(*a*) An *obliterating endarteritis*, characterized by a proliferation of the subendothelial tissue. The new growth lies within the elastic lamina, and may gradually fill the entire lumen; hence the term obliterating. The media and adventitia are also infiltrated with small cells. This form of endarteritis described by Heubner is not, however, characteristic of syphilis, and its presence alone in an artery could not be considered pathognomonic. If, however, there are gummata in other parts, or if the condition about to be described exists in adjacent arteries, the process may be regarded as syphilitic.

(*b*) *Gummatous Periarteritis.*—With or without involvement of the intima, nodular gummata may develop in the adventitia of the artery, producing globular or ovoid swellings, which may attain considerable size. They are not infrequently seen in the cerebral arteries, which seem to be specially prone to this affection. This form is specific and distinctive of syphilis. Reuter and Schmorl have found *Spirochæta pallida* in the syphilitic aortitis, and Benda in gummatous arteritis of the cerebral vessels.

6. *Renal Syphilis.*

(*a*) Gummata occasionally are found in the kidneys, particularly in cases in which there is extensive gummatous hepatitis. They are rarely numerous, and occasionally lead to scattered cicatrices. Clinically the affection is not recognizable.

(*b*) *Acute Syphilitic Nephritis.*—This condition has been carefully studied by the French writers and by Lafleur, of Montreal. It is estimated to occur in the secondary stage in about 3.8 per cent, and may occur in from three to six months, sometimes later, from the initial lesion. The outlook is good, though often the albuminuria may persist for months; more rarely chronic Bright's disease follows. In a few instances syphilitic nephritis has proved rapidly fatal in a fortnight or three weeks. The lesions are not specific, but are similar to those in other acute infections.

7. *Syphilitic Orchitis.*

This affection is of special significance to the physician, as its detection frequently clinches the diagnosis in obscure internal disorders. Syphilis occurs in the testes in two forms:

(*a*) The gummatous growth, forming an indurated mass or group of masses in the substance of the organ, and sometimes difficult to distinguish from tuberculous disease. The area of induration is harder and it affects the body of the testes, while tubercle more commonly involves the epididymis. It rarely tends to invade the skin, or to break down, soften, and suppurate, and is usually painless.

(*b*) There is an *interstitial orchitis* regarded as syphilitic, which leads to fibroid induration of the gland and gradually to atrophy. It is a slow,

120

progressive change, coming on without pain, usually involving one organ more than another.

DIAGNOSIS, TREATMENT, ETC.

General Diagnosis of Syphilis.—There is seldom any doubt concerning the existence of syphilitic lesions. Syphilis is common in the community, and is no respecter of age, sex, or station in life. It is possible that the primary sore may have been of trifling extent, or urethral and masked by a gonorrhœa, and the patient may not have had severe secondary symptoms, but such instances are extremely rare. Inquiries should be made into the history to ascertain if the patient has had skin rashes, sore throat, or if the hair has fallen out. Careful inspection should be made of the throat and skin for signs of old lesions. Scars in the groins, the result of buboes, are uncertain evidences of syphilitic infection. The cicatrices on the legs are often copper-colored, though this can not be regarded as peculiar to syphilis. The bones should be examined for nodes. In doubtful cases the scar of the primary sore may be found, or there may be signs of atrophy or of hardening of the testes. In women, special stress has been laid upon the occurrence of frequent miscarriages, which, in connection with other circumstances, are always suggestive.

In the congenital disease, the occurrence within the first three months of snuffles and skin rash is conclusive. Later, the characters of the syphilitic facies, already referred to, often give a clew to the nature of some obscure visceral lesion. Other distinctive features are the symmetrical development of nodes on the bones, and the interstitial keratitis.

The *Spirochæta pallida* may be studied from the fresh lesion. After cleaning carefully, serum is sucked out with a small Biers apparatus, and the living spirochetes may be seen in the special " dark field " apparatus used for the purpose.

Serum Diagnosis.—Wassermann's reaction has reached the clinical stage, and in good hands may be accepted as valuable aid in diagnosis. It is obtained in from 80 to 90 per cent of all cases of syphilis with manifestations. Observations are not altogether in accord, but such syphilographers as Neisser and Finger are convinced of its practical value. The results in tabes and dementia paralytica are very constant.

Therapeutic Test.—In a doubtful case, as, for example, an obstinate skin rash, or an obscure tumor in the abdomen, antisyphilitic treatment may prove successful, but this can not always be relied upon.

Prophylaxis.—Irregular intercourse has existed from the beginning of recorded history, and unless man's nature wholly changes—and of this we can have no hope—will continue. Resisting all attempts at solution, the social evil remains the great blot upon our civilization, and inextricably blended with it is the question of the prevention of syphilis. Two measures are available—the one personal, the other administrative.

Personal purity is the prophylaxis which we, as physicians, are especially bound to advocate. Continence may be a hard condition (to some harder than to others), but it can be borne, and it is our duty to urge this lesson upon young and old who seek our advice in matters sexual. Certainly it is better, as St. Paul says, to marry than to burn, but if the former is not feas-

121

ible there are other altars than those of Venus upon which a young man may light fires. He may practise at least two of the five means by which, as the physician Rondibilis counselled Panurge, carnal concupiscence may be cooled and quelled—hard work of body and hard work of mind. Idleness is the mother of lechery; and a young man will find that absorption in any pursuit will do much to cool passions which, though natural and proper, can not in the exigencies of our civilization always obtain natural and proper gratification.

To carry out successfully any administrative measures seems hopeless, at any rate, in our Anglo-Saxon civilization. The state accepts the responsibility of guarding citizens against small-pox or cholera, but in dealing with syphilis the problem has been too complex and has hitherto baffled solution. Inspection, segregation, and regulation are difficult, if not impossible, to carry out, and public sentiment is bitterly opposed to this plan. The compulsory registration of every case of gonorrhœa and syphilis, with greatly increased facilities for thorough treatment, offer a more acceptable alternative.

Treatment.—That the later stages which come under the charge of the physician are so common, results, in great part, from the carelessness of the patient, who, wearied with treatment, can not understand why he should continue to take medicine after all the symptoms have disappeared; but, in part, the profession also is to blame for not insisting more urgently that acquired syphilis is not cured in a few months, but takes at least three years, during which time the patient should be under careful supervision.

The discovery of the spirochete suggests prompt excision of the local breeding spot—the chancre—and in apes this may be done successfully within the first two weeks. Local treatment of the chancre with mercury will also prevent the development of the disease in the ape. Much more important is the fact that the virus is destroyed in the ape treated with atoxyl in from three to ten days after inoculation, so that the animal may be reinfected. These are practical points, the value of which in human practice will have to be tested. The atoxyl (metarœnic acid anilide) is strongly toxic to protozoan parasites, as its use in sleeping sickness has shown. It may be given intra-muscularly in doses of three grains every third day for ten days, and then resumed. Good results have been reported by Lambkin with it.

Mercury may be given by the mouth in the form of gray powder, the hydrargyrum cum cretâ, which Hutchinson recommends to be given in pills, one-grain doses with a grain of Dover's powder. One pill from four to six times a day will usually suffice. I warmly endorse the excellent results which are obtained by this method, under which the patient often gains rapidly in weight, and the general health improves remarkably. It may be continued for months without any ill effects. Other forms given by the mouth are the pilules of the biniodide (gr. $\frac{1}{16}$), or of the protiodide (gr. $\frac{1}{6}$), three times a day. " If mercury be begun as soon as the state of the sore permits of diagnosis, and continued in small but adequate doses, the patient will usually escape both sore throat and eruption " (Jonathan Hutchinson).

Inunction is a still more effective means. A drachm of the ordinary mercurial ointment is thoroughly rubbed into the skin every evening for six days; on the seventh a warm bath is taken, and on the eighth the mercurial course is resumed. At least half an hour should be given to each inunction. It is well to apply it at different places on successive days. The sides of the chest

122

and abdomen and the inner surfaces of the arms and thighs are the best positions.

The mercury may be given by direct injection into the muscles. If proper precautions are taken in sterilizing the syringe, and if the injections are made into the muscles, not into the subcutaneous tissue, abscesses rarely result. One-third of a grain of the bichloride in twenty drops of water may be injected once a week, or from one to two grains of calomel in glycerin (20 minims).

Still another method, greatly in vogue in certain parts of the Continent and in institutions, is fumigation. It may be carried out effectively by means of Lee's lamp. The patient sits on a chair wrapped in blankets, with the head exposed. The calomel is volatilized and deposited with the vapor on the patient's skin. The process lasts about twenty minutes, and the patient goes to bed wrapped in blankets without washing or drying the skin.

A patient under mercurial treatment should avoid stimulants and live a regular life, not necessarily abstaining from business. Green vegetables and fruit should not be taken. Salivation is to be avoided. The teeth should be cleansed twice a day, and if the gums become tender, the breath fetid, or the tongue swollen and indented, the drug should be suspended for a week or ten days.

In congenital syphilis the treatment of cases born with bullæ and other signs of the disease is not satisfactory, and the infants usually die within a few days or weeks. The child should be nursed by the mother alone, or, if this is not feasible, should be hand-fed, but under no circumstances should a wet-nurse be employed. The child is most rapidly and thoroughly brought under the influence of the drug by inunction. The mercurial ointment may be smeared on the flannel roller. This is not a very cleanly method, and sometimes rouses the suspicion of the mother. It is preferable to give the drug by the mouth, in the form of gray powder, half a grain three times a day. In the late manifestations associated with bone lesions, the combination of mercury and iodide of potassium is most suitable and is well given in the form of Gilbert's syrup, which consists of the biniodide of mercury (gr. j), of potassium iodide (℥ss.), and water (℥ij). Of this a dose for a child under three is from five to ten drops three times a day, gradually increased. Under these measures, the cases of congenital syphilis usually improve with great rapidity. The medication should be continued at intervals for many months, and it is well to watch these patients carefully during the period of second dentition and at puberty, and if necessary to place them on specific treatment.

In the treatment of the visceral lesions of syphilis, which come more distinctly within the province of the physician, iodide of potassium is of equal or even greater value than mercury. Under its use ulcers rapidly heal, gummatous tumors melt away, and we have an illustration of a specific action only equalled by that of mercury in the secondary stages, by iron in certain forms of anæmia, and by quinine in malaria. It is as a rule well borne in an initial dose of 10 grains; given in milk the patient does not notice the taste. It should be gradually increased to 30 or more grains three times a day. In syphilis of the nervous system it may be used in still larger doses. Seguin, who specially insisted upon the advantage of this plan, urged that the drug should be pushed, as good effects were not obtained with the moderate doses.

When syphilitic hepatitis is suspected the combination of mercury and iodide of potassium is most satisfactory. If there is ascites, Addison's pill (as it is often called) of calomel, digitalis, and squills will be found very useful. A patient of mine with recurring ascites, on whom paracentesis was repeatedly performed and who had an enlarged and irregular liver, took this pill for more than a year with occasional intermissions, and ultimately there was a complete disappearance of the dropsy and an extraordinary reduction in the volume of the liver. Occasionally the iodide of sodium is more satisfactory than the iodide of potassium. It is less depressing and agrees better with the stomach.

Syphilis and Marriage.—Upon this question the family physician is often called to decide. He should insist upon the necessity of two full years elapsing between the date of infection and the contracting of marriage. This, it should be borne in mind, is the earliest possible limit, and marriage should be allowed only if the treatment has been thorough and if at least a year has passed without any manifestation of the disease.

Syphilis and Life Insurance.—An individual with syphilis can not be regarded as a first-class risk unless he can furnish evidence of prolonged and thorough treatment and of immunity for two or three years from all manifestations. Even then, when we consider the extraordinary frequency of the cerebral and other complications in persons who have had this disease and who may even have undergone thorough treatment, the risk to the company is certainly increased (see Bramwell, Clinical Studies, vol. i).

XXXII. GONORRHŒAL INFECTION.

Gonorrhœa, one of the most widespread and serious of infectious diseases, presents many features for consideration. As a cause of ill-health and disability the gonococcus occupies a position of the very first rank among its fellows. While the local lesion is too often thought to be trifling, in its singular obstinacy, in the possibilities of permanent sexual damage to the individual himself and still more in the " grisly troop " which may follow in its train, gonorrhœal infection does not fall very far short of syphilis in importance.

The importance of the infection in children has been much dwelt upon of late, particularly as in them the severer systemic lesions are liable to occur, but more especially from the wide-spread and obstinate character of the epidemics in institutions. The gonococcus vaginitis and the ophthalmia are very serious diseases in children's hospitals and in infants' homes. The story of the gonococcus infection in the Babies' Hospital, New York, for the past eleven years, as told by Holt (N. Y. Med. Jour., March, 1905), illustrates the singular obstinacy of the infection. In spite of the greatest care and precaution, there were in 1903 65 cases of vaginitis, with 2 of ophthalmia and 12 of arthritis. In 1904 there were 52 cases of vaginitis, only 16 of which would have been recognized without the bacteriological examination. In all, in the eleven years, there were 273 cases of vaginitis, only 6 with ophthalmia and 26 with arthritis. Holt urges isolation and prolonged quarantine as the only measures to combat successfully the disease.

The immediate and remote effects of the gonococcus may be considered under—

syphilis

Reviewing the section on syph-
ilis in successive editions of Osler's *The Principles and Practice of Medicine*,
one is impressed with the promptness with which new knowledge of this
disease became incorporated into his text — joint tribute to Osler's thorough
scholarship and his long-standing interest in syphilis as a disease.

Three momentous developments occurred between
publication of the sixth and seventh editions: discovery of *Treponema pallidum,* transmission of the disease to apes, and development of the Wassermann test based on the fundamental investigations of Bordet and Gengou.
The great therapeutic breakthrough, the development of arsphenamine by
Ehrlich, was a year or two in the future, and of course penicillin was more
than 30 years away.

Osler's long service in Philadelphia and Baltimore and
his inquiring mind had made him a master clinical syphilologist, and it was to
be expected that the two laboratory tools added in quick succession illumi-
nated for him the highlights and shadows until many pieces of the clinical
puzzle fell into place.

Even so, one admires the clinical and epidemiological
astuteness which had identified so clearly most of the essential features of
syphilis as an infectious disease long before discovery of the etiological agent
and development of a test for the recognition of latent infection. For example,
the first edition as well as the sixth carries this short definition of the disease:
"a specific disease of slow evolution propagated by inoculation (acquired
syphilis), or by hereditary transmission (congenital syphilis)." In the seventh
edition only the phrase "caused by the *Spirochaeta pallida"* was added, a
definition still wholly accurate.

For centuries it had been recognized that syphilis is
commonly transmitted by sexual intercourse, but Osler's description of extra-
genital transmission is still valid, except that the wet-nurse, in whom the risk
of infection was high, has now gone out of fashion, at least in America.

Likewise, Osler's clinical descriptions of syphilis are,
as might be expected, excellent by present-day standards, although with
modern treatment it had been forgotten that neglected early syphilis can
partake of the characteristics of a severe subacute infection. A febrile course
was not uncommon, at times mimicking typhoid fever; profound anemia and
so-called syphilitic cachexia were observed, and jaundice and nephritis occasionally occurred. Already *T. pallidum* had been demonstrated in syphilitic
aortitis and in syphilitic arteritis of the cerebral vessels. It is natural that

125

Syphilis

much greater space was allotted to the description of late syphilis of the various systems that would be in a comparable modern text, simply because these presented everyday problems to the clinician, who rarely sees them today.

Nevertheless, the concept of subclinical or latent syphilis as we now know it does not emerge in the seventh edition, nor was the great value of the Wassermann test in differential diagnosis fully projected. Yet, Osler states, "Wassermann's reaction has reached the clinical stage, and in good hands may be accepted as valuable aid in diagnosis. It is obtained in from 80 to 90 percent of all cases of syphilis with manifestations. Observations are not altogether in accord, but such syphilographers as Neisser and Finger are convinced of its practical value. The results in tabes and dementia paralytica are very constant." These are wise and discriminating deductions from what must have been meager data available at the time.

There are, of course, other broad and important areas of the basic biology and clinical aspects of syphilis in which significant developments have occurred and of which no hint was given in the seventh edition.

For example, largely through the studies of Brown and Pearce, and Chesney in America, Matsumoto in Japan, Kolle in Germany, and their numerous associates, the basic elements of the host-parasite relationship in this slowly evolving chronic disease have been elucidated. Far from being something apart from the main stream of infectious processes the more that is learned about it the more it appears to follow the general pattern, save only in that the delicate balance existing between the parasite and host leads to a classic example of the nonequilibrium state, the saga of the foxes and the rabbits on an island being enacted in microcosmic fashion.

At the immunochemical level, in spite of the handicap posed by inability to cultivate virulent *T. pallidum* in vitro, investigators have searched, as yet with indifferent success, for antigenic components of the treponeme that will permit more specific serological tests, and perhaps induce immunity artificially. But one major contribution which has had a significant clinical and epidemiological impact was development of the Treponemal Immobilization Test by Nelson and Mayer in 1949. This test, based on an antibody hitherto only unsatisfactorily demonstrated, has led to the recognition and more certain identification of individuals with so-called biological false-positive serological tests.

The great gift of penicillin, which in a stroke toppled the complicated and uncertain therapeutic reign of the arsphenamines in the 1940s, is a familiar story to everyone, bringing the treatment of syphilis within the competence of most physicians and within the endurance of most patients.

126

Syphilis

Finally, along with the concept of One World, has come the realization that syphilis is but one component of a large spectrum of treponemal diseases, the so-called treponematoses. One or more of these diseases, syphilis, yaws, bejel, pinta, and numerous other less well-known syndromes, abound everywhere in the world. Their biological, clinical, and epidemiological relationships have been a major preoccupation of the author of this section and his associates, their studies showing beyond a doubt that there is strong biological and immunological overlap. Even more recently has come the discovery by Fribourg-Blanc and his associates that primates in the African jungles have positive serological tests for syphilis, including the TPI antibody. Reflecting on the now familiar story of yellow fever one may envision the jungle as the ultimate reservoir of treponemal infections.

Despite these revolutionary advances on one front, the story of syphilis has changed but little. Let the seventh edition tell it, for impressive as was Osler's penchant for critical evaluation of the recent medical and scientific literature, perhaps the most characteristic feature of the man is revealed in his broad humanistic approach to the question of the prevention of syphilis. The following passages appear in the first through the seventh edition: "Irregular intercourse has existed from the beginning of recorded history, and unless man's nature wholly changes — and of this we can have no hope — will continue. Resisting all attempts at solution, the social evil remains the great blot upon our civilization, and inextricably blended with it is the question of the prevention of syphilis. Two measures are available — the one personal, the other administrative.

"Personal purity is the prophylaxis which we, as physicians, are especially bound to advocate. Continence may be a hard condition (to some harder than to others), but it can be borne, and it is our duty to urge this lesson upon young and old who seek our advice in matters sexual. Certainly it is better, as St. Paul says, to marry than to burn, but if the former is not feasible there are other altars than those of Venus upon which a young man may light fires. He may practice at least two of the five means by which, as the physician Rondibilis counselled Panurge, carnal concupiscence may be cooled and quelled — hard work of body and hard work of mind. Idleness is the mother of lechery; a young man will find that absorption in any pursuit will do much to cool passions which, though natural and proper, can not in the exigencies of our civilization always obtain natural and proper gratification.

"To carry out successfully any administrative measures seems hopeless, at any rate, in our Anglo-Saxon civilization. The state accepts the responsibility of guarding citizens against small-pox or cholera, but in

127

Syphilis

dealing with syphilis the problem has been too complex and has hitherto baffled solution. Inspection, segregation, and regulation are difficult, if not impossible, to carry out, and public sentiment is bitterly opposed to this plan. The compulsory registration of every case of gonorrhoea and syphilis, with greatly increased facilities for thorough treatment, offer a more acceptable alternative."

Can much more be said today?

Thomas B. Turner

REFERENCES

Chesney, A.M. Acquired immunity in syphilis. The Harvey Lectures 1929-30. Baltimore, Maryland, 1931.

Ehrlich, P., and Hata, S. The Experimental Chemotherapy of Spirilloses. London, Rebman, Ltd., 1911.

Fribourg-Blanc, A., Niel, G., and Mollaret, H.H. Immunological aspects in African cynomolgous monkeys. Bull. Soc. Path. Exot., 56:474, 1963.

Mahoney, J.F., Arnold, R.C., and Harris, A. Penicillin treatment of early syphilis. Preliminary report. Vener. Dis. Information, 24:335, 1943.

Nelson, R.A., Jr., and Mayer, M.M. Immobilization of *Treponema pallidum* in vitro by antibody produced in syphilitic infection. J. Exp. Med., 89:369, 1949.

Turner, T.B., and Hollander, D.A. Biology of the Treponematoses. Geneva, World Health Organization, 1957.

gas bacilli are also met with. It is surprising in how many instances of arterio-sclerosis, of chronic heart disease, of Bright's disease, and particularly of cirrhosis of the liver in Flexner's series the fatal event was determined by an acute tuberculosis of the peritonæum or pleura.

The general terminal infections are somewhat less common. Of 85 cases of chronic renal disease in which Flexner found micro-organisms at autopsy, 38 exhibited general infections; of 48 cases of chronic cardiac disease, in 14 the distribution of bacteria was general. The blood-serum of persons suffering from advanced chronic disease was found by him to be less destructive to the staphylococcus aureus than normal human serum. Other diseases in which general terminal infection may occur are Hodgkin's disease, leukæmia, and chronic tuberculosis.

And, lastly, probably of the same nature is the terminal entero-colitis so frequently met with in chronic disorders.

XIX. RHEUMATIC FEVER.

Definition.—An acute, non-contagious fever, dependent upon an unknown infective agent, and characterized by multiple arthritis and a marked tendency to inflammation of the fibrous tissues.

Etiology.—DISTRIBUTION AND PREVALENCE.—It prevails in temperate and humid climates. Church has collected interesting statistics on this point. Oddly enough, the two countries with the highest admission in the British army per thousand of strength—Egypt, 7.02, and Canada, 6.26—have climates the most diverse. In 1903 in England and Wales 1,812 deaths were due to rheumatic fever (Tatham). The disease prevails more in the northern latitudes. In the Montreal General Hospital there were for the twelve years ending 1903, 2 deaths in 482 cases among 12,044 admissions; at the Royal Victoria Hospital, Montreal, for ten years ending 1903, 3 deaths in 285 cases among 9,286 admissions (John McCrae). At the Johns Hopkins Hospital for the fifteen years ending 1904, there were 360 admissions (330 patients) and 9 deaths (T. McCrae). The general impression is that the disease prevails more in the British Isles than elsewhere; but, as Church remarks, the returns are very imperfect (this holds good everywhere). In Norway, where cases of rheumatic fever are notified, there were for the four years 1888–'92 13,654 cases, with 250 deaths.

SEASON.—In London the cases reach the maximum in the months of September and October. In the Montreal General Hospital Bell's statistics of 456 cases show that the largest number was admitted in February, March, and April. And the same is true in Baltimore, 55 per cent of our cases were admitted in the first four months of the year (McCrae). The disease prevails most in the dry years or a succession of such, and is specially prevalent when the subsoil water is abnormally low and the temperature of the earth high (Newsholme).

AGE.—Young adults are most frequently affected, but the disease is by no means uncommon in children between the ages of ten and fifteen years. Sucklings are rarely attacked. Milton Miller has analyzed 19 undoubted cases. The cases have to be distinguished from a totally different affection, the pyogenic arthritis of infants. Of 456 cases admitted to the Montreal General Hospital there were, under fifteen years, 4.38 per cent; from fifteen to twenty-five years, 48.68 per cent; from twenty-five to thirty-five years, 25.87 per cent; from thirty-five to forty-five years, 13.6 per cent; above forty-five years, 7.4 per cent. Of our 360 admissions, 110 were in the third decade and 65 per cent below the thirtieth year of age (McCrae). Ten per cent of the cases had the first attack in the first decade. Of the 655 cases analyzed by Whipham for the Collective Investigation Committee of the British Medical Association, only 32 cases occurred under the tenth year and 80 per cent between the twentieth and fortieth years. These figures do not give the ratio of cases in children, in whom the milder types of arthritis are very common.

SEX.—If all ages are taken, males are affected oftener than females. Of our patients, 239 were males, 91 females. In the Collective Investigation Report there were 375 males and 279 females. Up to the age of twenty, however, females predominate. Between the ages of ten and fifteen girls are more prone to the disease.

HEREDITY.—It is a deeply grounded belief with the public and the profession that rheumatism is a family disease, but Church thinks the evidence is still imperfect. In 25 per cent of our cases there was a history of the disease in the family. The not rare occurrence in several members of the same family is used by those who believe in the infectious origin as an argument in favor of its being a house disease.

OCCUPATIONS which necessitate exposure to cold and great changes of temperature predispose strongly, and the disease is met with oftenest in drivers, servants, bakers, sailors, and laborers.

CHILL.—Exposure to cold, a wetting, or a sudden change of temperature are among the factors in determining the onset of an attack, but they were present in only 12 per cent of our cases.

Not only does an attack not confer IMMUNITY, but as in pneumonia predisposes the subject to the disease.

Rheumatic Fever as an Acute Infectious Disease.—(a) GENERAL EVIDENCE.—Rheumatic fever, as Newsholme has shown, occurs in epidemics without regular periodicity, recurring at intervals of three, four, or six years, and varying much in intensity. A severe epidemic is apt to be followed by two or three mild outbreaks. " The curves of the mortality statistics . . . approximate very closely to those of pyæmia, puerperal fever, and erysipelas, diseases which are certainly associated with specific micro-organisms " (Church). The constancy also of the seasonal variations is an additional support to this view.

(b) CLINICAL FEATURES.—Physicians have long been impressed with the striking similarity of the symptoms to those of septic infection. In the character of the fever, the mode of involvement of the joints, the tendency to relapse, the sweats, the anæmia, the leucocytosis, and, above all, the great liability to endocarditis and involvement of the serous membranes, the disease resembles pyæmia very closely, and may, indeed, be taken as the very type of an acute infection. But, as Stephen Mackenzie remarks, acute rheumatism should be considered not simply from the point of view of the rheumatic polyarthritis of the adult, but as a whole in its manifestations at different periods of life; yet even from this standpoint the multiform manifestations of the rheumatic poison in childhood and young adults may very reasonably be referred to the effect of the toxins of micro-organisms.

(*c*) SPECIAL EVIDENCE.—The bacteriology of the disease is still under discussion. Many organisms have been described, a special bacillus by Achalme, forms of streptococci, and a diplococcus by Wasserman, which is probably the same as that described in England by Poynton and Payne, Ainley Walker, Shaw and Beattie. This latter, which has been called the *Micrococcus rheumaticus*, has been isolated from the throat, joints, and exudates in persons suffering with rheumatic fever. Poynton, Payne, and others have produced with this organism, injected into rabbits, endocarditis, arthritis, and subcutaneous nodules. In a series of cases in my clinic Cole could not confirm these results, studying blood cultures and the effusion into the joints. On the other hand, he was able with strains of streptococci from various sources to produce experimentally endocarditis and arthritis. A view very commonly held is that the organism producing the disease is an attenuated streptococcus. Beattie, in a recent paper, claims that the results obtained by injecting streptococci are different from those produced by *Micrococcus rheumaticus*. A point of great interest is that Ainley Walker has obtained formic acid from the cultures of this germ. The problem is one of great difficulty and of the first importance, in view of the suffering and incapacity caused by rheumatic fever.

There is considerable evidence against the view that it is simply a mild pyogenic infection. Salicylates have no effect on the ordinary streptococcus infections, and the clinical course in the streptococcus arthritis is very different; moreover, rheumatic joints never suppurate. The isolation of streptococci may simply indicate the presence of secondary streptococcus invaders such as occur in scarlet fever and small-pox.

Other views as to the nature of rheumatism are the *metabolic* or *chemical:* that it depends upon a morbid material produced within the system in defective processes of assimilation. It has been suggested that this material is lactic acid (Prout) or certain combinations with lactic acid (Latham).

A *nervous theory of acute rheumatism* was advocated by the late J. K. Mitchell, of Philadelphia, who believed that the nerve centres were primarily affected by cold and that the local lesions were really trophic in character.

Morbid Anatomy.—There are no changes characteristic of the disease. The affected joints show hyperæmia and swelling of the synovial membranes and of the ligamentous tissues. There may be slight erosion of the cartilage. The fluid in the joint is turbid, albuminous in character, and contains leucocytes and a few fibrin flakes. Pus is very rare in uncomplicated cases. Rheumatic fever rarely proves fatal, except when there are serious complications, such as pericarditis, endocarditis, myocarditis, pleurisy, or pneumonia. The conditions found show nothing peculiar, nothing to distinguish them from other forms of inflammation. In death from hyperpyrexia no special changes are found. The blood usually contains an excessive amount of fibrin. In the secondary rheumatic inflammations, as pleurisy and pericarditis, various pus organisms have been found, possibly the result of a mixed infection.

Symptoms.—As a rule, the disease sets in abruptly, but it may be preceded by irregular pains in the joints, slight *malaise*, sore throat, and particularly by tonsillitis. A definite rigor is uncommon; more often there is slight chilliness. The fever rises quickly, and with it one or more of the joints become painful. Within twenty-four hours from the onset, the disease is fully manifest. The temperature range is from 102° to 104°. The pulse is frequent, soft, and usually above 100. The tongue is moist, and rapidly becomes covered with a white fur. There are the ordinary symptoms associated with an acute fever, such as loss of appetite, thirst, constipation, and a scanty, highly acid, highly colored urine. In a majority of the cases there are profuse, very acid sweats, of a peculiar sour odor. Sudaminal and miliary vesicles are abundant, the latter usually surrounded by a minute ring of hyperæmia. The mind is clear, except in the cases with hyperpyrexia. The affected joints are painful to move, soon become swollen and hot, and present a reddish flush. The order of frequency of involvement of the joints in our series was knee, ankle, shoulder, wrist, elbow, hip, hand, foot. The joints are not attacked together, but successively. For example, if the knee is first affected, the redness may disappear from it as the wrists become painful and hot. The disease is seldom limited to a single articulation. The amount of swelling is variable. Extensive effusion into a joint is rare, and much of the enlargement is due to the infiltration of the periarticular tissues with serum. The swelling may be limited to the joint proper, but in the wrists and ankles it sometimes involves the sheaths of the tendons and produces great enlargement of the hands and feet. Corresponding joints are often affected. In attacks of great severity every one of the larger joints may be involved. The vertebral, sterno-clavicular, and phalangeal articulations are less often inflamed in acute than in gonorrhœal rheumatism. Perhaps no disease is more painful than acute polyarthritis. The inability to change the posture without agonizing pain, the drenching sweats, the prostration and utter helplessness, combine to make it one of the most distressing of febrile affections. A special feature of the disease is the tendency of the inflammation to subside in one joint while increasing with great intensity in another.

The temperature range in an ordinary attack is between 102° and 104°. In only 18 of our cases did the temperature rise above 104°. In 100 it reached 103° or over. It is peculiarly irregular, with marked remissions and exacerbations, depending very much upon the intensity and extent of the articular inflammation. Defervescence is usually gradual. The profuse sweats materially influence the temperature curve. If a two-hourly chart is made and observations upon the sweats are noted, the remissions will usually be found coincident with the sweats. The perspiration is sour-smelling and acid at first; but, when persistent, becomes neutral or even alkaline.

The blood is profoundly altered in acute rheumatism. There is, indeed, no acute febrile disease in which an anæmia occurs with greater rapidity. The average leucocyte count in our cases was about 12,000 per c.mm.

With the high fever a murmur may often be heard at the apex region. Endocarditis is also a common cause of an apex *bruit*. The heart should be carefully examined at the first visit and subsequently each day.

The urine is, as a rule, reduced in amount, of high density and high color. It is very acid, and, on cooling, deposits urates. The chlorides may be greatly diminished or even absent. Formic acid is present (Walker). Febrile albuminuria is not uncommon.

The saliva may become acid in reaction and is said to contain an excess of sulphocyanides.

Subacute Rheumatism.—This represents a milder form of the disease, in which all the symptoms are less pronounced. The fever rarely rises above 101°; fewer joints are involved; and the arthritis is less intense. The cases may drag on for weeks or months, and the disease may finally become chronic. It should not be forgotten that in children this mild or subacute form may be associated with endocarditis or pericarditis.

Complications.—These are important and serious.

(1) HYPERPYREXIA.—The temperature may rise rapidly a few days after the onset, and be associated with delirium; but not necessarily, for the temperature may rise to 108° or, as in one of Da Costa's cases, 110°, without cerebral symptoms. Hyperpyrexia is most common in first attacks, 57 of 107 cases (Church). It is most apt to occur during the second week. Delirium may precede or follow its onset. As a rule, with the high fever, the pulse is feeble and frequent, the prostration is extreme, and finally stupor supervenes. In our series there was no instance of hyperpyrexia, which seems rare in the United States.

(2) CARDIAC AFFECTIONS.—(*a*) *Endocarditis,* the most frequent and serious complication, occurs in a considerable percentage of all cases. Of 889 cases, 494 had signs of old or recent endocarditis (Church). The liability to endocarditis diminishes as age advances. The incidence of organic disease in our cases was more than double in patients who had had their first attack below the age of twenty years, compared with those with the first attack over twenty years of age. It increases directly with the number of attacks. Of 116 cases, in the first attack 58.1 per cent had endocarditis, 63 per cent in the second attack, and 71 per cent in the third attack (Stephen Mackenzie). Thirty-five per cent of our cases showed organic valve lesions, in 96 per cent the mitral was involved, in 27 per cent the aortic, and in 23 per cent both the lesions were combined. The mitral segments are most frequently involved and the affection is usually of the simple, verrucose variety. Ulcerative endocarditis is very rare. Of 209 cases of this disease which I analyzed, in only 24 did the symptoms of a severe endocarditis arise during the progress of acute or subacute rheumatism. The valvulitis in itself is rarely dangerous, producing few symptoms, and is usually overlooked. Unhappily, though the valve at the time may not be seriously damaged, the inflammation starts changes which lead to sclerosis and retraction of the segments, and so to chronic valvular disease. Venous thrombosis is an occasional complication..

(*b*) *Pericarditis* may occur independently of or together with endocarditis. It may be simple fibrinous, sero-fibrinous, or in children purulent. Clinically we meet it more frequently in connection with this disease than in any other acute affection. It was present in 20 cases of our series—6 per cent—in only four of which did effusion occur. The physical signs are very characteristic. The condition will be fully described under its appropriate section. A peculiar form of delirium may develop during the progress of rheumatic pericarditis.

(*c*) *Myocarditis* is most frequent in connection with endo-pericardial changes. As Sturges insisted, the term *carditis* is applicable to many cases. The anatomical condition is a granular or fatty degeneration of the heart-muscle, which leads to weakening of the walls and to dilatation. It is not, I think, nearly so common as the other cardiac affections. S. West has reported instances of acute dilatation of the heart in rheumatic fever, in one of which marked fatty changes were found in the heart-fibres.

(3) PULMONARY AFFECTIONS.—Pneumonia and pleurisy occurred in 9.94 per cent of 3,433 cases (Stephen Mackenzie). They frequently accompany the cases of endo-pericarditis. According to Howard's analysis of a large number of cases, there were pulmonary complications in only 10.5 per cent of cases of rheumatic endocarditis; in 58 per cent of cases of pericarditis; and in 71 per cent of cases of endo-pericarditis. Congestion of the lung is occasionally found, and in several cases has proved rapidly fatal.

(4) NERVOUS COMPLICATIONS.—These are due, in part, to the hyperpyrexia and in part to the special action upon the brain of the toxic agent of the disease. They may be grouped as follows: (a) *Delirium*, associated with the hyperpyrexia or the toxæmia, may be active and noisy in character; more rarely a low muttering delirium, passing into stupor and coma. It was present in only five of our 307 cases, and in four of these we thought the salicylates at fault. A peculiar delirium occurs in connection with rheumatic pericarditis. It may be excited by the salicylate of soda, either shortly after its administration, or more commonly a few days later. (b) *Coma*, which is more serious, may occur without preliminary delirium or convulsions, and may prove rapidly fatal. Certain of these cases are associated with hyperpyrexia; but Southey has reported the case of a girl who, without previous delirium or high fever, became comatose, and died in less than an hour. A certain number of such cases, as those reported by Da Costa, have been associated with marked renal changes and were evidently uræmic. The coma may supervene during the attack, or after convalescence has set in. (c) *Convulsions* are less common, though they may precede the coma. Of 127 observations cited by Besnier, there were 37 of delirium, only 7 of convulsions, 17 of coma and convulsions, 54 of delirium, coma, and convulsions, and 3 of other varieties (Howard). (d) *Chorea*. The relations of this disease and rheumatism will be subsequently discussed. It is sufficient here to say that in only 88 out of 554 cases which I have analyzed from the Infirmary for Diseases of the Nervous System, Philadelphia, were chorea and rheumatism associated. It is most apt to develop in the slighter attacks in childhood. (e) *Meningitis* is extremely rare, though undoubtedly it does occur. It must not be forgotten that in ulcerative endocarditis, which is occasionally associated with acute rheumatism, meningitis is frequent. (f) *Polyneuritis* has been described. I saw a remarkable case which followed hyperpyrexia. Free venesection saved the patient's life. After many months the patient recovered, but with a remarkable ataxia.

(5) CUTANEOUS AFFECTIONS.—Sweat-vesicles have already been mentioned as extremely common. A red miliary rash may also develop. Scarlatiniform eruptions are occasionally seen. Purpura, with or without urticaria, may occur, and various forms of erythema. It is doubtful whether the cases of extensive purpura with urticaria and arthritis—peliosis rheumatica—belong truly to acute rheumatism.

(6) RHEUMATIC NODULES.—These curious structures, described originally by Meynet, occur in the form of small subcutaneous nodules attached to the tendons and fasciæ. Barlow and Warner, in England, and T. B. Futcher, in the United States, have paid special attention to their varieties and impor-

tance. They vary in size from a small shot to a large pea, and are most numerous on the fingers, hands, and wrists. They also occur about the elbows, knees, the spines of the vertebræ, and the scapulæ. They are not often tender. They are more common after the decline of the fever and in the children with mitral valve disease. In only 5 of our patients were they present during the acute attack. The nodules may grow with great rapidity and usually last for weeks or months. They are more common in children than in adults, and in the former their presence may be regarded as a positive indication of rheumatism. They have been noted particularly in association with chronic rheumatic endocarditis. Subcutaneous nodules occur also in migraine, gout, and arthritis deformans. Histologically they are made up of round and spindle-shaped cells. In addition to these firm, hard nodules, there occur in rheumatism and in chronic vegetative endocarditis remarkable bodies, which have been called by Féréol " nodosités cutanées éphémères." In a case of chronic vegetative endocarditis (without arthritis), which I saw with Dr. J. K. Mitchell, there were, in addition to occasional elevated spots resembling urticaria, areas of infiltration in the skin, from two to three lines in diameter, not elevated, but pale pink, and exquisitely tender and painful even without being touched.

The *course* of acute rheumatism is extremely variable. It is, as Austin Flint first showed, a self-limited disease, and it is not probable that medicines have any special influence upon its *duration* or *course*. Gull and Sutton, who likewise studied a series of 62 cases without special treatment, arrived at the same conclusion.

Prognosis.—Rheumatic fever is the most serious of all diseases with a low death-rate. The mortality is rarely above 2 or 3 per cent. Only 9 of our 330 patients died, 2.7 per cent, all with endocarditis and 6 with pericarditis.

Sudden death in rheumatic fever is due most frequently to myocarditis. Herringham has reported a case in which on the fourteenth day there was fatty degeneration and acute inflammation of the myocardium. In a few rare cases it results from embolism. I saw one case at the Montreal General Hospital in which we thought possibly the sudden death was due to Fuller's alkaline treatment, which had been kept up by mistake. There was slight endocarditis but no myocardial changes. Alarming symptoms of depression sometimes follow excessive doses of the salicylate of soda.

Diagnosis.—Practically, the recognition of acute rheumatism is very easy; but there are several affections which, in some particulars, closely resemble it.

(1) MULTIPLE SECONDARY ARTHRITIS.—Under this term may be embraced the various forms of arthritis which come on or follow in the course of the infective diseases, such as gonorrhœa, scarlet fever, dysentery, and cerebro-spinal meningitis. Of these the gonorrhœal form will receive special consideration and is the type of the entire group.

(2) SEPTIC ARTHRITIS, which occurs in the course of pyæmia from any cause, and particularly in puerperal fever. No hard and fast line can be drawn between these and the cases in the first group; but the inflammation rapidly passes on to suppuration and there is more or less destruction of the joints. The conditions under which the arthritis occurs give a clew at once to the nature of the case. Under this section may also be mentioned:

(*a*) *Acute necrosis* or *acute osteo-myelitis*, occurring in the lower end of the femur, or in the tibia, and which may be mistaken for acute rheumatism.

Sometimes, too, it is multiple. The greater intensity of the local symptoms, the involvement of the epiphyses rather than the joints, and the more serious constitutional disturbances are points to be considered. The condition is unfortunately often mistaken for acute arthritis, and, as the treatment is essentially surgical, the error is one which may cost the life of the patient.

(*b*) *The acute arthritis of infants* must be distinguished from rheumatism. It is a disease which is usually confined to one joint (the hip or knee), the effusion in which rapidly becomes purulent. The affection is most common in sucklings and is undoubtedly pyæmic in character. It may also occur in the gonorrhœal ophthalmia or vaginitis of the new-born, as pointed out by Clement Lucas.

(3) GOUT.—While the localization in a single, usually a small, joint, the age, the history, and the mode of onset are features which enable us to recognize acute gout, there are everywhere many cases of 'acute arthritis, called rheumatic fever, which are in reality gout. The involvement of several of the larger joints is not so infrequent in gout, and unless tophi are present, or unless a very accurate analysis of the urine is made, the diagnosis may be difficult.

(4) ACUTE ARTHRITIS DEFORMANS.—In several cases I have mistaken this form for rheumatic fever. It may come on with fever and multiple arthritis, and for weeks there may be no suspicion of the true nature of the disease. Gradually the fever subsides, but the periarticular thickening persists. As a rule, however, in the acute febrile cases the involvement of the smaller joints, the persistence and the early changes in the articulations suggest arthritis deformans.

Treatment.—The bed should have a smooth, soft, yet elastic mattress. The patient should wear a flannel night-gown, which may be opened all the way down the front and slit along the outer margin of the sleeves. Three or four of these should be made, so as to facilitate the frequent changes required after the sweats. He may wear also a light flannel cape about the shoulders. He should sleep in blankets, not in sheets, so as to reduce the liability to catch cold and obviate the unpleasant clamminess consequent upon heavy sweating. Chambers insisted that the liability to endocarditis and pericarditis was much reduced when the patients were in blankets.

Milk is the most suitable diet. It may be diluted with alkaline mineral waters. Lemonade and oatmeal or barley water should be freely given. The thirst is usually great and may be fully satisfied. There is no objection to broths and soups if the milk is not well borne. The food should be given at short and stated intervals. As convalescence is established a fuller diet may be allowed, but meat should be used sparingly.

The local treatment is of the greatest importance. It often suffices to wrap the affected joints in cotton. If the pain is severe, hot cloths may be applied, saturated with Fuller's lotion (carbonate of soda, 6 drachms; laudanum, 1 oz.; glycerine, 2 oz.; and water, 9 oz.). Tincture of aconite or chloral may be employed in an alkaline solution. Chloroform liniment is also a good application. Fixation of the joints is of great service in allaying the pain. I have seen, in a German hospital, the joints enclosed in plaster of Paris, apparently with great relief. Splints, padded and bandaged with moderate firmness, will often be found to relieve pain. Friction is rarely well borne in an acutely inflamed joint. Cold compresses are much used in Germany. The application of blisters above and below the joint often relieves the pain. This method, which was used so much a few years ago, is not to be compared with the light application of the Paquelin thermo-cautery.

The drug treatment of acute rheumatism is still far from satisfactory, though the introduction of the salicyl compounds has been a great boon. Pribram's exhaustive consideration of the question, extending over some 67 pages (Nothnagel's Handbuch, Bd. v), in which he discusses some 75 drugs and measures, indicates perhaps better than anything else that the therapeutics of the disease are still far from satisfactory.

TREATMENT WITH THE SALICYL COMPOUNDS.—Salicin, introduced in 1876 by Maclagan, may be used in doses of 20 grains every hour or two until the pain is relieved. It has the advantage of being less depressing than the salicylate of soda. It is also perhaps the best drug to use for children. Salicylic acid, 15 to 20 grains, may be given every two hours in acute cases until the pain is relieved. It is best given in capsules. Salicylate of soda, 20-grain doses every two hours, is perhaps the best of the drugs for general use in the acute rheumatism of adults. After the pain has been relieved, the drug should be given every four or five hours until the temperature begins to fall. The potassium bicarbonate may be given with it. Oil of wintergreen, 20 minims every two hours in milk, may be used if the salicylate of soda disagrees. There are many other salicyl compounds introduced of late, but the best results are obtained from the use of one or other of the above-named preparations. There can be no question as to their efficacy in relieving the pain in the disease. A majority of observers agree that they also protect the heart, shorten the course, and render relapse less likely.

THE ALKALINE TREATMENT.—Potassium bicarbonate may be given in half-drachm doses every three hours with the salicylic acid or salicin. Fuller's plan was to give a drachm and a half of the sodium bicarbonate with half a drachm of potassium acetate in three ounces of water, rendered effervescent at the time of administration by half a drachm of citric acid or an ounce of lemon-juice. When the urine is alkaline the amount may be reduced.

The heart should be watched carefully during the administration of full doses of the alkalies.

A wide-spread popular belief attributes marvellous efficacy to bee-stings in all sorts of rheumatism, and a formic-acid treatment has been introduced. A 2½ per cent solution is injected in the neighborhood of the painful joints. Ainley Walker has collected (B. M. J., October 10, 1908) an interesting literature on the subject.

To allay the pain opium may be given in the form of Dover's powder, or morphia hypodermically. Antipyrin, antifebrin, and phenacetin are useful sometimes for the purpose. During convalescence iron is indicated in full doses, and quinine is a useful tonic. Of the complications, hyperpyrexia should be treated by the cold bath or the cold pack. The treatment of endocarditis and pericarditis and the pulmonary complications will be considered under their respective sections.

To prevent and arrest endocarditis Caton urges the use of a series of small blisters along the course of the third, fourth, fifth, and sixth intercostal nerves of the left side, applied one at a time and repeated at different points. Potassium or sodium iodide is given in addition to the salicylates. The patients are kept in bed for about six weeks.

XX. CHOLERA ASIATICA.

Definition.—A specific, infectious disease, caused by the comma bacillus of Koch, and characterized clinically by violent purging and rapid collapse.

Historical Summary.—Cholera has been endemic in India from a remote period, but only within the last century did it make inroads into Europe and America. An extensive epidemic occurred in 1832, in which year it was brought in immigrant ships from Great Britain to Quebec. It travelled along the lines of traffic up the Great Lakes, and finally reached as far west as the military posts of the upper Mississippi. In the same year it entered the United States by way of New York. There were recurrences of the disease in 1835–'36. In 1848 it entered the country through New Orleans, and spread widely up the Mississippi Valley and across the continent to California. In 1849 it again appeared. In 1854 it was introduced by immigrant ships into New York and prevailed widely throughout the country. In 1866 and in 1867 there were less serious epidemics. In 1873 it again appeared in the United States, but did not prevail widely. In 1884 there was an outbreak in Europe, and again in 1892 and 1893. Although occasional cases have been brought by ship to the quarantine stations in this country, the disease has not gained a foothold here since 1873. It has prevailed in the Philippines, but is now, 1904, well under control.

Etiology.—In 1884 Koch announced the discovery of the specific organism of this disease. Subsequent observations have confirmed his statement that the comma bacillus, as it is termed, occurs constantly in the true cholera, and in no other disease. It has the form of a slightly bent rod, which is thicker, but not more than about half the length of the tubercle bacillus, and sometimes occurs in corkscrew-like or S forms. It is not a true bacillus, but really a spirochæte. The organisms grow upon a great variety of media and display distinctive and characteristic appearances. Koch found them in the water-tanks in India, and they were isolated from the Elbe water during the Hamburg epidemic of 1892. During epidemics virulent bacilli may be found in the fæces of healthy persons. The bacilli are found in the intestine, in the stools from the earliest period of the disease, and very abundantly in the characteristic rice-water evacuations, in which they may be seen as an almost pure culture. They very rarely occur in the vomit. Post mortem, they are found in enormous numbers in the intestine. In acutely fatal cases they do not seem to invade the intestinal wall, but in those with a more protracted course they are found in the depths of the glands and in the still deeper tissues. Experimental animals are not susceptible to cholera germs administered per os. But if introduced after neutralization of the gastric contents, and if kept in contact with the intestinal mucosa by controlling peristalsis with opium, guinea-pigs succumb after showing cholera-like symptoms. The intestines are filled with thin, watery contents, containing comma bacilli in almost pure culture.

CHOLERA TOXIN.—Koch in his studies of cholera failed to find the spirilla in the internal organs. He concluded that the constitutional symptoms of

138

rheumatic fever

Osler's description reflects to a remarkable degree the broad outlines of our current views on rheumatic fever and points up many of the dilemmas that are still posed by the disease. The major single development since this was written — and one which provides an explanation for certain patterns of the disease and at the same time substantially affects its management — is the recognition of the etiological significance of infections with group A hemolytic streptococci. The streptococci to which Osler refers in his discussion of the bacteriological evidence for considering rheumatic fever to be an acute infectious disease were not members of serological group A but organisms of the viridans or indifferent variety to which no primary pathogenic significance can currently be ascribed. The state of knowledge of streptococcal disease in the early years of this century is indicated by the sentence: "The isolation of streptococci may simply indicate the presence of secondary streptococcus invaders such as occur in scarlet fever and small-pox." One is inclined to forget that the primary role of streptococci in scarlet fever did not gain general acceptance until the second quarter of this century.

A number of developments were required for acceptance of the concept that rheumatic fever follows as a sequela of the common streptococcal sore throat. The clinical association of streptococcal disease and rheumatic fever had been noted (and, indeed, this is alluded to indirectly in the quotation from Church that "the curves of mortality statistics . . . approximate very closely to those of pyemia, puerperal fever, and erysipelas"), but demonstration of a direct relationship between the two in individual cases depended on more specific bacteriological and immunological information. Thus, such developments as the introduction of methods for the serological identification and differentiation of streptococci by Lancefield and the description of a technique for measurement of antibody to a streptococcal antigen (streptolysin O) by Todd were of primary importance. The association between precursory streptococcal infection and rheumatic fever was well documented before penicillin became available, but the clear demonstration by Rammelkamp and his colleagues that rheumatic fever can be prevented by effective treatment of streptococcal sore throat with this bactericidal agent added decisive proof.

Among those features of rheumatic fever which are explained by the streptococcal etiology are certain epidemiological characteristics, such as the seasonal incidence and the observation that an attack of the disease, rather than conferring immunity, appears to predispose the patient to subsequent attacks. With regard to the first of these features, it is now clear that the epidemiology of rheumatic fever is essentially the same

139

as that of streptococcal disease. The problem of lack of immunity in rheumatic fever was clarified by bacteriological studies which showed that there are a large number of specific types of group A streptococci. The type-specific antigens are associated with virulence of the organism, and immunity is largely dependent on production of antibodies to these antigens. Thus, infection with a given group of A streptococcus will result in immunity to reinfection with that specific type but will not affect susceptibility to the numerous other types that exist in nature. As a result, a child may have many different streptococcal infections during his school years — sometimes three or more in a single year — and in the case of an individual susceptible to rheumatic fever these are frequently associated with recurrences of the disease.

The mechanism by which the streptococcal infection initiates the rheumatic process remains uncertain, so that recognition of the relationship has not helped in treatment of the established disease. The use of penicillin, for example, appears to do little to affect the course of rheumatic fever when administered after onset. Nonetheless, the use of antibacterial drugs is clearly influencing the natural history of the disease. This is most evident in the prevention of recurrences by the prophylactic use of sulfonamides or penicillin to prevent streptococcal infection. Today, in areas where prophylaxis is effectively practiced, second attacks of rheumatic fever are rare rather than the rule as they were twenty-five years ago. It is less easy to judge to what extent first attacks of the disease are being reduced by the appropriate treatment of streptococcal sore throat.

Some changes that have occurred in the disease since Osler's day have no clear relation to the use of antibiotics. There has been a steady decline in fatality rate, and also probably in incidence, which began prior to the introduction of antibacterial agents. With regard to incidence, however, it is still true that "the returns are very imperfect (this holds good everywhere)." Rather curiously, a change in age incidence has taken place. Osler stated that young adults are most frequently affected, but for many years the peak incidence in this country has been during the school years, predominantly ages 5 to 15. Only in certain special epidemiological situations, as in military establishments, has there been a high incidence among young adults, and this has been uniformly associated with a high incidence of streptococcal infection for this age group.

Aside from the fact that salicylate is now most commonly used as the acetyl derivative and that corticosteroids have been added to the armamentarium, there has been no very great advance in the drug therapy of rheumatic fever. It remains uncertain whether these agents do more than suppress the inflammatory response to the disease process, and there is difference of opinion on their possible beneficial effect on the development of permanent cardiac damage. Osler himself was faced with a similar divergence of opinion and stated at one point that "it is not probable that medicines have any special influence upon its *duration* or *course*," and yet in discussing salicylates he was forced to point out: "A majority of observers agree that they also protect the heart, shorten the course, and render relapse less likely." The latter is probably no longer a majority view and has no sound basis in fact.

Many of the other aspects of treatment discussed by Osler, such as special bedclothes, diet, and the alkaline treatment, represent medical fashions of the time which lack scientific rationale and have largely been discarded.

Osler's account conveys well the great variability in the manifestations and course of rheumatic fever. It is difficult to agree today with his statement that "the recognition of acute rheumatism is very easy." The manifestations vary in intensity as well as in kind, and there is still no specific diagnostic test to assist the clinician in doubtful cases. The only significant advance in laboratory diagnosis of the disease depends on the demonstration of an increase in titer of antibodies to certain streptococcal antigens as evidence for a recent infection with group A streptococci. While these tests are useful, they fall short of conclusively establishing the diagnosis.

Maclyn McCarty

REFERENCES

Markowitz, M., and Kuttner, A.G. Rheumatic Fever: Diagnosis, Management and Prevention. Philadelphia, W. B. Saunders Co., 1965.

McCarty, M. Rheumatic fever. In Cecil and Loeb Textbook of Medicine, 11th ed. Edited by Beeson, P., and McDermott, W. Philadelphia, W. B. Saunders Co., 1963.

McCarty, M. Missing links in the streptococcal chain leading to rheumatic fever. Circulation, 29:488, 1964.

Paul, J.R. The Epidemiology of Rheumatic Fever. New York, The American Heart Association, 1957.

The mortality is slight, only about 2 per cent. There are no characteristic morbid lesions. Malta fever can now be readily differentiated from enteric fever and malaria. The *prophylaxis* is self-evident, and the brilliant work of the commission has already reduced the incidence of the disease to a minimum,

Treatment.—General measures suitable to typhoid fever are indicated. Fluid food should be given during the febrile period. Hydrotherapy, either the bath or the cold pack, should be used every third hour when the temperature is above 103° F. Otherwise the treatment is symptomatic. No drugs appear to have any special influence on the fever. A change of climate seems to promote convalescence.

XXV. BERI-BERI.

Definition.—An endemic and epidemic multiple neuritis of unknown etiology, occurring in tropical and subtropical countries, characterized by motor and sensory paralysis and anasarca.

History.—The disease is believed to be of great antiquity in China, and is possibly mentioned in the oldest known medical treatise. In the early years of the nineteenth century it attracted much attention among the Anglo-Indian surgeons, and we may date the modern scientific study of the disease from Malcolmson's monograph, published in Madras in 1835. The opening of Japan gave an opportunity to the European physicians holding university positions, particularly Anderson, Baelz, Scheube, and more recently Grimm, to investigate the disease. The studies of the native Japanese physicians, particularly Miura and Takagi, and of the Dutch physicians in the East, have contributed much to our knowledge. An added interest has been given to the subject by the discovery of the disease among the Cape Cod fishermen, and by the recurring outbreaks of endemic neuritis at the Richmond Asylum in Dublin and at the State Insane Hospital at Tuscaloosa, Ala.

Distribution.—Beri-beri, Kakke, or endemic neuritis prevails most extensively in the Malay Archipelago; in certain of the Dutch colonies the mortality among the coolies is simply frightful. It is widely distributed in China, Japan, and the Philippine Islands. In the Philippines the admissions to the Government hospitals for the year ending June 30, 1903, were 626, nearly all among the Philippine scouts. In India it has become less common, but is still prevalent in parts of Burma. Localized outbreaks have occurred in Australia. It prevails extensively in parts of South America and in the West Indies, and from the ports of these countries cases occasionally reach the United States, and it occurs also among the Chinese and Japanese in California. Birge, of Provincetown, and J. J. Putnam encountered beri-beri among the fishermen on the Newfoundland Banks. Birge writes (March 10, 1898) that he has seen 47 cases of both the wet and the dry form. The disease is not entirely confined to the fishermen on the Grand Banks, but occurs occasionally among those living on shore or making " shore trips." In 1895–'96 a remarkable outbreak of epidemic neuritis occurred at the State Insane Hospital at Tuscaloosa, Ala., which has been described fully by E. D. Bondurant. Between February, 1895, and October, 1896, in a population of 1,200 there were 71 cases with 21 deaths. None occurred among the 200 employees of the hospital. The negroes were relatively less affected than the whites. The chief symptoms were " muscular weakness, tenderness, pain, paræsthesiæ, loss of deep reflexes, followed by atrophy of muscles and the electrical reaction of degeneration, accompanied by rise of temperature, gastro-intestinal disturbance, general anasarca, and tachycardia." At the Arkansas State Insane Asylum at Little Rock, in 1895, there was an outbreak of between 20 and 30 cases possibly of beri-beri.

In Great Britain the disease is not infrequent at the seaports.

At the Richmond Asylum, Dublin, there have been extensive outbreaks in the years 1894, 1896, 1897, under conditions of overcrowding.

Etiology.—Two main views prevail as to the nature of the disease—that it is an infection, and that it is a toxæmia caused by food.

1. BERI-BERI AS AN ACUTE INFECTION.—Baelz and Scheube, with many of the Dutch physicians, hold that the disease is due to a germ. In favor of this view, Scheube refers to the fact that strong, well-nourished young people are attacked, that the disease has definite foci in which it prevails, definite seasonal relations, and has of late years spread in some countries as an epidemic without any special change in the diet of the inhabitants. So far as seasonal and telluric influences are concerned, it is a disease which resembles malaria, with which, in fact, some authors have confounded it. It is probably not directly contagious. On the other hand, Scheube, Manson and others bring forward evidence to show that beri-beri may probably be conveyed from one district to another. Many bacteriological studies have been made in the disease, particularly by Dutch physicians, but there is no unanimity as to the results, and we may say that no specific organism has as yet been determined upon.

Hamilton Wright, who has made a prolonged study of the disease in the Malay States, describes a specific duodenitis, a primary bacterial lesion, from which the poison is evolved, just as it is from the throat in diphtheria.

2. FOOD THEORY.—This theory is widely held in Japan, some believing that it is due to the eating of bad rice, and others that it is associated with the use of certain fish. In favor of the dietetic view of its origin is adduced the extraordinary change which has taken place in the Japanese navy since the introduction by Takagi of an improved diet, allowing a larger portion of nitrogenous food, and forbidding the use of fresh fish altogether. Subsequent to this there has certainly been the most remarkable diminution in the number of cases—a reduction from about a fourth of the entire strength attacked annually to a practical abolition of the disease.

Many of the Dutch physicians in Java regard rice as the important cause of the disease. It is stated that in the prisons of Java the proportion of cases is 1 to 39 when the rice is eaten completely shelled, 1 to 10,000 when the grain is eaten with its pericarp; in some places the disease has disappeared when the unshelled rice has been substituted for the shelled. Miura, with whose studies of the disease all readers of Virchow's Archiv are familiar, regards beri-beri as a form of chronic poisoning due to the use of the flesh of certain fish eaten raw or improperly prepared. Grimm, in his monograph, regards the immunity of Europeans as in great part owing to the fact that they do not follow the Japanese custom of eating various kinds of raw fish.

Among the most important factors are the following: Overcrowding, as in ships, jails, and asylums, hot and moist seasons, and exposure to wet. Europeans under good hygienic conditions rarely contract the disease in beri-beri regions. The natives and the imported coolies are most often attacked. Males are more subject to the disease than females. Young men from sixteen to twenty-five are chiefly affected.

Symptoms.—The incubation period is unknown, but it probably extends over several months. The following forms of the disease are recognized by Scheube:

1. THE INCOMPLETE OR RUDIMENTARY FORM which often sets in with catarrhal symptoms, followed by pains and weakness in the limbs and a lowering of the sensibility in the legs, with the occurrence of paræsthesiæ. Slight œdema sometimes appears. After a time paræsthesiæ are felt in other parts of the body, and the patient may complain of palpitation of the heart, uneasy sensations in the abdomen, and sometimes shortness of breath. There may be weakness and tenderness of the muscles. After lasting from a few days to many months, these symptoms all disappear, but with the return of the warm weather there may be a recurrence. One of Scheube's patients suffered in this way for twenty years.

2. THE ATROPHIC FORM sets in with much the same symptoms, but the loss of power in the limbs progresses more rapidly, and very soon the patient is no longer able to walk or to move the arms. The atrophy, which is associated with a good deal of pain, may extend to the muscles of the face. The œdematous symptoms and heart troubles play a minor *rôle* in this form, which is known as the dry or paralytic variety.

3. THE WET OR DROPSICAL FORM.—Setting in as in the rudimentary variety, the œdema soon becomes the most marked feature, extending over the whole subcutaneous tissue, and associated with effusions into the serous sacs. The atrophy of the muscles and disturbance of sensation are not such prominent symptoms. On the other hand, palpitation and rapid action of the heart and dyspnœa are common. The wasting may not be apparent until the dropsy disappears.

4. THE ACUTE, PERNICIOUS, OR CARDIAC FORM is characterized by threatenings of an acute cardiac failure, coming on rapidly after the existence of slight symptoms, such as occur in the rudimentary form. In the most acute type death may follow within twenty-four hours; more commonly the symptoms extend over several weeks.

The mortality of the disease varies greatly, from 2 or 3 per cent to 40 or 50 per cent among the coolies in certain of the settlements of the Malay Archipelago.

Morbid Anatomy.—The most constant and striking features are changes in the peripheral nerves and degenerative inflammation involving the axis cylinder and medullary sheaths. In the acute cases this is found not only in the peripheral nerves, but also in the pneumogastric and in the phrenic. The fibres of the voluntary muscles, as well as of the myocardium, are also much degenerated. Hamilton Wright has described an acute duodenitis.

Diagnosis.—In tropical countries there is rarely any difficulty in the diagnosis. In cases of peripheral neuritis, associated with œdema, coming from tropical ports, the possibility of this disease should be remembered. Scheube states that rarely any difficulty offers in the diagnosis of the different forms.

144

Treatment.—Much has been done to prevent the disease, particularly in Japan. There is no more remarkable triumph of modern hygiene than that which followed Takagi's dietetic reforms in the Japanese navy. In beri-beri districts Europeans should use a diet rich in nitrogenous ingredients. In the dietary of prisons and asylums the experience of the Javanese physicians with reference to the remarkable diminution of the disease with the use of unshelled rice should be borne in mind. In ships, prisons, and asylums the disease has rarely occurred except in connection with overcrowding, an element which prevailed both at the Richmond Asylum and at the State Hospital for the Insane at Tuscaloosa.

Baelz recommends in early cases a free use of the salicylates, 15 or 20 grains four or five times a day. Others favor early free purgation. In very severe acute cases, both Anderson and Baelz advise blood-letting. The more chronic cases demand, in addition to dietetic measures, drugs to support the heart and treatment of the atrophied muscles with electricity and massage.

XXVI. ANTHRAX.

(Splenic Fever; Charbon; Wool-sorter's Disease.)

Definition.—An acute infectious disease caused by *Bacillus anthracis*. It is a wide-spread affection in animals, particularly in sheep and cattle. In man it occurs sporadically or as a result of accidental inoculations with the virus.

Etiology.—The infectious agent is a non-motile, rod-shaped organism, *Bacillus anthracis*, which has, by the researches of Pollender, Davaine, Koch, and Pasteur, become the best known perhaps of all pathogenic microbes. The bacillus has a length of from 2 to 25 μ; the rods are often united. The bacilli themselves are readily destroyed, but the spores are very resistant, and survive after prolonged immersion in a 5-per-cent solution of carbolic acid, or withstand for some minutes a temperature of 212° Fahr. They are capable also of resisting gastric digestion. Outside the body the spores are in all probability very durable.

IN ANIMALS.—Geographically and zoölogically the disease is the most widespread of all infectious disorders. It is much more prevalent in Europe and in Asia than in America. Its ravages among the herds of cattle in Russia and Siberia, and among sheep in certain parts of Europe, are not equalled by any other animal plague. In the United States anthrax is not very widespread. Mohler, of the Bureau of Animal Industry, informs me that since 1900 it has been reported in cattle from sixteen States. It is not very uncommon in Delaware, New Jersey, and Pennsylvania.

A protective inoculation with a mitigated virus was introduced by Pasteur, and has been adopted in certain anthrax regions. Mendez describes excellent results from his antitoxin (1904).

The disease is conveyed sometimes by direct inoculation, as by the bites and stings of insects, by feeding on carcasses of animals which have died of the disease, but more commonly by grazing in pastures in which the germs have been preserved. Pasteur believes that the earthworm plays an important part in bringing to the surface and distributing the bacilli which have

145

beriberi

The very notion of vitamin deficiency diseases was caught in an occluded front in the meterology of ideas during the period which spanned the time from the first edition of Osler's textbook until well after 1909, the year of the edition considered here. One of the hardest ideas for the intellect to grasp is that a lack may cause disaster even though starvation, thirst, and the noxious effects of high altitudes are axioms of human experience. It took decades for many of the details of careful experiments as well as the codification of folk ideas about nutrition to gain acceptance. Perhaps not till the 1940s when pellagra, beriberi, and riboflavin deficiency were largely explained did vitamins and trace minerals come into their own. In fact vitamins came to function as placebos and panaceas before a sensible recoil from vitamania began to put them in proper therapeutic perspective.

Osler was in the mainstream of contemporary medicine which was moving little or none in its nutritional part, though some current was stirring the calm of meandering estuaries. Part of the long, intermittently forgotten history of nutrition Osler knew; some he quoted. But the tone of discussion suggests that he did not accept some of the information confidently. He shared in the prevailing fact-blindness in this area. Such a state is almost inevitable, even for the best physician, where his personal experience is small or nil and he must depend on secondary sources. Clearly Osler was not familiar with beriberi. Examples he might have seen would have been classed as toxic polyneuritis.

In his textbook, Osler contrasted the food theory with the infection theory. He thought of beriberi as a poisoning, perhaps analogous to ergotism which results from eating rye grain or flour spoiled by ergot. In referring to Takaki, whose name he spelled "Takagi," Osler agreed with him in ascribing the eradication of beriberi from the Japanese Navy to the increase in the amount of nitrogenous food in the diet. Polished rice as the main source of calories was inadequate. When the ration was changed the Japanese sailors became healthy. Before 1884 when legumes and meat were substituted for some of the polished rice, beriberi had affected from 23 to 40 percent of the naval manpower every year. Osler said, "Subsequent to this there has certainly been a most remarkable diminution in the number of cases — a reduction from about a fourth of the entire strength attacked annually to a practical abolition of the disease."

Despite this evidence of familiarity with this experience we find in the 1909 edition that the chapter on beriberi is included in the section entitled "Specific Infectious Diseases." It is sandwiched between

146

Malta fever and anthrax. In the discussion of both of these infections, the specific causative organism is described. This location is no improvement over the situation in the first edition when Osler described beriberi as "Endemic Neuritis" in the section entitled "Disease of the Nervous System."

It is very simple by aftersight to take a dim view of the foresight of our predecessors. During a time of rapid progress a medical generation can look back on its immediate or more distant forebears with the illusion that current superiority makes the past look pretty stupid. The great conserving instincts of clinical medicine have been necessary to hold the dikes against the perennially rising tides of quackery, fraud, and much more often simple confusion or error established and sanctified by authoritarian repetition. From our stance today it is simple enough to look down as we look back.

It would be very difficult to find any portion of clinical medicine in which advances have been more dramatic than those which followed establishing the conception of deficiency disease. Biochemists and experimental nutritionists, working with animals or microorganisms, have provided physicians with one after another of the mysterious and almost explosively multiplying elements of what was originally thought to be a single "vitamine" by Casimir Funk. Later it divided into a water soluble and a fat soluble component; and by now "water soluble vitamin B" has expanded into a family of more than a dozen. In fact, the functions of some of the elements presumed essential have to be looked for in crafty experiments designed to find out what trouble a specific deficiency causes when in natural diets that particular substance is never the limiting factor. For instance, other deficiencies produce disease, disability, and finally death before pantothenic acid deficiency causes any recognized clinical damage.

The capital observations James Lind made on scurvy constitute one of the most brilliant examples of clinical investigation. In his book published in 1753, he merely described the exact curcumstances under which scurvy was produced, the precise method for its alleviation, and the very simple procedure for its prevention.

Lind's classic treatise on scurvy gives the details of his experiments. He died 41 years later and nothing had been done about it officially. The year of his death a naval ship sailing to Madras had lemons aboard, issued and used regularly. Not a single case of scurvy occurred. Two years after this the Royal Navy, after a lapse of 43 years, came around to adopting this program of dietary prophylaxis.

Beriberi

So it was some forty years after Lind reported this magnificent discovery in an elegantly simple and definitive study, the Lords of the British Admiralty got around to acting on his observations and recommendations. This resulted in the complete elimination of scurvy from the British Navy and Merchant Marine. What we call lemons were called "limes," whence the nickname "limey" for the British sailor. This was a term of derogation whose significance was missed by competing navies when Britain really ruled the waves and ran rings around its numerous competitors on the high seas, in no small measure because of the startling discovery of Lind.

In Italy near Milan in 1795, at almost exactly the time that the Royal Navy took advantage of Lind's discovery, Giuseppe Cerri used as subjects 10 peasants who had typical pellagra; he improved their diet. He continued the program into the succeeding year and had the satisfaction of seeing their general condition greatly improve. In no instance did pellagra develop though previously it had been an annual event. One of Cerri's patients was violently assailed with pellagra. He changed his occupation and became a family servant. Straightaway he recovered. He considered himself well and after a time returned to his former occupation. Again his diet consisted mainly of polenta, or cornmeal mush. Pellagra recurred. He resumed his work as a servant, eating the food of the well-to-do, and recovered. Once more he went back to labor in the field and developed pellagra again. Finally he was convinced that he could not live the life of a peasant. He returned to his job as a servant, regained his health, and lived to the age of 86. Thus the relationship of diet to pellagra was established. But the cause continued to be argued, in a strange eclipse of the intellect.

The rise of Japan as a naval power certainly was accelerated if not indeed made possible by the changes introduced by the Surgeon General Takaki. Then Eijkman's studies in Java in 1897, and those of Grijns, his successor, were particularly helpful in establishing the significance of experimental beriberi in fowls fed on a diet of polished rice. Beriberi developed spontaneously in the chickens cooped in the laboratory very early in the course of work undertaken to demonstrate the infectious nature of the disease. Changing the diet cured or prevented the disorder if it had not advanced too far. Fletcher's studies at Quala Lumpur in 1905 were classical in their simplicity and in their results. In an asylum for the insane where epidemic beriberi had been a major problem, he numbered the patients sequentially and divided them, the odd ones going to one ward, the even ones to another. Patients in the first ward were fed on white polished rice. The others had unpolished brown rice. Nearly half of the 153 patients eating white rice developed beriberi. Not one of the 154 controls did. This information was resisted by those who believed in toxic causes of beriberi.

Beriberi

In conclusion, the medical world was not ready to make the bold intellectual jump required to establish the doctrine of severe human illness produced by deficiency of dietary factors needed for health. Clinical medicine had a large blind spot. Osler was not in advance of his time in collecting and applying facts which existed, scattered about in many books and journals. Indeed, it took several more decades for many of the puzzles of human nutrition to approach solution.

William B. Bean

REFERENCES

Eijkman, C. Note sur la prophylaxie du béribéri. Janus, 2:23, 1897.

Fletcher, W. Rice and beriberi. J. Trop. Med. Hyg., 12:127, 1909.

Funk, C. Die Vitamine. Wiesbaden, J.F. Bergmann, 1914.

Grijns, G. Polyneuritis gallinarum. Geneesk. Tijdschr. Nederl.-Indië, 41:3, 1901.

Harris, H.F. Pellagra. New York, The Macmillan Company, 1919, p. 51.

Takaki, K. Prevention of kakke in Japanese Navy. Sei-i-K-wai, August, 1885, and April, 1886.

Williams, R.R., and Spies, T.D. Vitamin B$_1$. New York, The Macmillan Company, 1938.

CONSTITUTIONAL DISEASES.

I. ARTHRITIS DEFORMANS.

Definition.—A chronic disease of the joints of doubtful etiology, characterized by changes in the synovial membranes and peri-articular structures, and in some cases by atrophic and hypertrophic changes in the bones.

Long believed to be intimately associated with gout and rheumatism (whence the names rheumatic gout and rheumatoid arthritis), this close relationship seems now very doubtful, since in a majority of the cases no history of either affection can be determined. By the studies of the Boston orthopedic surgeons (Bradford, Goldthwaite, and Lovett) and of Strangeways and his pupils at Cambridge (England) we are gradually getting a very accurate knowledge of the anatomical and clinical forms of this common disease.

Etiology.—*Age.*—A majority of the cases are between the ages of thirty and fifty. In A. E. Garrod's analysis of 500 cases there were only 25 under twenty years of age. In my series of 170 cases studied by T. McCrae, in one half the onset was before the age of thirty years.

Sex.—Among Garrod's 500 cases there were 411 in women. More than half in my series were in males. In James Stewart's report of 40 cases from the Royal Victoria Hospital only 20 were in females. In women its close association with the menopause has been noted. It seems to be more frequent, too, in those who have had ovarian or uterine trouble or who are sterile.

Predisposition.—In 216 cases in Garrod's series there was a family history of joint troubles. About one-third of my series gave a family history of arthritis. Two or three children in a family may be affected. In America the incidence in the negro is much less than in the white.

Rheumatism and Gout.—In nearly a third of Garrod's cases there was a history of gout in the family; of rheumatism in only 64 cases.

Exposure to cold, wet and damp, errors in diet, worry and care, and local injuries are all spoken of as possible exciting causes.

At present two chief views prevail as to the etiology of arthritis deformans —one that it is of nervous origin, the other that it is a chronic infection.

THE RELATION OF ARTHRITIS DEFORMANS TO DISEASES OF THE NERVOUS SYSTEM.—Various forms of arthritis may occur with lesions of the spinal cord, and it has been held by J. K. Mitchell (Sr.) that changes in the nervous system are the cause of the joint lesions. This does not seem to be supported by recent work, which rather supports the view that the disease is the result of a chronic infection. The rapid muscular atrophy, the associated neuritis,

150

the pain, the increase in the reflexes, and the nutritional disturbances suggest a change in the nervous system, but this may be secondary to an infective or toxic process.

ARTHRITIS DEFORMANS AS A CHRONIC INFECTION.—In recent years this view has been gaining ground, although as yet positive bacteriological evidence is lacking. The infection may be with a specific organism or perhaps with various ones. Bannatyne, Poynton and Payne, Chauffard, and others have obtained organisms from the joints, and suggestive results have followed the injection of the cultures in animals. But no constant association with any organism has been proved. The influence of various infections such as gonorrhœa, influenza, etc., is important. Some writers have reported a large proportion of cases with a previous history of gonorrhœa, but this was given in only 13 per cent of my series.

The acute onset with fever, the polyarthritis, the presence of enlarged glands, and the frequent enlargement of the spleen are all suggestive of an infection. In a small number cardiac complications occur. The attack may subside, leaving more or less damage, to recur later with the same features.

And, lastly, a consideration of the form in children described by Still lends weight to this view, particularly in the wide-spread enlargement of the lymph-glands and the swelling of the spleen. A number of the very best students of the disease, as Bäumler, of Freiburg, have accepted the infective theory of origin, which is gaining adherents, though it still lacks demonstration.

Morbid Anatomy.—The changes in the joints differ essentially from those of gout in the absence of deposits of urate of soda, and from chronic rheumatism in the existence of extensive structural alterations, particularly in the cartilages. We are largely indebted to the magnificent work of Adams for our knowledge of the anatomy of this disease.

The usual descriptions are of the late stages of the disease when extensive damage has occurred. There have been few opportunities to study the early changes, although more frequent operations should extend our knowledge. The radiographs have aided much in the study of the disease. There are three main types: (1) With lesions principally in the synovial membranes and peri-articular tissues, (2) with atrophic changes in the cartilage and bones predominating, and (3) with hypertrophy and overgrowth of bone. The first and second are seen especially in the joints of the extremities, the third in the spine. Whether these are distinct processes or different manifestations of the same disease it is difficult to say. The synovial membrane is usually thickened, and may form large fringes and villi. The peri-articular tissues show infiltration and swelling. The enlargement is more often due to swelling about the joint than to bony changes. The cartilage may become soft and gradually be absorbed or thinned. This seems to begin opposite the point of greatest involvement of the synovial membrane. The ends of the bones may become smooth and eburnated, which is usually found in long-standing cases and in old persons. With this there may be marked atrophy of the shaft of the bone. Proliferation of bone usually occurs at the margins of the joints in the form of irregular nodules—the osteophytes. On the knuckles these are known as Haygarth's nodosities. These may lock the joint. The formation of bone may also occur in the ligaments, especially in the spine, which may be converted into a rigid bony column. Bony anchylosis rarely occurs in the peripheral joints, but is common in the spine.

There may be extensive secondary changes. Muscular atrophy is common and may appear with great rapidity. Subluxation may occur, especially in the knee and finger joints. The hands often show great deformity, especially ulnar deflection. Contractures may follow and the joint become fixed in a flexed position. Neuritis and trophic disturbances may be associated. The neuritis is sometimes due to direct extension of the inflammatory process. Subcutaneous fibroid nodules are occasionally met with.

The radiographs of arthritis deformans are very instructive. The changes in the bones are very evident. The thinning due to atrophy and the bony overgrowth can be readily recognized. Erosion of the cartilages is easily seen. In the type with predominant peri-articular changes the bones show little alteration.

Symptoms.—For convenience the forms may be described as those with Heberden's nodes, general progressive arthritis, the mono-articular form, the vertebral form, and the arthritis deformans of children.

HEBERDEN'S NODES.—In this form the fingers are affected, and " little hard knobs" develop gradually at the sides of the distal phalanges. They are much more common in women than in men. They begin usually between the thirtieth and fortieth year. The subjects may have had digestive troubles or gout. Heberden, however, says " they have no connection with gout, being found in persons who never had it." In the early stage the joints may be swollen, tender, and slightly red, particularly when knocked. The attacks of pain and swelling may come on in the joints at long intervals or follow indiscretion in diet. The little tubercles at the sides of the dorsal surface of the second phalanx increase in size, and give the characteristic appearance to the affection. The cartilages also become soft, and the ends of the bones eburnated. Urate of soda is never deposited (Charcot). The condition is not curable; but there is this hopeful feature—the subjects of these nodosities rarely have involvement of the larger joints. They have been regarded, too, as an indication of longevity. Charcot states that in women with these nodes cancer seems more frequent.

GENERAL PROGRESSIVE FORM.—This occurs in two varieties, acute and chronic. The *acute* form may resemble, at its outset, ordinary rheumatic fever. There is involvement of many joints; swelling, particularly of the synovial sheaths and bursæ; not often redness; but there is moderate fever. Howard describes this condition as most frequent in young women from twenty to thirty years of age, often in connection with recent delivery, lactation, or rapid child-bearing. Acute cases may occur at the menopause. It may also come on in children. " These patients suffer in their general health, become weak, pale, depressed in spirits, and lose flesh. In several cases of this form marked intervals of improvement have occurred; the local disease has ceased to progress, and tolerable comfort has been experienced perhaps until pregnancy, delivery, or lactation again determines a fresh outbreak of the disease" (Howard).

The *chronic* form is by far the most common. Most of these have had at some time an acute attack. The joints are usually involved symmetrically. The first symptoms are pain on movement and slight swelling, which may be in the joint itself or in the peri-articular sheaths. In some cases the effusion is marked, in others slight. The local conditions vary greatly, and periods of improvement alternate with attacks of swelling, redness, and pain. At first only one or two joints are affected; usually the joints of the hands, then the knees and feet; gradually other articulations are involved, and in extreme cases every joint in the body is affected. Pain is an extremely variable symptom. Some cases proceed to the most extreme deformity without it; in others the suffering is very great, particularly at night and during exacerbations of the disease. There are cases in which pain of an agonizing character is an almost constant symptom, requiring for years the use of morphia.

Gradually the shape of the joints is greatly altered, partly by the presence of osteophytes, partly by the great thickening of the capsular ligaments, and still more by the retraction of the muscles. In moving the affected joint crepitation can be felt, due to the eburnation of the articular surfaces. Ultimately the joints become completely locked, not by a true bony anchylosis, it may be by the osteophytes which form around the articular surfaces, like ringbone in the horse, but is more often due to adhesions and peri-articular thickenings. The muscles about the joints undergo important changes. Atrophy from disuse gradually supervenes, and contractures tend to flex the thigh upon the abdomen and the leg upon the thigh. There are cases with rapid muscular wasting, symmetrical involvement of the joints, increased reflexes, and trophic changes, which strongly suggest a central origin. Numbness, tingling, pigmentation or glossiness of the skin, and onychia may be present. In extreme cases the patient is completely helpless, and lies on one side with the legs drawn up, the arms fixed, and all the articulations of the extremities locked. Fortunately, it often happens in these severe general cases that the joints of the hand are not so much affected, and the patient may be able to knit or to write, though unable to walk or to use the arms. In many cases, after involving two or three joints, the disease becomes arrested, and no further development occurs. It may be limited to the wrists, or to the knees and wrists, or to the knees and ankles. A majority of the patients finally reach a quiescent stage, in which they are free from pain and enjoy excellent health, suffering only from the inconvenience and crippling necessarily associated with the disease. Coincident affections are not uncommon. In the active stage the patients are often anæmic and suffer from dyspepsia, which may recur at intervals. A small percentage show cardiac lesions. The pulse rate is frequently higher than normal.

The PARTIAL or MONO-ARTICULAR form affects chiefly old persons, and is seen particularly in the hip, the knee, the spinal column, or shoulder. It is, in its anatomical features, identical with the general disease. In the hip and shoulder the muscles early show wasting, and in the hip the condition ultimately becomes that already described as *morbus coxæ senilis.* These cases seem not infrequently to follow an injury. They differ from the polyarticular form in occurring chiefly in men and at a later period of life.

THE VERTEBRAL FORM.—There is a progressive anchylosis of the vertebræ, causing rigidity of the spine—" poker-back "—*spondylitis deformans.* There are two varieties. In one (von Bechterew), in which the disease may follow trauma or be hereditary, the spine alone is involved, and there are pronounced nerve-root symptoms—pain, anæsthesia, atrophy of muscles, and ascending degeneration in the cord; in the other—Strümpell-Marie type—the hip and shoulder joints may be involved (*spondylose rhizomélique*), and the nervous symptoms are less prominent. I believe they are both forms of arthritis deformans, and should neither be regarded nor described as separate diseases. The cases are more frequent in males than in females; the onset may be in the upper or in the lower part of the spine. The involvement of the spine in the lumbar region may cause sciatica. It may be limited to the neck. There is gradually induced complete immobility, with some kyphosis. The other joints may not be affected, or the hips and shoulders may be anchylosed. The ribs are fixed, the thorax immobile, and the breathing abdominal. Pressure on the nerve-roots may cause great pain, paræsthesia, and atrophy of muscles. Von Bechterew thinks that it begins as a meningitis, leads to compression of the nerve-roots, loss of function of the spinal muscles, atrophy of the intervertebral disks, and gradually anchylosis of the spines. Seguin reported three children in one family with the disease.

ARTHRITIS DEFORMANS IN CHILDREN.—Some cases resemble closely the disease in adults, in others there are very striking differences. A very interesting variety has been differentiated by George F. Still, in which the general enlargement of the joints is associated with swelling of the lymph-glands and of the spleen. He has studied 22 cases of this character. The following are among the more striking peculiarities: The onset is almost always before the second dentition. Girls are more frequently affected than boys. The symptoms complained of are usually slight stiffness in one or two joints; gradually others become involved. The onset may be more acute with fever, or even with chills. The enlargement of the joints is due rather to a general thickening of the soft tissues than to a bony enlargement. There is no bony grating. The limitation of movement may be extreme, owing to the fixation of the joints, and there may be much muscular wasting. The enlargement of the lymph-glands is most striking, and may be general; even the supratrochlear glands may be as large as hazel-nuts. They increase with the fever. The edge of the spleen can usually be felt below the costal margin. Sweating is often profuse and there may be anæmia, but heart complications are rare. The children look puny and generally show arrest of development.

Diagnosis.—The early stages may be difficult to diagnose from acute rheumatism. The involvement of the smaller joints and the persistence of the condition in a joint when once attacked are important points. In an advanced stage it can rarely be mistaken for either rheumatism or gout. Late cases are difficult or impossible to distinguish from chronic rheumatism. It is important to distinguish from the mono-articular form the local arthritis of the shoulder-joint which is characterized by pain, thickening of the capsule and of the ligaments, wasting of the shoulder-girdle muscles, and sometimes by neuritis. This is an affection which is quite distinct from arthritis deformans, and is, moreover, in a majority of cases curable.

Treatment.—Once established, the disease is rarely curable. After attacking two or three joints it may be arrested. Too often it is a slow, but progressive, crippling of the joints, with a disability that makes the disease one of the most terrible of human afflictions.

154

In the acute febrile form, usually mistaken for rheumatic fever, moderate doses of the salicylates should be given, and the joints require the local measures mentioned in the section on acute rheumatism.

The treatment of the ordinary form may be considered under:

(1) MEDICINAL.—No single remedy is of special value. General tonics are indicated. Arsenic in full doses is helpful in some cases. The syrup of the iodide of iron is useful, alternating with arsenic. Potassium iodide is useful in the form with much periarthritis.

(2) GENERAL HYGIENE AND DIET.—The disease is one of progressive debility, and measures of a supporting character are indicated. Fresh air and careful attention to personal hygiene are most essential. The question of diet is of the first importance. There is one rule—let the patient eat all the good food she can digest. So many persons are afflicted not only with the disease, but reduced by dieting, that I often find "full diet" the best prescription. One has to remember that gastro-intestinal disturbances are common in the disease.

(3) HYDROTHERAPY.—The Hot Springs, Bath County, Va., and the Hot Springs, Ark., in the United States, and those of Bath, England, sometimes give very good results. Many of our cases seem to have been made much worse by the treatment at Spas, largely, I believe, from over-use of baths and a reducing diet. Much may be effected at home by hot-air baths, hot baths, and compresses at night to the tender joints.

(4) LOCAL TREATMENT.—Vigorous measures should be taken early. It is a disease to be fought actively at every stage. Massage, carefully given, reduces the peri-articular infiltrations, increases the mobility of stiffened joints, and, most important of all, prevents the atrophy of the muscles adjacent to the affected joints. The hot-air treatment, thoroughly carried out, helps many cases, and should be given a trial. Systematic exercises by the patients are very useful.

And lastly, surgical measures may be needed. The thermo-cautery is most useful in relieving the pain and in lessening the ligamentous thickening. Repeated applications are helpful along the spine in the spondylitis deformans. The jacket is useful in the spinal cases until the acute symptoms are past. Goldthwaite and others have reported good results from the breaking up of adhesions and the use of orthopædic appliances.

II. CHRONIC RHEUMATISM.

Etiology.—This affection may follow an acute or subacute attack, but more commonly comes on insidiously in persons who have passed the middle period of life. In my experience it is extremely rare as a sequence of acute rheumatism. It is most common among the poor, particularly washerwomen, day-laborers, and those whose occupation exposes them to cold and damp.

Morbid Anatomy.—The synovial membranes are injected, but there is usually not much effusion. The capsule and ligaments of the joints are thickened, and the sheaths of the tendons in the neighborhood undergo similar alterations, so that the free play of the joint is greatly impaired. In long-standing cases the cartilages also undergo changes, and may show erosions.

Even in cases with the severest symptoms, the joint may be very slightly altered in appearance. Important changes take place in the muscles and nerves adjacent to chronically inflamed joints, particularly in the mono-articular lesions of the shoulder or hip. Muscular atrophy supervenes partly from disuse, partly through nervous influences, either centric or reflex (Vulpian), or as a result of peripheral neuritis. In some cases when the joint is much distended the wasting may be due to pressure, either on the muscles themselves or on the vessels supplying them.

Symptoms.—Stiffness and pain are the chief features of chronic rheumatism. The latter is very liable to exacerbations, especially during changes in the weather. The joints may be tender to the touch and a little swollen, but are seldom reddened. As a rule, many joints are affected; but there are instances in which the disease is confined to one shoulder, knee, or hip. The stiffness and pain are more marked after rest, and as the day advances the joints may, with exertion, become much more supple. The general health may not be seriously impaired. The disease is not immediately dangerous. Anchylosis may occur, and ultimately the joints may become much distorted. In many instances, particularly those in which the pain is severe, the general health may be seriously involved and the subjects become anæmic and very apt to suffer with neuralgia and dyspepsia. Valvular lesions, due to slow sclerotic changes, are not uncommon. They are associated with, not dependent upon, the articular disease.

Prognosis.—The prognosis is not favorable, as a majority of the cases resist all methods of treatment. It is, however, a disease which persists indefinitely, and does not necessarily shorten life.

Treatment.—Internal remedies are of little service. It is important to maintain the digestive functions and to keep the general health at a high standard. Potassium iodide, sarsaparilla, and guaiacum are sometimes beneficial. The salicylates are useless.

Local treatment is very beneficial. "Firing" with the Paquelin cautery relieves the pain, and it is perhaps the best form of counter-irritation. Massage, with passive motion, helps to reduce swelling, and prevents anchylosis. It is particularly useful in cases which are associated with atrophy of the muscles. Electricity is not of much benefit. Climatic treatment is very advantageous. Many cases are greatly helped by prolonged residence in southern Europe or Southern California or by spending the winters in Egypt. Rich patients should always winter in the South, and in this way avoid the cold, damp weather.

Hydrotherapeutic measures are specially beneficial. Great relief is afforded by wrapping the affected joints in cold cloths, covered with a thin layer of blanket, and protected with oiled silk. The Turkish bath is useful, but the full benefit of this treatment is rarely seen except at bathing establishments. The hot alkaline waters are particularly useful, and a residence at Bath, England, the Hot Springs of Virginia, Arkansas, or Santa Rosalia, Mexico, or at Banff, in the Rocky Mountains, on the Canadian Pacific Railway, will sometimes cure even obstinate cases.

III. MUSCULAR RHEUMATISM (Myalgia).

Definition.—A painful affection of the voluntary muscles and of the fasciæ and periosteum to which they are attached. The affection has received various names, according to its seat, as torticollis, lumbago, pleurodynia, etc.

Etiology.—The attacks follow cold and exposure. It is by no means certain that the muscular tissues are the seat of the disease. Many writers claim, perhaps correctly, that it is a neuralgia of the sensory nerves of the muscles. Until our knowledge is more accurate, however, it may be considered under the rheumatic affections.

It is most commonly met with in men, particularly those exposed to cold and whose occupations are laborious. It is apt to follow exposure to a draught of air, as from an open window in a railway carriage. A sudden chilling after heavy exertion may also bring on an attack of lumbago. Persons of a rheumatic or gouty habit are certainly more prone to this affection. One attack renders an individual more liable to another. It is usually acute, but may become subacute or even chronic.

Symptoms.—The affection is entirely local. The constitutional disturbance is slight, and, even in severe cases, there may be no fever. Pain is a prominent symptom. It may be constant, or may occur only when the muscles are drawn into certain positions. It may be a dull ache, like the pain of a bruise, or sharp, severe, and cramp-like. It is often sufficiently intense to cause the patient to cry out. Pressure on the affected part usually gives relief. As a rule, myalgia is a transient affection, lasting from a few hours to a few days. Occasionally it is prolonged for several weeks. It is very apt to recur.

The following are the principal varieties:

(1) LUMBAGO, one of the most common and painful forms, affects the muscles of the loins and their tendinous attachments. It occurs chiefly in workingmen. It comes on suddenly, and in very severe cases completely incapacitates the patient, who may be unable to turn in bed or to rise from the sitting posture.

(2) STIFF NECK or TORTICOLLIS affects the muscles of the antero-lateral region of the neck. It is very common, and occurs most frequently in the young. The patient holds the head in a peculiar manner, and rotates the whole body in attempting to turn it. Usually the attack is confined to one side. The muscles at the back of the neck may also be affected.

(3) PLEURODYNIA involves the intercostal muscles on one side, and in some instances the pectorals and serratus magnus. This is, perhaps, the most painful form of the disease, as the chest can not be at rest. It is more common on the left than on the right side. A deep breath, or coughing, causes very intense pain, and the respiratory movements are restricted on the affected side. There may be pain on pressure, sometimes over a very limited area. It may be difficult to distinguish from intercostal neuralgia, in which affection, however, the pain is usually more circumscribed and paroxysmal, and there are tender points along the course of the nerves. It is sometimes mistaken for pleurisy, but careful physical examination readily distinguishes between the two affections.

(4) Among other forms which may be mentioned are CEPHALODYNIA, affecting the muscles of the head; SCAPULODYNIA, OMODYNIA, and DORSODYNIA, affecting the muscles about the shoulder and upper part of the back. Myalgia may also occur in the abdominal muscles and in the muscles of the extremities.

Treatment.—Rest of the affected muscles is of the first importance. Strapping the side will sometimes completely relieve pleurodynia. No belief is more wide-spread among the public than in the efficacy of porous plasters for muscular pains of all sorts, particularly those about the trunk. If the pain is severe and agonizing, a hypodermic of morphia gives immediate relief. For lumbago acupuncture is, in acute cases, the most efficient treatment. Needles of from three to four inches in length (ordinary bonnet-needles, sterilized, will do) are thrust into the lumbar muscles at the seat of the pain, and withdrawn after five or ten minutes. In many instances the relief is immediate, and I can corroborate fully the statements of Ringer, who taught me this practice, as to its extraordinary and prompt efficacy in many instances. The constant current is sometimes very beneficial. In many forms of myalgia the thermo-cautery gives great relief. In obstinate cases blisters may be tried. Hot fomentations are soothing, and at the outset a Turkish bath may cut short the attack. In chronic cases potassium iodide may be used, and both guaiacum and sulphur have been strongly recommended. Persons subject to this affection should be warmly clothed, and avoid, if possible, exposure to cold and damp. In gouty persons the diet should be restricted and the alkaline mineral waters taken freely. Large doses of nux vomica are sometimes beneficial.

IV. GOUT (Podagra).

Definition.—A nutritional disorder, one factor of which is an excess of uric acid in the circulating blood, characterized clinically by attacks of acute arthritis, by the gradual deposition of sodium biurate in and about the joints, and by the occurrence of irregular constitutional symptoms.

Etiology.—The precise nature of the disturbance in metabolism is not known. There is probably defective oxidation of the foodstuffs, combined with imperfect elimination of the waste products of the body.

(1) PREDISPOSING ETIOLOGICAL FACTORS.—*Hereditary Influences.*—Statistics show that in from 50 to 60 per cent of all cases the disease existed in the parents or grandparents. The transmission is supposed to be more marked from the male side. Cases with a strong hereditary taint have been known to occur before puberty. The disease has been seen even in infants at the breast. Males are more subject to the disease than females. It rarely is seen before the thirtieth year, and in a large majority of the cases the first manifestations appear before the age of fifty.

Alcohol is the most potent factor in the etiology of the disease. Fermented liquors favor its occurrence much more than distilled spirits, and it prevails most extensively in countries like England and Germany, which consume the most beer and ale. The lighter beers used in this country are much less liable to produce gout than the heavier English and Scotch ales. Many cases occur in bartenders and brewery men.

158

rheumatoid arthritis

When the student of rheumatic disease, vintage 1966, reviews Osler's description of these diseases in 1909, the result is encouragement laced with a liberal component of humility. Encouragement stems from the fact that as a result of careful clinical, pathological, and radiological descriptions the general characteristics of the pathological processes affecting the joints and adjacent tissues are much better understood than in Osler's time. Humility stems from realization that the underlying etiological and pathogenetic mechanisms are not much better understood than they were 58 years ago and that treatment is still largely empirical and often leaves much to be desired.

Probably the most important advance has been in understanding the nature and location of pathological changes affecting the joints and contiguous structures. Osler's classification depended largely on recognizable distortion of joint structure and function, often relatively late in the evolution of the disease. It is now possible to separate more clearly actual disease of the joints from various forms of nonarticular rheumatism, and to classify intrinsic joint disease according to the predominant pathological process, either inflammatory or degenerative.

One can fairly clearly separate out from Osler's "Arthritis Deformans" the statements which apply to the most common form of chronic inflammatory arthritis. The designation of *rheumatoid arthritis* became widely accepted in the 1930s, largely to avoid the ambiguity of previous terminology. It is now accepted that the disease is seen more frequently in women (ratio about 2:1), that the peak incidence of onset is between 20 and 40 although it may occur at any age, and that familial predisposition is not the primary determining factor.

Theories regarding etiology are of particular interest. Apparently in 1909 Osler felt that the infectious theory of origin was the most plausible possibility. Such thinking dominated much of the investigative work on the etiology of rheumatoid arthritis for the next 30 years. It would be quite accurate to say that the currently popular concept of autoimmunity in the pathogenesis of the disease is "gaining in adherents, although it still lacks demonstration." Interest has been reawakened, however, in the possibility that some microorganisms, difficult to culture and identify, may be involved in the pathogenesis of the disease, in some way setting off a self-perpetuating type of immunological reaction.

Osler's description of the symptoms and findings in the "general progressive form" would require no modification to be incorporated into a current textbook describing the classical features of rheumatoid arth-

Rheumatoid arthritis

ritis. He emphasized the constitutional nature of the disease, its variable and unpredictable course, and generally progressive nature. His description of arthritis deformans in children was a clear portrayal of that variety of juvenile rheumatoid arthritis which still goes under the eponym of Still's disease. Current thinking emphasizes that rheumatoid arthritis in children is essentially the same disease as seen in adults, with certain features modified by the state of development.

In considering arthritis of the spine, Osler, in common with most authors of his time, made a distinction between von Bechterew's disease, which was believed to start in the cervical spine and progress downward, and the Strümpell-Marie type, believed to start in the lower spine and progress upward. Most modern students of the disease regard the rare von Bechterew type of involvement as very likely a degenerative disease of the cervical spine, perhaps complicated by disc disease which accounts for its predominant neurological complications. The much more common Strümpell-Marie type, or ankylosing spondylitis, is now recognized as a variant of rheumatoid arthritis, and may be diagnosed at a much earlier stage due to appreciation of the importance of early x-ray changes in the sacroiliac joints.

Under differential diagnosis, Osler recognized that monoarticular involvement of the shoulder joint is quite distinct from arthritis deformans and has a much more favorable prognosis; such conditions now would undoubtedly be classified as a form of nonarticular rheumatism, such as subacromial bursitis or adhesive capsulitis of the shoulder.

It is convenient to view Osler's comments on therapy as applying to the disease which we would now call rheumatoid arthritis. His statement that "No single remedy is of special value" still holds today. Modern students of the disease emphasize the importance of an individualized program, with emphasis on rest, the use of analgesics, attention to orthopedic principles to prevent deformities, the use of physical therapy to maintain joint function, and careful attention to all the factors which may be brought to bear to improve the general health of the patient. Some of these measures were considered by Osler under the heading of "General Hygiene and Diet." Considerably greater reliance is now placed on the use of analgesics such as salicylates. Worthy of note is the emphasis that Osler placed on what would now be termed physical therapy, and the importance of local treatment. Present thinking would place much less emphasis on the use of massage, and much more on the use of heat followed by therapeutic exercises. Methods employing counterirritants, apparently quite popular in 1909, have been recognized as giving only brief and inconsistent symptomatic relief.

Rheumatoid arthritis

It is clear that under the heading of "Arthritis Deformans," Osler included, in addition to what would now be classified as rheumatoid arthritis, those forms of degenerative joint disease which produce palpably or radiographically recognizable distortion of joint structure. One can distinguish the following entities which now would be classified as osteoarthritis: Heberden's nodes, degenerative arthritis in the hip, those cases in which degenerative changes are superimposed on a joint previously damaged by an inflammatory process, and very likely some types of osteoarthritis of the spine.

His succinct description of the clinical findings of Heberden's nodes needs no additions. Subsequent work has emphasized the importance of genetic factors in the development of this form of degenerative arthritis of the terminal interphalangeal joints, but has not substantiated the suggested association of these nodes with malignant disease.

It is more difficult to recognize, in modern terminology, the conditions described under the heading of "Chronic Rheumatism." At the present time, the physician would not be satisfied with this diagnosis but would attempt to differentiate those cases which were due either to conditions which now would be recognized as less obvious forms of degenerative joint disease, to localized forms of nonarticular rheumatism (particularly those due to affections of the periarticular structures around the shoulder), or possibly to some of the less severe forms of rheumatoid arthritis and its variants.

Under the heading of "Muscular Rheumatism" the symptom complex described as lumbago would at present be recognized as due to mechanical spinal difficulties, particularly intervertebral disc disease. Torticollis would still be classified as a form of muscular rheumatism. Pleurodynia, at least in its epidemic forms, has only recently been identified as a manifestation of infection with a Coxsackie virus.

It is noteworthy that Osler seems to have used acute rheumatism (acute rheumatic fever) as the prototype of inflammatory disease, and gout as the reference point for more chronic inflammatory and degenerative disease of the joints. This reflects the fact that the classical forms of these two entities were clearly recognized, accurately described, and identified long before the more chronic types of joint disease were well understood. A disease with dramatic onset, which runs its course in a period of several days to a few weeks undoubtedly attracts the attention of both the patient and the physician much more than conditions which require months or years

Rheumatoid arthritis

to evolve and develop. Much of our increased understanding of the disease processes concerned, imperfect as it is, has resulted from observation of these chronic diseases over periods of years.

William D. Robinson

REFERENCES

Bennett, G.A., Waine, H., and Bauer, W. Changes in the Knee Joint at Various Ages. New York, The Commonwealth Fund, 1942.

Decker, J.L., Bollet, A.J., Duff, I.F., Shulman, L.E., and Stollerman, G.H. Primer on the rheumatic diseases, J.A.M.A. 190:127, 425, 509, 741, 1964.

Short, C.L., Bauer, W., and Reynolds, W.E. Rheumatoid Arthritis. Cambridge, Mass., Harvard University Press, 1957.

(4) Among other forms which may be mentioned are CEPHALODYNIA, affecting the muscles of the head; SCAPULODYNIA, OMODYNIA, and DORSODYNIA, affecting the muscles about the shoulder and upper part of the back. Myalgia may also occur in the abdominal muscles and in the muscles of the extremities.

Treatment.—Rest of the affected muscles is of the first importance. Strapping the side will sometimes completely relieve pleurodynia. No belief is more wide-spread among the public than in the efficacy of porous plasters for muscular pains of all sorts, particularly those about the trunk. If the pain is severe and agonizing, a hypodermic of morphia gives immediate relief. For lumbago acupuncture is, in acute cases, the most efficient treatment. Needles of from three to four inches in length (ordinary bonnet-needles, sterilized, will do) are thrust into the lumbar muscles at the seat of the pain, and withdrawn after five or ten minutes. In many instances the relief is immediate, and I can corroborate fully the statements of Ringer, who taught me this practice, as to its extraordinary and prompt efficacy in many instances. The constant current is sometimes very beneficial. In many forms of myalgia the thermo-cautery gives great relief. In obstinate cases blisters may be tried. Hot fomentations are soothing, and at the outset a Turkish bath may cut short the attack. In chronic cases potassium iodide may be used, and both guaiacum and sulphur have been strongly recommended. Persons subject to this affection should be warmly clothed, and avoid, if possible, exposure to cold and damp. In gouty persons the diet should be restricted and the alkaline mineral waters taken freely. Large doses of nux vomica are sometimes beneficial.

IV. GOUT (Podagra).

Definition.—A nutritional disorder, one factor of which is an excess of uric acid in the circulating blood, characterized clinically by attacks of acute arthritis, by the gradual deposition of sodium biurate in and about the joints, and by the occurrence of irregular constitutional symptoms.

Etiology.—The precise nature of the disturbance in metabolism is not known. There is probably defective oxidation of the foodstuffs, combined with imperfect elimination of the waste products of the body.

(1) PREDISPOSING ETIOLOGICAL FACTORS.—*Hereditary Influences.*—Statistics show that in from 50 to 60 per cent of all cases the disease existed in the parents or grandparents. The transmission is supposed to be more marked from the male side. Cases with a strong hereditary taint have been known to occur before puberty. The disease has been seen even in infants at the breast. Males are more subject to the disease than females. It rarely is seen before the thirtieth year, and in a large majority of the cases the first manifestations appear before the age of fifty.

Alcohol is the most potent factor in the etiology of the disease. Fermented liquors favor its occurrence much more than distilled spirits, and it prevails most extensively in countries like England and Germany, which consume the most beer and ale. The lighter beers used in this country are much less liable to produce gout than the heavier English and Scotch ales. Many cases occur in bartenders and brewery men.

Food plays a *rôle* equal in importance to that of alcohol. Overeating without active bodily exercise is regarded as a very special predisposing cause. A form of gouty dyspepsia has been described. A robust and active digestion is, however, often met in gouty persons. Gout is by no means confined to the rich. In England the combination of poor food, defective hygiene, and an excessive consumption of malt liquors makes the " poor man's gout " a common affection.

Lead.—Garrod has shown that workers in lead are specially prone to gout. In 30 per cent of the hospital cases the patients had been painters or workers in lead. The association is probably to be sought in the production by this poison of arterio-sclerosis and chronic nephritis. In the United States, chronic lead-poisoning is frequently associated with arterio-sclerosis and con- tracted kidneys, but lead-gout is comparatively rare. Gouty deposits are, however, to be found in the big-toe joint and in the kidneys in cases of chronic plumbism.

The colored race does not escape. Of 59 cases of gout admitted to the medical wards of the Johns Hopkins Hospital up to April 1, 1905, 3 were in negroes. In two the diagnosis was confirmed at autopsy and in the third by the presence of tophi in the ears. Only 2 of the 59 were females.

(2) EXCITING CAUSES.—Worry or a sudden mental shock may bring on an attack within ten or twelve hours. In susceptible persons a slight injury or an accident of any sort or a surgical operation may be followed by an acute arthritis.

(3) METABOLIC CAUSES.—The nature of gout is unknown. That there is faulty metabolism, associated in some very special way with the chemistry of uric acid, we know, but nothing more. The remainder is theory, awaiting refutation or confirmation. Notwithstanding attempts to minimize the im- portance of uric acid as a factor, until more convincing evidence to the con- trary is advanced we must adhere to the uric acid theory. The conditions of life favorable to the development of gout are present in too many of us after the middle period of life—more fuel in the form of meat and drink than the machine needs—the condition which Francis Hare describes as hyper- pyræmia. G. B. Balfour puts it well when he says: " The gouty diathesis is only a comprehensive term for all those changes in the character and com- position of the blood induced by the evils of civilization—deficient exercise and excess of nutriment. . . . Gout, on the other hand, is the name given to all those modifications of our metabolism caused by the gouty diathesis, as well as to all the symptoms to which those modifications give rise."

The views regarding uric acid and its relation to gout are very numerous.

Although we are still ignorant of the actual seat of formation of uric acid, yet its source has been pretty accurately determined. It constitutes one of the " purin " bodies of Fischer, the xanthin or nuclein bases comprising the re- mainder. All are closely related chemically. Horbaczewski and others have demonstrated that uric acid is largely, if not entirely, derived from nuclein resulting from nuclear disintegration. According to Burian and Schur, the uric acid formed in the system is from two sources. The " endogenous " uric acid is derived from the nucleins of the body, while the " exogenous " uric acid is formed from the nucleins of the ingested food. The uric acid derived from the intake of exogenous oxypurins (nucleo-proteids) constitutes from 40 to

60 per cent of the total purin content of the body. We do not know in what form uric acid exists in the circulating blood. It is not as uric acid itself. Bence Jones and Roberts held that it occurs as a very soluble quadriurate consisting of a molecule of uric acid in loose combination with an acid urate molecule. Many think that such a compound is not capable of existing in a medium with a composition such as the blood has. Minkowski claims that it exists normally in the blood in organic combination with nucleotin-phosphoric acid. Garrod was the first to point out that there was an excess of uric acid in the blood. This is about the only feature of the disease on which there seems general agreement. Magnus-Levy made 34 analyses in 17 cases of gout and found the uric acid in the blood to range between 0.021 and 0.10 grams in 1,000 cc. It has not been definitely established that the amount is increased during the acute attack. Of the three possible causes for this increase—increased formation, diminished destruction or oxidation, and diminished excretion—the balance of evidence favors the latter. Schmoll found that there is a nitrogen retention in gout, which supports this view. Minkowski and His believe that in gouty individuals the uric acid circulates in the blood in a different organic combination than in the blood of healthy persons, and that consequently the kidneys are functionally incapable of eliminating it as in normal conditions. The studies of the alkalinity of the blood, even with the most modern methods, are very conflicting. Magnus-Levy's investigations seem to show that there is no constant diminution in the alkalinity of the blood in gout, also that there is no greater diminution in the alkalinity during the acute attacks than in the intervals. The methods of determining the alkalinity of the blood are notoriously inaccurate. It has been held that the uric acid excess in the blood is due to deficient alkalinity, thus preventing solubility and easy excretion of the uric acid. There is now no evidence to support this view. The recent electro-potential measurements of Fakkas, Fraenkel, and Hoeber seem to show that the reaction of the blood normally is neutral and not alkaline.

The excretion of uric acid by a healthy individual on an average mixed diet ranges normally between 0.4 and 1.0 gramme daily. Hammarsten gives the average as 0.7 gramme. Of the total purin or alloxuric bodies of the urine, nine-tenths exist as uric acid and one-tenth as the purin or xanthin bases. Quantitative determinations show that the excretion of uric acid in gout is usually far below the lower limit for normal in the intervals between attacks, particularly just before an acute exacerbation. With the onset of an acute attack the excretion gradually increases until in three or four days the amount of uric acid may reach or occasionally exceed the upper limit for normal. The cause of this increase is not clear. Quantitative determinations of uric acid in the blood show no constant increase in the uric acid during the acute attacks, nor has there been found any constant variation in the chemical reaction of the blood at this time.

Garrod holds that with lessened alkalinity of the blood there is an increase in the uric acid, due chiefly to diminished elimination. He attributes the deposition of the sodium urate to the diminished alkalinity of the plasma, which is unable to hold it in solution. In an acute paroxysm there is an accumulation of the urates in the blood, and the inflammation is caused by their sudden deposit in crystalline form about the joint.

Haig thinks that there is no increased formation of uric acid in gout, but that the blood is less alkaline than normal, and less able to hold the uric acid or its salts in solution.

According to Sir William Roberts, owing to deficient elimination the soluble quadriurate accumulates in the blood. This quadriurate, circulating in a medium rich in sodium carbonate, takes on an additional atom of the base and becomes converted into the insoluble biurate, which becomes deposited in the tissues, particularly about the joints.

Ebstein thinks that the first change is a nutritive tissue disturbance, which leads to necrosis, and in the necrotic areas the urates are deposited—a view which has been modified by von Noorden, who holds that a special ferment leads to the tissue change, to which the deposit of the urates is secondary. Ebstein designates these as " primary joint-gout " cases. Most cases belong to this group. He also describes what he terms " primary kidney-gout " cases. Owing to primary disease of the kidneys the uric acid is not properly eliminated and secondary joint manifestations ensue. These cases are rare, and he states that they must not be confused with the secondary nephritis.

Cullen held that gout was primarily an affection of the nervous system. On this nervous theory of gout there is a basic, arthritic stock—a diathetic habit, of which gout and rheumatism are two distinct branches. The gouty diathesis is expressed in (a) a neurosis of the nerve-centres, which may be inherited or acquired; and (b) " a peculiar incapacity for normal elaboration within the whole body, not merely in the liver or in one or two organs, of food, whereby uric acid is formed at times in excess, or is incapable of being duly transformed into more soluble and less noxious products " (Duckworth). The explosive neuroses and the influence of depressing circumstances, physical or mental, point strongly to the part played by the nervous system in the disease. For a full discussion of the various theories and an elaborate consideration of the clinical chemistry of the subject the reader is referred to von Noorden's Treatise on Diseases of Metabolism (English edition) and to Futcher's article in my System of Medicine.

Morbid Anatomy.—The *blood* is stated to have an excess of uric acid. It may be obtained from the blood-serum by the method known as Garrod's uric-acid thread experiment, or from the serum obtained from a blister. To ℥ ij of serum add ♏ v–vj of acetic acid in a watch-glass. A thread immersed in this may show in a few hours an incrustation of uric acid. The experiment is rarely successful even in cases of manifest gout. This excess, also, is not peculiar to gout, but occurs in leukæmia and chlorosis.

The " perinuclear basophilic granules " about the nuclei of the leucocytes, described by Neusser in 1894 and regarded by him as practically pathognomonic of gout or a gouty diathesis, were subsequently shown to be artifacts produced during the process of staining. The red cells in the " lead-gout " cases may show basophilic granular staining.

The important changes are in the articular tissues. The first joint of the great toe is most frequently involved; then the ankles, knees, and the small joints of the hands and wrists. The deposits may be in all the joints of the lower limbs and absent from those of the upper limbs (Norman Moore). If death takes place during an acute paroxysm, there are signs of inflammation, hyperæmia, swelling of the ligamentous tissues, and of effusion into the joint.

166

The primary change, according to Ebstein, is a local necrosis, due to the presence of an excess of urates in the blood. This is seen in the cartilage and other articular tissues in which the nutritional currents are slow. His and Mordhorst hold that the deposition of the urates is primary, and that the tissue necrosis takes place as a result of this deposit. In these areas of coagulation necrosis the reaction is always acid and the neutral urates are deposited in crystalline form, as insoluble acid urate. The articular cartilages are first involved. The gouty deposit may be uniform, or in small areas. Though it looks superficial, the deposit is invariably interstitial and covered by a thin lamina of cartilage. The deposit is thickest at the part most distant from the circulation. The ligaments and fibro-cartilage ultimately become involved and are infiltrated with biurate deposits, the so-called chalk-stones, or tophi. These are usually covered by skin; but in some cases, particularly in the metacarpo-phalangeal articulations, this ulcerates and the chalk-stones appear externally. The synovial fluid may also contain crystals. In very long-standing cases, owing to an excessive deposit, the joint becomes immobile. The marginal outgrowths in gouty arthritis are true exostoses (Wynne). The cartilage of the ear may contain tophi, which are seen as whitish nodules at the margin of the helix. The cartilages of the nose, eyelids, and larynx are less frequently affected. Somewhat analogous to these tophi in man are the deposits characterizing the " guanin gout " of hogs. Under certain conditions in pigs one sees in the muscles, ligaments, and articular tissues small whitish deposits which are made up of guanin. These are frequently seen in the Smithfield and Westphalian hams.

Of changes in the internal organs, those in the renal and vascular systems are the most important. The kidney changes believed to be characteristic of gout are: (*a*) A deposit of urates chiefly in the region of the papillæ. This, however, is less common than is usually supposed. Norman Moore found it in only 12 out of 80 cases. The apices of the pyramids show lines of whitish deposit. On microscopical examination the material is seen to be largely in the intertubular tissue. In some instances, however, the deposit seems to be both in the tissue and in the tubules. Ebstein has described and figured areas of necrosis in both cortex and medulla, in the interior of which were crystalline deposits of urate of soda. The presence of these uratic concretions at the apices of the pyramids is not a positive indication of gout. (*b*) An interstitial nephritis, either the ordinary " contracted kidney " or the arterio-sclerotic form, neither of which is in any way distinctive. It is not possible to say in a given case that the condition has been due to gout unless marked evidences of the disease coexist.

The metatarso-phalangeal joint of the big toe should be carefully examined, as it may show typical lesions of gout without any outward token of arthritis.

Arterio-sclerosis is a very constant lesion. With it the heart, particularly the left ventricle, is found hypertrophied. According to some authors, concretions of urate of soda may occur on the valves. Myocarditis is a frequent occurrence in chronic cases.

Changes in the respiratory system are rare. Deposits have been found in the vocal cords, and uric-acid crystals have been met in the sputa of a gouty patient (J. W. Moore). Emphysema is a very constant condition in old cases.

Symptoms.—Gout is usually divided into acute, chronic, and irregular forms.

ACUTE GOUT.—Premonitory symptoms are common—twinges of pain in the small joints of the hands or feet, nocturnal restlessness, irritability of

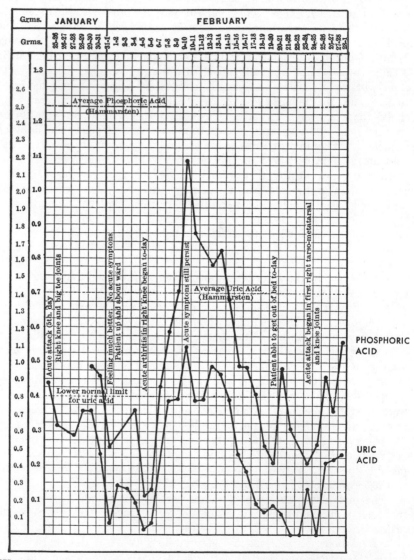

CHART XIV.—SHOWING URIC ACID AND PHOSPHORIC ACID OUTPUT IN CASE OF ACUTE GOUT.

temper, and dyspepsia. The urine is acid, scanty, and high-colored. It deposits urates on cooling, and there may be, according to Garrod, transient albuminuria. There may be traces of sugar (gouty glycosuria). Before an attack the output of uric acid is low and is also diminished in the early part of the paroxysm. The relation of uric and phosphoric acids to the acute attacks is well represented in Chart XIV, prepared by Futcher. Both were extremely low in the intervals, but reached within normal limits shortly after the onset of the acute symptoms. The phosphoric acid and uric acid show almost parallel curves. The patient was on a very light fixed diet at the time the determinations were made. Bain holds that the phosphoric acid excretion varies directly with that of the uric acid. Watson claims that there is no relationship between the two. In some instances the throat is sore, and there may be asthmatic symptoms. The attack sets in usually in the early morning hours. The patient is aroused by a severe pain in the metatarso-phalangeal articulation of the big toe, and more commonly on the right than on the left side. The pain is agonizing, and, as Sydenham says, " insinuates itself with the most exquisite cruelty among the numerous small bones of the tarsus and metatarsus, in the ligaments of which it is lurking." The joint swells rapidly, and becomes hot, tense, and shiny. The sensitiveness is extreme, and the pain makes the patient feel as if the joint were being pressed in a vise. There is fever, and the temperature may rise to 102° or 103°. Toward morning the severity of the symptoms subsides, and, although the joint remains swollen, the day may be passed in comparative comfort. The symptoms recur the next night, and the fit, as it is called, usually lasts for from five to eight days, the severity of the symptoms gradually abating. There is usually a moderate leucocytosis during the acute manifestations. Occasionally other joints are involved, particularly the big toe of the opposite foot. The inflammation, however intense, never goes on to suppuration. With the subsidence of the swelling the skin desquamates. After the attack the general health may be much improved. As Aretæus remarks, a person in the interval has won the race at the Olympian games. Recurrences are frequent. Some patients have three or four attacks in a year; others suffer at longer intervals.

The term *retrocedent* or *suppressed* gout is applied to serious internal symptoms, coincident with a rapid disappearance or improvement of the local signs. Very remarkable manifestations may occur under these circumstances. The patient may have severe gastro-intestinal symptoms—pain, vomiting, diarrhœa, and great depression—and death may occur during such an attack. Or there may be cardiac manifestations—dyspnœa, pain, and irregular action of the heart. In some instances in which the gout is said to attack the heart, an acute pericarditis proves fatal. So, too, there may be marked cerebral manifestations—delirium or coma, and even apoplexy—but in a majority of these instances the symptoms are, in all probability, uræmic.

Gout in America.—While not so common as in England and Germany, the disease is by no means infrequent, and is perhaps on the increase. It is only one-third less frequent at the Johns Hopkins Hospital than at Saint Bartholomew's Hospital. It is more common among the lower classes, who drink beer, than among the well-to-do, who have become of late much more temperate. Among about 18,000 cases in my wards there were 59 cases of gout. All were whites but three, and all males but two (Futcher).

CHRONIC GOUT.—With increased frequency in the attacks, the articular symptoms persist for a longer time, and gradually many joints become affected. Deposits of urates take place, at first in the articular cartilages and then in the ligaments and capsular tissues; so that in the course of years the joints become swollen, irregular, and deformed. The feet are usually first affected, then the hands. In severe cases there may be extensive concretions about the elbows and knees and along the tendons and in the bursæ. The tophi appear in the ears. Finally, a unique clinical picture is produced which can not be mistaken for that of any other affection. The skin over the tophi may rupture or ulcerate, and about the knuckles the chalk-stones may be freely exposed. Patients with chronic gout are usually dyspeptic, often of a sallow complexion, and show signs of arterio-sclerosis. The pulse tension is increased, the vessels are stiff, and the left ventricle is hypertrophied. The urine is increased in amount, is of low specific gravity, and usually contains a slight amount of albumin, with a few hyaline casts. Severe cramps involving the calf, abdominal, and thoracic muscles may occur. Intercurrent attacks of acute polyarthritis may develop, in which the joints become inflamed, and the temperature ranges from 101° to 103°. There may be pain, redness, and swelling of several joints without fever. Uræmia, pleurisy, pericarditis, peritonitis, and meningitis are common terminal affections. The victim of gout may show remarkable mental and even bodily vigor. Certain of the most distinguished members of our profession have been terrible sufferers from this disease, notably the elder Scaliger, Jerome Cardan, and Sydenham, whose statement that "more wise men than fools are victims of the affection" still holds good.

IRREGULAR GOUT.—This is a motley, ill-defined group of symptoms, manifestations of a condition of disordered nutrition, to which the terms *gouty diathesis* or *lithæmic state* have been given. Cases are seen in members of gouty families, who may never themselves have suffered from the acute disease, and in persons who have lived not wisely but too well, who have eaten and drunk largely, lived sedentary lives, and yet have been fortunate enough to escape an acute attack. It is interesting to note the various manifestations of the disease in a family with marked hereditary disposition. The daughters often escape, while one son may have gouty attacks of great severity, even though he lives a temperate life and tries in every way to avoid the conditions favoring the disorder. Another son has, perhaps, only the irregular manifestations and never the acute articular affection. While the irregular features are perhaps more often met with in the hereditary affection, they are by no means infrequent in persons who appear to have acquired the disease. The tendency in some families is to call every affection gouty. Even infantile complaints, such as scald-head, naso-pharyngeal vegetations, and enuresis, are often regarded, without sufficient grounds, I believe, as evidences of the family ailment. Among the commonest manifestations of irregular gout are the following:

(*a*) *Cutaneous Eruptions.*—Garrod and others have called special attention to the frequent association of eczema with the gouty habit. The French in particular insist upon the special liability of gouty persons to skin affections, the *arthritides,* as they call them.

(*b*) *Gastro-intestinal Disorders.*—Attacks of what is termed biliousness, in which the tongue is furred, the breath foul, the bowels constipated, and the action of the liver torpid, are not uncommon in gouty persons. A gouty parotitis is described.

(*c*) *Cardio-vascular Symptoms.*—With the lithæmia, arterio-sclerosis is frequently associated. The blood tension is persistently high, the vessel walls become stiff, and cardiac and renal changes gradually occur. In this condition the manifestations may be renal, as when the albuminuria becomes more marked, or dropsical symptoms supervene. The manifestations may be cardiac, when the hypertrophy of the left ventricle fails and there are palpitation, irregular action, and ultimately a condition of asystole. Or, finally, the manifestations may be vascular, and thrombosis of the coronary arteries may cause sudden death. Aneurism may occur and prove fatal, or, as most frequently happens, a blood-vessel gives way in the brain, and the patient dies of apoplexy. It makes but little difference whether we regard this condition as primarily an arterio-sclerosis, or as a gouty nephritis; the point to be remembered is that the nutritional disorder with which an excess of uric acid is associated induces in time increased tension, arterio-sclerosis, chronic interstitial nephritis, and changes in the myocardium. Pericarditis is not an infrequent terminal complication of gout. Phlebitis occasionally occurs.

(*d*) *Nervous Manifestations.*—Headache and megrim attacks are not infrequent. Haig attributes them to an excess of uric acid. Neuralgias are not uncommon; sciatica and paræsthesias may develop. A common gouty manifestation, upon which Duckworth has laid stress, is the occurrence of hot or itching feet at night. Plutarch mentions that Strabo called this symptom " the lisping of the gout." Cramps in the legs may also be very troublesome. Hutchinson has called attention to hot and itching eyeballs as a frequent sign of masked gout. Associated or alternating with this symptom there may be attacks of episcleral congestion. Apoplexy is a common termination of gout. Meningitis may occur, usually basilar.

(*e*) *Urinary Disorders.*—The urine is highly acid and high-colored, and may deposit on standing crystals of uric acid. Transient and temporary increase in this ingredient can not be regarded as serious. In many cases of chronic gout the amount may be diminished, and increased only at certain periods, forming the so-called uric-acid showers. The chart on page 402 illustrates this very well. A sediment of uric acid in a urine does not necessarily mean an excess. It is often dependent on the inability of the urine to hold it in solution. Sugar is found intermittently in the urine of gouty persons—gouty glycosuria. It may pass into true diabetes, but is usually very amenable to treatment. Oxaluria may also be present. Gouty persons are specially prone to calculi, Jerome Cardan to the contrary, who reckoned freedom from stone among the chief of the *dona podagræ*. Minute quantities of albumin are very common in persons of gouty dyscrasia, and, when the renal changes are well established, tube-casts. Urethritis, with a purulent discharge, may arise, so it is stated, usually at the end of an attack. It may occur spontaneously, or follow a pure connection.

(*f*) *Pulmonary Disorders.*—There are no characteristic changes, but, as Greenhow has pointed out, chronic bronchitis occurs with great frequency in persons of a gouty habit.

(*g*) Of eye affections, iritis, glaucoma, hæmorrhage retinitis, and suppurative panophthalmitis have been described.

Diagnosis.—Recurring attacks of arthritis, limited to the big toe and to the tarsus, occurring in a member of a gouty family, or in a man who has lived too well, leave no question as to the nature of the trouble. There are many cases of gout, however, in which the feet do not suffer most severely. After an attack or two in one toe, other joints may be affected, and it is just in such cases of polyarthritis that the difficulty in diagnosis is apt to arise. We have had of late years several cases admitted for the third or fourth time with involvement of three or more of the larger joints. The presence of tophi has settled the nature of a trouble which in the previous attacks had been regarded as rheumatic. The following are suggestive points in such cases: (1) The patient's habits and occupation. In the United States the brewery men and barkeepers are often affected. (2) The presence of tophi. The ears should always be inspected in a case of polyarthritis. The diagnosis may rest with a small tophus. The student should learn to recognize on the ear margin, Woolner's tip, fibroid nodules, and small sebaceous tumors. The last are easily recognized microscopically. The needle-shaped sodium biurate crystals are distinctive of the tophi. (3) The condition of the urine. As shown in Chart XIV, the uric-acid output is usually very low during the intervals of the paroxysm. At the height of the attack the elimination, as a rule, is greatly increased. The ratio of the uric acid to the urea excretion is disturbed in gouty cases, and may fall as low as 1 to 100 or 1 to 150. (4) The gouty polyarthritis may be afebrile. A patient with three or four joints red, swollen, and painful in acute rheumatism has fever, and, while pyrexia may be present and often is in gout, its absence is, I think, a valuable diagnostic sign. Many cases go a-begging for a diagnosis. A careful study of the patient's habits as to beer drinking, of the location of the initial arthritic attacks, and the examination for tophi in the ears will prevent many cases being mistaken for rheumatism or arthritis deformans.

Treatment.—HYGIENIC.—Individuals who have inherited a tendency to gout, or who have shown any manifestations of it, should live temperately, abstain from alcohol, and eat moderately. An open-air life, with plenty of exercise and regular hours, does much to counteract an inborn tendency to the disease. The skin should be kept active: if the patient is robust, by the morning cold bath with friction after it; but if he is weak or debilitated the evening warm bath should be substituted. An occasional Turkish bath with active shampooing is very advantageous. The patient should dress warmly, avoid rapid alterations in temperature, and be careful not to have the skin suddenly chilled.

DIETETIC.—With few exceptions, persons over forty eat too much, and the first injunction to a gouty person is to keep his appetite within reasonable bounds, to eat at stated hours, and to take plenty of time at his meals. In the matter of food, quantity is a factor of more importance than quality with many gouty persons. As Sir William Roberts well says, " Nowhere perhaps is it more necessary than in gout to consider the man as well as the ailment, and very often more the man than the ailment."

Very remarkable differences of opinion exist as to the most suitable diet in this disease, some urging warmly a vegetable diet, others allowing a very liberal amount of meat. On the one hand, the author just quoted says: " The most trustworthy experiments indicate that fat, starch, and sugar have not the least direct influence on the production of uric acid; but as the free consumption of these articles naturally operates to restrict the intake of the nitrogenous food, their use has indirectly the effect of diminishing the average production of uric acid." On the other hand, W. H. Draper says: "The conversion of azotized food is more complete with a minimum of carbohydrates than it is with an excess of them; in other words, one of the best means of avoiding the accumulation of lithic acid in the blood is to diminish the carbohydrates rather than the azotized foods." The weight of opinion leans to the use of a modified nitrogenous diet, without excess in starchy and saccharine articles of food. Animal foods rich in nuclear material, such as sweetbreads, liver, kidneys, and brain, should be avoided. Beef extracts are injurious, owing to their richness in extractives belonging to the xanthin group. Milk and eggs are particularly useful, owing to their not containing any nuclein. Fresh vegetables and fruits may be used freely, but among the latter strawberries and bananas should be avoided.

Ebstein urges strongly the use of fat in the form of good fresh butter, from $2\frac{1}{2}$ to $3\frac{1}{2}$ ounces in the day. He says that stout gouty subjects not only do not increase in weight with plenty of fat in the food, but that they actually become thin and the general condition improves very much. Hot bread of all sorts and the various articles of food prepared from Indian corn should, as a rule, be avoided. Roberts advises gouty patients to restrict as far as practicable the use of common salt with their meals, since the sodium biurate very readily crystallizes out in tissues with a high percentage of sodium salts.

In this matter of diet each individual case must receive separate consideration.

There are very few conditions in the gouty in which stimulants of any sort are required. Whenever indicated, whisky will be found perhaps the most serviceable. While all are injurious to these patients, some are much more so than others, particularly malted liquors, champagne, port, and a very large proportion of all the light wines.

MINERAL WATERS.—All forms may be said to be beneficial in gout, as the main element is the water, and the ingredients are usually indifferent. Much of the humbuggery in the profession still lingers about mineral waters, more particularly about the so-called lithia waters.

The question of the utility of alkalies in the treatment of gout is closely connected with this subject of mineral waters. This deep-rooted belief in the profession was rudely shaken a few years ago by Sir William Roberts, who claims to have shown conclusively that alkalescence as such has no influence whatever on the sodium biurate. The sodium salts are believed by this author to be particularly harmful, but, in spite of all the theoretical denunciation of the use of the sodium salts in gout, the gouty from all parts of the world flock to those very Continental springs in which these salts are most predominant. Bain urges the use of potassium salts.

Of the mineral springs best suited for the gouty may be mentioned, in the United States, those of Saratoga, Bedford, and the White Sulphur; Buxton and Bath, in England; in France, Aix-les-Bains and Contrexéville; and in Germany, Carlsbad, Wildbad, and Homburg.

The efficacy in reality is in the water, in the way it is taken, on an empty stomach, and in large quantities; and, as every one knows, the important accessories in the modified diet, proper hours, regular exercise, with baths, douches, etc., play a very important *rôle* in the "cure."

MEDICINAL TREATMENT.—In an acute attack the limb should be elevated and the affected joint wrapped in cotton-wool. Warm fomentations, or Fuller's lotion, may be used. The local hot-air treatment may be tried. A brisk mercurial purge is always advantageous at the outset. The wine or tincture of colchicum, in doses of 20 to 30 minims, may be given every four hours in combination with the citrate of potash or the citrate of lithium. The action of the colchicum should be carefully watched. It has, in a majority of the cases, a powerful influence over the symptoms—relieving the pain, and reducing, sometimes with great rapidity, the swelling and redness. It should be promptly stopped so soon as it has relieved the pain. In cases in which the pain and sleeplessness are distressing and do not yield to colchicum, morphia is necessary. The patient should be placed on a diet chiefly of milk and barley-water, but if there is any debility, strong broths may be given, or eggs. It is occasionally necessary to give small quantities of stimulants. During convalescence meats and fish and game may be taken, and gradually the patient may resume the diet previously laid down.

In some of the subacute intercurrent attacks of arthritis in old, deformed joints, the sodium salicylate is occasionally useful, but its administration must be watched in cases of cardiac and renal insufficiency. It is also much advocated by Haig in the uric-acid habit.

The chronic and irregular forms of gout are best treated by the dietetic and hygienic measures already referred to. Potassium iodide is sometimes useful, and preparations of guaiacum, quinine, and the bitter tonics combined with alkalies are undoubtedly of benefit.

Piperazin has been much lauded as an efficient aid in the solution of uric acid. The clinical results, however, are very discordant. It may be employed in doses of from 15 to 30 grains in the day, and is conveniently given in aërated water containing 5 grains to the tumblerful. Piperazin, as a uric acid solvent, was rapidly followed by lysidin, urotropin, urea, and urol among others—a sure indication of their therapeutic worthlessness.

Albu speaks favorably of lemon-juice as a remedy. The vegetable acids are converted in the system into alkaline carbonates, thus enabling the blood to keep the uric acid compounds in solution, and consequently facilitating their elimination by the kidneys.

Where the arthritic attacks are confined to one joint, such as the great-toe joint, surgical interference may be considered. Riedel reports two successful cases in which he removed the entire joint capsule of the big-toe joint, with permanent relief.

V. DIABETES MELLITUS.

Definition.—A disorder of nutrition, in which sugar accumulates in the blood and is excreted in the urine, the daily amount of which is greatly increased.

For a case to be considered one of diabetes mellitus it is necessary that the form of sugar eliminated in the urine be grape sugar, that it must be eliminated for weeks, months, or years, and that the excretion of sugar must take place after the ingestion of moderate amounts of carbohydrates.

gout

Osler's chapter on gout in the seventh edition of *The Principles and Practice of Medicine* antedates the development of reliable methods for quantitative measurements of uric acid in body fluids and the extensive application of the roentgen ray in medical diagnosis. The scientific basis of medicine was largely pathological anatomy, and Osler's own first-hand experience in pathology was such as to make possible vivid descriptions of the morbid anatomy of disease in a way unusual for a clinician. This faculty is in clear evidence in this section. His clinical descriptions need very little updating, though today one would stress more strongly the incidence and significance of urolithiasis in gout. In portraying the acute attack Osler too found it impossible to improve on Sydenham and joined a still lengthening succession of writers who quote the modern Hippocrates. Osler's description now needs amplification chiefly in the areas of x-ray findings, biochemical understanding, and new therapeutic measures.

One of the remarkable features of the early editions of Osler's textbook was his skepticism toward many of the accepted therapeutic regimens of the day. The effect upon the profession, and especially upon the student, was a salutary one indeed. This skepticism toward medical dogma is well exemplified in this chapter also. Osler dismissed the contemporary preoccupation with diminished alkalinity of the blood in gout ("The methods of determining the alkalinity of the blood are notoriously inaccurate") as a cause of renal retention of uric acid ("There is now no evidence to support this view"). Regarding the fad of spas, Osler wryly observed that "All forms may be said to be beneficial in gout, as the main element is the water [taken] in large quantities." In other sections, one is now surprised at the range of manifestations attributed rather uncritically to gout, or to the gouty diathesis in members of gouty families who may never themselves have suffered an acute attack, but "Who have lived not wisely but too well." Although Osler recognized "The tendency in some families to call every affliction gouty," he seemed to do the same in his section on "Irregular Gout," when including various manifestations, such as eczema, attacks of "biliousness," headache, itching feet, leg cramps, and chronic bronchitis as among those of the gouty habit.

In his first edition (1892), Osler characterized gout as "A nutritional disorder associated with an excessive formation of uric acid . . . most probably . . . [secondary to] defective oxidation of nitrogenous foodstuffs." In his second edition (1895) he began to emphasize the additional factor of underexcretion by the kidney ("A nutritional disorder, one factor of

Gout

which is an excessive formation of uric acid. . . . There is probably defective oxidation of the food-stuffs, combined with imperfect elimination of the waste products of the body."). In the sixth edition and in the seventh, he listed three possible causes for the hyperuricemia — increased formation, diminished destruction or oxidation, and diminished excretion — and concluded that "the balance of evidence favors the latter." Osler was aware that urinary urate excretion is usually normal or low in gout, despite hyperuricemia, but there is no clue that he considered the renal handling of urate apart from that of other excretory products, and the idea of a specific defect of urate transport as distinguished from a general retention of nitrogenous compounds does not appear to have been developed at that time. The question of whether uric acid exists in a different physiochemical state in the blood of gouty subjects, rendering it difficult for the kidney to excrete, has only recently been discarded.

Advances since 1909 have greatly broadened our understanding of primary gout as a genetically determined inborn error of metabolism and of secondary gout as an acquired disease, a distinction not made by Osler. Uric acid was only established as a purine compound by Emil Fischer in 1898, and knowledge of its relationship to the purine bases of nucleic acids dates from that time. The first reliable method for determination of uric acid in blood and urine was introduced by Folin and Denis in 1913. In that same year Folin and Lyman first recorded asymptomatic hyperuricemia in a man in whose family gout occurred. Extensive studies of the distribution of hyperuricemia in families of gouty families followed in the 1940s and 1950s, with an average finding of 20 percent hyperuricemic relatives. Studies of the distribution of uric acid values in the general population in this and other countries, as well as in gouty families, have led to divergent views of the genetic mode of transmission, the uncertainty involving theories of a single autosomal dominant gene versus multifactorial inheritance. The weight of evidence favors the latter view in the population as a whole, with single specific gene differences possibly occurring in any given family.

In the 1940s the metabolic origins of the various atoms of the purine ring were established, and in the 1950s the individual reactions of purine synthesis and degradation were defined. Studies of uric acid turnover, and of rates of incorporation of labeled precursors (chiefly glycine) into urinary uric acid, established that all gouty subjects who excrete excessive quantities of uric acid in urine (20 to 25 percent of the total) have "increased formation" of uric acid. In addition about two thirds of the group with normal urinary uric acid values also show evidence of overincorporation of isotopic precursors into uric acid. For a time it was believed that the hyperuricemia

176

of primary gout was attributable to overproduction in all subjects. It is now believed that most gouty subjects show both overproduction and underexcretion of uric acid.

Uric acid exists in true solution in blood as sodium biurate and is thought to be freely filtrable at the glomerulus in the gouty subject as in the normal. The bulk of the filtered urate is now thought to be reabsorbed, and the excreted urate is believed to arise in part or in total by a tubular secretory process, evidence for which is largely indirect in man. The rate of uric acid excretion at any given plasma urate level is less in the gouty subject than in the normal. These results confirm the "diminished excretion" theory and are in agreement with the long-standing observation that about 75 percent of gouty subjects excrete normal quantities of uric acid each day despite elevated plasma levels and, in many cases, normal glomerular function. Thus the pendulum of thought regarding the metabolic defects of gout has swung through several arcs.

After a period of years in which a direct role of uric acid in the acute attack was doubted, the acute attack is once again thought to be triggered by crystals of sodium urate, which may form from supersaturated body fluids when a local pH gradient develops between blood and tissue. Ammonium chloride administration may precipitate attacks in gouty subjects. Thus the role of "alkalinity of the blood" re-emerges in another form. The phenomenon of crystal-induced synovitis has proved to be a rediscovery of observations made by Freudweiler in 1899. Apparently his papers escaped Osler's attention, as they did that of others for so many years.

A number of substances are known which interfere with tubular secretion of urate, among them the lactate and β-hydroxybutyrate ions. Metabolism of ethanol leads indirectly to elevation of plasma lactate levels, at least in inebriated subjects. However, this hardly provides an explanation for the association of gout with beer drinking, especially of the "heavier English and Scottish ales," rather than with drinking of distilled spirits. Perhaps this axiom should be subjected to critical test, as should Osler's contention that the "well-to-do . . . have become of late much more temperate."

The advent of well-tolerated uricosuric agents has revolutionized the outlook for the gouty patient. More recently the development of xanthine oxidase inhibitors, such as Allopurinol, has added another dimension to the armamentarium of the physician, who though always well advised to view claims for new nostrums and remedies with some skepticism, has in

Gout

these two groups of agents a rational approach to therapy exceeding that available in many other disorders. The chalkstones about the knuckles that ulcerate and drain are today a preventable or treatable aspect of this disease.

Some insight into the action of that interesting drug colchicine exists at long last, and other agents, such as phenylbutazone and indocin, have broadened the range of choices for handling the acute attack. The victim need no longer relive the Sydenham experience with each return of the gout.

The disease retains its special connotations. Formerly a sign of intemperate living, it is today a hallmark of superior intelligence and academic or executive success. Medical students who rejoice in the reading of this classic will be reassured to know that they are statistically well represented within the hyperuricemic group.

James B. Wyngaarden

REFERENCES

Seegmiller, J.E., Laster, L., and Howell, R.R. Biochemistry of uric acid and its relation to gout. New Eng. J. Med., 268:712, 1963.

Wyngaarden, J.B. Gout. in The Metabolic Basis of Inherited Disease, 2nd ed. Stanbury, J.B., Wyngaarden, J.B. and Fredrickson, D.S., ed. New York, McGraw-Hill Book Company, 1966.

MEDICINAL TREATMENT.—In an acute attack the limb should be elevated and the affected joint wrapped in cotton-wool. Warm fomentations, or Fuller's lotion, may be used. The local hot-air treatment may be tried. A brisk mercurial purge is always advantageous at the outset. The wine or tincture of colchicum, in doses of 20 to 30 minims, may be given every four hours in combination with the citrate of potash or the citrate of lithium. The action of the colchicum should be carefully watched. It has, in a majority of the cases, a powerful influence over the symptoms—relieving the pain, and reducing, sometimes with great rapidity, the swelling and redness. It should be promptly stopped so soon as it has relieved the pain. In cases in which the pain and sleeplessness are distressing and do not yield to colchicum, morphia is necessary. The patient should be placed on a diet chiefly of milk and barley-water, but if there is any debility, strong broths may be given, or eggs. It is occasionally necessary to give small quantities of stimulants. During convalescence meats and fish and game may be taken, and gradually the patient may resume the diet previously laid down.

In some of the subacute intercurrent attacks of arthritis in old, deformed joints, the sodium salicylate is occasionally useful, but its administration must be watched in cases of cardiac and renal insufficiency. It is also much advocated by Haig in the uric-acid habit.

The chronic and irregular forms of gout are best treated by the dietetic and hygienic measures already referred to. Potassium iodide is sometimes useful, and preparations of guaiacum, quinine, and the bitter tonics combined with alkalies are undoubtedly of benefit.

Piperazin has been much lauded as an efficient aid in the solution of uric acid. The clinical results, however, are very discordant. It may be employed in doses of from 15 to 30 grains in the day, and is conveniently given in aerated water containing 5 grains to the tumblerful. Piperazin, as a uric acid solvent, was rapidly followed by lysidin, urotropin, urea, and urol among others—a sure indication of their therapeutic worthlessness.

Albu speaks favorably of lemon-juice as a remedy. The vegetable acids are converted in the system into alkaline carbonates, thus enabling the blood to keep the uric acid compounds in solution, and consequently facilitating their elimination by the kidneys.

Where the arthritic attacks are confined to one joint, such as the great-toe joint, surgical interference may be considered. Riedel reports two successful cases in which he removed the entire joint capsule of the big-toe joint, with permanent relief.

V. DIABETES MELLITUS.

Definition.—A disorder of nutrition, in which sugar accumulates in the blood and is excreted in the urine, the daily amount of which is greatly increased.

For a case to be considered one of diabetes mellitus it is necessary that the form of sugar eliminated in the urine be grape sugar, that it must be eliminated for weeks, months, or years, and that the excretion of sugar must take place after the ingestion of moderate amounts of carbohydrates.

Etiology.—*Incidence.*—According to recent statistics diabetes appears about as frequent in the United States as in European countries. The last census gave 9.3 deaths per 100,000 population in the former compared with from 5 to 14 in the latter. In England and Wales the death-rate from diabetes in 1903 was 8.7 per 100,000 of population. The death-rate has been gradually on the increase in Paris during the last three or four decades, reaching 14 to the 100,000 of population in 1891. The disease is gradually on the increase in the United States. The statistics for 1870 gave 2.1; for 1880, 2.8; for 1890, 3.8; and for 1900, 9.3 deaths to the 100,000 population. This apparent increase may be in part due to more accurate vital statistics records. In this region the incidence of the disease may be gathered from the fact that among 99,000 patients admitted to the medical wards and medical dispensary of the Johns Hopkins Hospital in nearly sixteen years there were 226 cases of diabetes, or 0.22 per cent. Among 18,000 ward cases there were 147 diabetics.

Hereditary influences play an important *rôle,* and cases are on record of its occurrence in many members of the same family. Morton, who calls the disease *hydrops ad matulam* (Phthisiologia, 1689) records a remarkable family in which four children were affected, one of whom recovered on a milk diet and diascordium. An analysis of the cases in my series gave only 6 cases with a history of diabetes in relatives (Pleasants). Naunyn obtained a family history of diabetes in 35 out of 201 private cases, but in only 7 of 157 hospital cases. There are instances of the coexistence of the disease in man and wife. Among 516 married pairs collected by Senator, in which either husband or wife was diabetic, in 18 cases the second partner had become diabetic. It is not easy to explain this conjugal diabetes. The suggestion of contagion seems scarcely tenable.

Sex.—Men are more frequently affected than women, the ratio being about three to two. Up to April 1, 1905, 226 cases of diabetes had been treated in the medical wards and medical dispensary of the Johns Hopkins Hospital, 131 of which were in males and 95 in females (Futcher). It is a disease of adult life; a majority of the cases occur from the third to the sixth decade. Of the 226 cases, the largest number—63, or 27 per cent—occurred between fifty and sixty years of age. These figures agree fairly closely with those of Frerichs, Seegen, and Pavy, all of whom found the largest number of cases in the sixth decade, their percentages being 26, 30, and 30.7 respectively. It is rare in childhood, but cases are on record in children under one year of age.

In the above series there were no cases in the first hemi-decade, 2 in the second, 7 in the third, and 6 in the fourth.

Persons of a neurotic *temperament* are often affected. It is a disease of the higher classes. Von Noorden states that the statistics for London and Berlin show that the number of cases in the upper ten thousand exceeds that in the lower hundred thousand inhabitants.

Race.—Hebrews seem especially prone to it; one-fourth of Frerichs' patients were of the Semitic race. I have been much impressed with the frequency of the disease among them. Diabetes is comparatively rare in the colored race, but not so uncommon as was formerly supposed. Of the series of 226 cases, 23, or 11.3 per cent, were in negroes. The ratio of males to

28

females affected is almost exactly the reverse of that in the white race; 15 of the 23 were in females and 8 in males.

Obesity.—In a considerable proportion of the cases of diabetes the subjects have been excessively fat at the beginning of, or prior to, the onset of the disease. A slight trace of sugar is not very uncommon in obese persons. This so-called lipogenic glycosuria is not of grave significance, and is only occasionally followed by true diabetes. On the other hand, as von Noorden has shown, there may be a " diabetogenous obesity," in which diabetes and obesity develop in early life, and these cases are very unfavorable. There are instances on record in which obesity with diabetes has occurred in three generations. Diabetes is more common in cities than in country districts. Gout, syphilis, and malaria have been regarded as predisposing causes.

Nervous Influences.—Mental shock, severe nervous strain, and worry precede many cases. In one case the symptoms came on suddenly after the patient had been nearly suffocated by smoke from having been confined in a cell of a burning jail. Shock and the toxic effects of the smoke may both have been factors in this case. The combination of intense application to business, over-indulgence in food and drink, with a sedentary life, seems particularly prone to induce the disease. Glycosuria may set in during pregnancy, and in rare instances may only occur at this period. Trousseau thought that the offspring of phthisical parents were particularly prone to diabetes.

Injury to or disease of the spinal cord or brain has been followed by diabetes. In the carefully analyzed cases of Frerichs there were 30 instances of organic disease of these parts. The medulla is not always involved. In only 4 of his cases, which showed organic disease, was there sclerosis or other anomaly of this part. An irritative lesion of Bernard's diabetic centre in the medulla is an occasional cause. I saw with Reiss, at the Friedrichshain, Berlin, a woman who had anomalous cerebral symptoms and diabetes, and in whom there was found post mortem a cysticercus in the fourth ventricle. Glycosuria sometimes occurs in tumors of the hypophysis such as accompany acromegaly. Ebstein has recorded 4 cases in which there was a coincident occurrence of epilepsy and diabetes mellitus. He thinks that in the majority of cases the two diseases are dependent on a common cause. He believes that the association would be found much more commonly in Jacksonian epilepsy than has been the case heretofore, if more careful and systematic examinations of the urine were made. A transitory glycosuria occasionally follows cerebral hæmorrhage and also severe gall-stone colic.

The disease has occasionally followed the *infectious fevers.* Cases have been recorded as occurring during or immediately after diphtheria, influenza, rheumatism, enteric fever, and syphilis.

Experimental Diabetes.—Leo believes that diabetes is due to a toxic agent. He has produced glycosuria in dogs by administering both fresh and fermented diabetic urine. In 1901, Blum reported that the subcutaneous injection of an aqueous solution of adrenalin produced glycosuria in 22 out of 25 animals experimented upon. Herter confirmed these results, and found that the direct application of the solution to the surface of the pancreas caused a marked glycosuria. Adrenalin is a powerful reducing substance, and Herter thinks that the glycosuria results from interference with normal oxidation processes in the pancreatic cells. Phloridzin administered internally or hypodermically produces a marked temporary glycosuria. There is no accompanying hyperglycæmia. The phloridzin acts primarily on the renal epithelium, destroying its power of keeping back the sugar. Naunyn and Klemperer hold the view that there is a renal form of diabetes.

Metabolism in Diabetes.—Our ignorance of the metabolic disturbances in diabetes has been largely due to the fact that we have not known how the carbohydrates are eventually disposed of in the body in health. Normally the carbohydrates of the food are stored in the liver and muscles as glycogen. Pavy holds that a part of the ingested carbohydrates is converted by the villi of the intestinal mucosa into fat and carried thence by the lacteals to the blood. By a splitting-off process another portion is incorporated with nitrogenous matters and carried away in the form of proteid. He thinks that only a portion of the carbohydrates reaches the liver as glucose, where the hepatic cells convert this monosaccharid into the polysaccharid glycogen. Glycogen can also be formed from the proteids of the food; and under certain circumstances sugar can be directly formed from the body proteids. In health the amount of glucose in the circulating blood ranges between 0.1 and 0.2 per cent. If it were not for the reservoir action of the liver and muscles in storing up the excess of carbohydrates after a meal as glycogen, we would have more than 0.2 per cent of glucose in the blood, a hyperglycæmia would occur and a glycosuria ensue. In health the glycogen is reconverted into glucose, which is distributed to the muscles by the circulating blood and there burnt up, producing heat and energy.

The manner in which this final combustion is effected has hitherto not been known. Cohnheim's (Jr.) published researches in 1903 and 1904 throw much light on this subject. By a specially constructed press he obtained the juice from the pancreas and muscles of dogs and cats. Each juice added independently to solutions of glucose was inert. When, however, the pancreatic juice was added to a mixture of muscle juice and glucose there was a rapid breaking up of the latter into alcohol and carbonic acid. Cohnheim holds that this remarkable effect is analogous to Pavlow's observation that trypsinogen is only made active for proteid digestion by being converted into trypsin by the " enterokinase " of the succus entericus. He believes that the muscles produce a proenzyme which is only made active for carbohydrate combustion by the action of another substance produced in the pancreas and conveyed to the muscles by the blood stream. He showed that the glycolytic substance produced by the pancreas is not a true ferment but a body closely related in its characteristics with other well-known constituents of internal secretions as adrenalin and iodothyrin. He also found that when too large a quantity of the juice of the pancreas is used carbohydrate combustion is retarded or even stopped. The pancreas juice is supposed to supply the amboceptors and the muscle juice the complement. The retarding action of an excess of pancreas juice is believed to be due to an overabundance of amboceptors. According to these researches the carbohydrates normally are burnt up in the muscles, producing heat and energy, by the combined action of two glycolytic bodies, one· produced in the muscles and the other in the pancreas. This important work awaits confirmation.

When the percentage of glucose in the circulating blood exceeds 0.2 **per** cent a glycosuria occurs. This may theoretically be produced as follows:

(*a*) By functional or organic disease of the islands of Langerhans in the pancreas. These islands of cells probably produce a glycolytic ferment or body. This substance seems necessary for the proper burning up of the carbohydrates. If the islands be diseased the ferment is not produced, glucose accumulates in the blood, and glycosuria results. This substance may act on the carbohydrates independently, or, as Cohnheim believes, is necessary to render active a pro-ferment manufactured by the muscle cells.

(*b*) By the sudden ingestion of a greater quantity of carbohydrates than can for the time being be stored up in the liver as glycogen. A healthy person can take from 180 to 250 grams of glucose on an empty stomach without glycosuria occurring. Larger amounts will produce a so-called alimentary glycosuria, or glycosuria e saccharo. In a healthy person no amount of carbohydrates in the form of starch will produce a glycosuria owing to the comparative slowness of its transformation into glucose. If, however, the person's "assimilation limit," or power of warehousing carbohydrates, be lowered, a glycosuria e amylo may occur.

(*c*) By changes in the liver function: (1) Changes in the circulation under nervous influences. Puncture of the medulla, lesions of the cord, and central irritation of various kinds are followed by glycosuria, which is attributed to a vasomotor paralysis induced by these causes, resulting in a greater quantity of blood flowing through the liver. On this view the disease is a neurosis. (2) Instability of the glycogen, owing either to imperfect formation or to conditions in the cells which render it less stable.

Morbid Anatomy.—Saundby (Lectures on Diabetes, 1891) has given a good summary of the anatomical changes:

The *nervous system* shows no constant lesions. In a few instances there have been tumors or sclerosis in the medulla, or, as in the case above mentioned, a cysticercus has pressed on the floor. Cysts have been met with in the white matter of the cerebrum and perivascular changes have been described. A secondary multiple neuritis is not rare, and to it the so-called diabetic tabes is probably due. R. T. Williamson has found changes in the posterior columns of the cord similar to those which occur in pernicious anæmia.

In the sympathetic system the ganglia have been enlarged and in some instances sclerosed. The *blood* may contain as high as 0.4 per cent of sugar instead of 0.15 per cent. The plasma is usually loaded with fat, the molecules of which may be seen as fine particles. When drawn, a white creamy layer coats the coagulum, and there may be lipæmic clots in the small vessels. There are no special changes in the red or white corpuscles. The polynuclear leucocytes contain glycogen. Glycogen can occur in normal blood, but it is here extracellular. It has been also found in the polynuclear leucocytes in leukæmia. The *heart* is hypertrophied in some cases. Endocarditis is very rare. Arterio-sclerosis is common. The *lungs* show important changes. Acute broncho-pneumonia or croupous pneumonia (either of which may terminate in gangrene) and tuberculosis are common. The so-called diabetic phthisis is always tuberculous and results from a caseating broncho-pneumonia. In rare cases there is a chronic interstitial pneumonia, non-tuberculous. Fat embolism of the pulmonary vessels has been described in connection with diabetic coma.

The *liver* is usually enlarged; fatty degeneration is common. In the so-called diabetic cirrhosis—the *cirrhose pigmentaire*—the liver is enlarged and sclerotic, and a cachexia develops with melanoderma. This condition is probably identical with hæmochromatosis. Dilatation of the stomach is common.

The Pancreas in Diabetes.—Our scientific knowledge of the relationship of the pancreas to glycosuria dates from 1889, when Minkowski and von Mering published the results of their experiments on extirpation of the pancreas in animals. The present status may be thus summarized: (*a*) Extirpation of the gland in dogs (and occasionally in man—W. T. Bull) is followed by glycosuria. If a small portion remains, sugar does not appear. (*b*) In a considerable percentage of cases of diabetes lesions of the pancreas are found; 50 per cent (Hansemann, Williamson) show a chronic interstitial inflammation. (*c*) In view of the experimental work, it is reasonable to infer that the diabetes is secondary to the pancreatic lesion. The organ has, like the liver, a double secretion—an external, which is poured into the intestines, and an internal, of the nature either of a ferment or of a body similar in chemical characteristics to those of adrenalin or iodothyrin, as Cohnheim claims, which seems necessary for the proper combustion of glucose in the muscles. Disease of the pancreas causes diabetes by preventing the formation of this glycolytic body. The fact that if a small portion of the gland is left, in the experiments upon dogs, diabetes does not occur, is analogous to the remarkable circumstance that a small fragment of the thyroid is sufficient to prevent the occurrence of artificial myxœdema.

It is probable that the observations of Opie from Dr. Welch's laboratory, confirmed by those of Weichselbaum and Stange, give a key to the problem. Imbedded in the gland are the peculiar bodies known as the islands of Langerhans, composed of polygonal cells arranged in irregular columns, between which are wide anastomosing capillaries. The lumina of the ducts do not enter the islands, which are in reality ductless glands, like the para-thyroid, the thyroid, the pituitary, etc. The intimate relation of the columns of cells to the rich network of blood-vessels suggests, as advanced by Schäfer, that they furnish the internal secretion of the gland. It is probable that the glycolytic body found by Cohnheim is produced by these specialized cells. Experimental evidence is defective, but changes in the islands have been found in diabetes. In a diabetic woman, aged twenty-four, from my wards, dead of tuberculosis of the lungs, Opie found the glandular tissue of the pancreas well preserved and healthy, but the islands of Langerhans were everywhere "represented by a sharply circumscribed hyaline structure composed of particles of homogeneous material." In two other cases lesions of the islands were found, but there was also chronic pancreatitis (Opie, Jour. Exper. Med., vol. v). Hoppe-Seyler has recently described a clinical form of pancreatic diabetes due to arterio-sclerosis of the pancreatic vessels. These arterial changes were found in a series of autopsies.

Of 15 autopsies from my own 27 cases, in 9 on gross examination the pancreas was found to be atrophic. In one of these fat necroses, and in another calculi, were present.

The *kidneys* show usually a diffuse nephritis with fatty degeneration. A hyaline change occurs in the tubal epithelium, particularly of the descending limb of the loop of Henle, and also in the capillary vessels of the tufts.

Symptoms.—*Acute* and *chronic* forms are recognized, but there is no essential difference between them, except that in the former the patients are younger, the course is more rapid, and the emaciation more marked. Acute cases may occur in the aged. I saw with Sowers in Washington a man aged seventy-three in whom the entire course of the disease was less than three weeks.

It is also possible to divide the cases into (1) *lipogenic* or *dietetic,* which includes the transient glycosuria of stout persons; (2) *neurotic,* due to injuries or functional disorders of the nervous system; and (3) *pancreatic,* in which there is a lesion of the pancreas. It is, however, by no means easy to discriminate in all cases between these forms. Attempts have been made to separate a clinical variety analogous to experimental pancreatic diabetes. Hirschfeld, from Guttman's clinic, has described cases running a rapid and severe course usually in young and middle-aged persons. The polyuria is less common or even absent, and there is a striking defect in the assimilation of the albuminoids and fats, as shown by the examination of the fæces and urine. In 4 of 7 cases autopsies were made and the pancreas was found atrophic in two, cancerous in one, and in the fourth exceedingly soft.

The *onset* of the disease is gradual, and either frequent micturition or inordinate thirst first attracts attention. Very rarely it sets in rapidly, after a sudden emotion, an injury, or after a severe chill. When fully established the disease is characterized by great thirst, the passage of large quantities of saccharine urine, a voracious appetite, and, as a rule, progressive emaciation.

Among the *general symptoms* of the disease *thirst* is one of the most distressing. Large quantities of water are required to keep the sugar in solution and for its excretion in the urine. The amount of fluid consumed will be found to bear a definite ratio to the quantity excreted. Instances, however, are not uncommon of pronounced diabetes in which the thirst is not excessive; but in such cases the amount of urine passed is never large. The thirst is most intense an hour or two after meals. As a rule, the digestion is good and the appetite inordinate. The condition is sometimes termed *bulimia* or *polyphagia.* Lumbar pain is common.

The tongue is usually dry, red, and glazed, and the saliva scanty. The gums may become swollen, and in the later stages aphthous stomatitis is common. Constipation is the rule.

In spite of the enormous amount of food consumed a patient may become rapidly emaciated. This loss of flesh bears some ratio to the polyuria, and when, under suitable diet, the sugar is reduced, the patient may quickly gain in flesh. The skin is dry and harsh, and sweating rarely occurs, except when phthisis coexists. Drenching sweats have been known to alternate with excessive polyuria. General pruritus or pruritus pudendi may be very distressing, and occasionally is one of the earliest symptoms. The temperature is often subnormal; the pulse is usually frequent, and the tension increased. Many diabetics, however, do not show marked emaciation. Patients past the middle period of life may have the disease for years without much

185

disturbance of the health, and may remain well nourished. These are the cases of the *diabète gras* in contradistinction to *diabète maigre.*

THE URINE.—The amount varies from 3 to 4 litres in mild cases to 15 to 20 litres in very severe cases. In rare instances the quantity of urine is not much increased. Under strict diet the amount is much lessened, and in intercurrent febrile affections it may be reduced to normal. The specific gravity is high, ranging from 1.025 to 1.045; but in exceptional cases it may be low, 1.013 to 1.020. The highest specific gravity recorded, so far as I know, is by Trousseau—1.074. Very high specific gravities—1.070 + —suggest fraud. The urine is pale in color, almost like water, and has a sweetish odor and a distinctly sweetish taste. The reaction is acid. Sugar is present in varying amounts. In mild cases it does not exceed $1\frac{1}{2}$ or 2 per cent, but it may reach from 5 to 10 per cent. The total amount excreted in the twenty-four hours may range from 10 to 20 ounces (320 to 640 grammes) and in exceptional cases from 1 to 2 pounds. The following are the most satisfactory tests:

Fehling's Test.—The solution consists of sulphate of copper (grs. $90\frac{1}{2}$), neutral tartrate of potassium (grs. 364), solution of caustic soda (fl. ozs. 4), and distilled water to make up 6 ounces. Put a drachm of this in a test-tube and boil (to test the reagent); add an equal quantity of urine and boil again, when, if sugar is present, the yellow suboxide of copper is thrown down. The solution must be freshly prepared, as it is apt to decompose.

Trommer's Test.—To a drachm of urine in a test-tube add a few drops of a dilute sulphate-of-copper solution and then as much *liquor potassæ* as urine. On boiling, the copper is reduced if sugar be present, forming the yellow or orange-red suboxide. There are certain fallacies in the copper tests. Thus, a substance called glycuronic acid is met with in the urine after the use of certain drugs—chloral, phenacetin, morphia, chloroform, etc.—which reduces copper. Alcaptonuria may also be a source of error (see Alcaptonuria).

Fermentation Test.—This is free from all doubt. Place a small fragment of yeast in a test-tube full of urine, which is then inverted over a glass vessel containing the same fluid. There are now specially devised fermentation tubes. If sugar is present, fermentation goes on with the formation of carbon dioxide, which accumulates in the upper part of the tube and gradually expels the urine. In doubtful cases a control test should always be used.

Polariscope Test.—For laboratory work the polariscope test is of great value. Glucose is dextro-rotatory. The percentage of sugar can be quickly estimated by the degree of rotation, and for quantitative determination is the most serviceable method. The presence of β-oxybutyric acid, which is lævo-rotatory, will neutralize some of the dextro-rotatory action of the glucose.

Nylander's Bismuth Test.—Nylander's solution is prepared by dissolving 4 grammes of Rochelle salt in 100 cc. of 10 per cent caustic soda solution and adding 2 grammes of bismuth subnitrate and digesting on the water-bath until as much of the bismuth salt is dissolved as possible. To 10 cc. of urine add 1 cc. of the Nylander's solution and boil for a few minutes. If glucose be present a black deposit of bismuth occurs.

Of other ingredients in the urine, the urea is increased, the uric acid does not show special changes, and the phosphates may be greatly in excess. The calcium salts are markedly increased. The same holds true for the ammonia in all severe cases, and particularly in diabetic coma. Ralfe has described a great increase in the phosphates, and in some of these cases, with an excessive excretion, the symptoms may be very similar to those of diabetes, though the sugar may not be constantly present. The term phosphatic diabetes has sometimes been applied to them. *Acetone* and acetone-forming substances are not infrequently present. Lieben's test is as follows: .The urine is distilled and a few cubic centimetres of the distillate are rendered alkaline with liquor potassæ. A few drops of Lugol's solution are then added, when, if acetone be present, the distillate assumes a turbid yellow color, due to the formation of iodoform, which is recognized by its odor and by the formation of minute hexagonal and stellate crystals. *Diacetic acid* is sometimes present, and may be recognized from the fact that a solution of the chloride of iron yields a beautiful Bordeaux-red color. Other substances, as formic, carbolic, and salicylic acids, give the same reaction in both fresh and previously boiled urine, while diacetic acid does not give the reaction in urine previously boiled. In testing for diacetic acid perfectly fresh urine should be used, as it rapidly becomes broken up into acetone and carbonic acid. β-oxybutyric acid, the recognized cause of coma, should be tested for in all severe cases. As it is lævo-rotatory, its presence is indicated by lævo-rotation in completely fermented urine, as well as by the greater percentage of sugar demonstrable with Fehling's than with the polariscopic method. The occurrence of acetone and diacetic acid in the urine, both derivative products of β-oxybutyric acid, is conclusive evidence that β-oxybutyric acid is being produced in the body.

Bremer finds that diabetic urine has the power of dissolving gentian violet, whereas normal urine fails to do so. Unfortunately, the urine in diabetes insipidus and in certain forms of polyuria reacts similarly. Fröhlich has recently devised a test based on the fact that diabetic urine has the property of decolorizing solutions of methylene blue.

Glycogen has also been described as present in the urine.

Albumin is not infrequent. It occurred in nearly 37 per cent of the examinations made by Lippman at Carlsbad.

Pneumaturia, the formation of gas in the urine, due to fermentative processes in the bladder, is occasionally met with.

Cammidge found glycerine in the urine in one case of pancreatic diabetes. This results from fat necroses due to the action of a fat-splitting ferment.

Fat may be passed in the urine in the form of a fine emulsion (lipuria).

BLOOD IN DIABETES.—In true diabetes hyperglycæmia is constant. As coma supervenes, β-oxybutyric acid occurs. Polycythæmia, with the red cells between 6,000,000 and 8,000,000 per cmm., is not uncommon in the desiccated cases with marked polyuria. Coma is accompanied by a moderate leucocytosis. Lipæmia occurs in a certain number of cases. It is recognized by the presence of innumerable dancing particles between the red cells in a fresh preparation, and by the creamy appearance of the serum of centrifugalized blood. Normal blood contains between 0.16 to 0.325 per cent of fat (Becquerel and Rodier). Fraser found 16.44 per cent of fat in the blood of a diabetic. Opinions vary as to the source of the fat.

DIABETES IN CHILDREN.—Stern has analyzed 117 cases in children. They usually occur among the better classes.. Six were under one year of age. Hereditary influences were marked. The course of the disease is, as a rule, much more rapid than in adults. The shortest duration was two days. In 7 cases it did not last a month. One case is mentioned of a child apparently born with the glycosuria, who recovered in eight months.

Complications.—(*a*) CUTANEOUS.—Boils and carbuncles are extremely common. Painful onychia may occur. Eczema is also met with, and at times an intolerable itching. In women the irritation of the urine may cause the most intense pruritus pudendi, and in men a balanitis. Rarer affections are xanthoma and purpura. Gangrene is not uncommon, and is associated usually with arterio-sclerosis. William Hunt has analyzed 64 cases. In 50 the localities were as follows: Feet and legs, 37; thigh and buttock, 2; nucha, 2; external genitals, 1; lungs, 3; fingers, 3; back, 1; eyes, 1. Perforating ulcer of the foot may occur. Bronzing of the skin (*diabète bronzé*) occurs in certain cases in which the diabetes arises as a late event in the disease known as hæmochromatosis, which is further characterized by pigmentary cirrhosis of the liver and pancreas. With the onset of severe complications the tolerance of the carbohydrates is much increased. Profuse sweats may occur.

(*b*) PULMONARY.—The patients are not infrequently carried off by *acute pneumonia,* which may be lobar or lobular. *Gangrene* is very apt to supervene, but the breath does not necessarily have the foul odor of ordinary gangrene. Abscess following lobar pneumonia occurred in one of my cases.

Tuberculous broncho-pneumonia is very common. It was formerly thought, from its rapid course and the limitation of the disease to the lung, that this was not a true tuberculous affection; but in the cases which have come under my notice the bacilli have been present, and the condition is now generally regarded as tuberculous.

(*c*) RENAL.—*Albuminuria* is a tolerably frequent complication. The amount varies greatly, and, when slight, does not seem to be of much moment. Œdema of the feet and ankles is not an infrequent symptom. General anasarca is rare, however, owing to the marked polyuria. It is sometimes associated with arterio-sclerosis. It occasionally precedes the occurrence of the diabetic coma. Occasionally cystitis develops.

(*d*) NERVOUS SYSTEM.—(1) *Diabetic coma,* first studied by Kussmaul, comes on in a considerable proportion of all cases, particularly in the young. Stephen Mackenzie states that of the fatal cases of diabetes at the London Hospital, all under the age of twenty-five, with but one exception, had died in coma. In Naunyn's 44 fatal cases it occurred in 12. It preceded death in 28 of Williamson's 40 cases. It occurred in 15 of 27 fatal cases in my series. Frerichs recognized three groups of cases: (a) Those in which after exertion the patients were suddenly attacked with weakness, syncope, somnolence, and gradually deepening unconsciousness; death occurring in a few hours. (β) Cases with preliminary gastric disturbance, such as nausea and vomiting, or some local affection, as pharyngitis, phlegmon, or a pulmonary complication. In such cases the attack begins with headache, delirium, great distress, and dyspnœa, affecting both inspiration and expiration, a condition called by Kussmaul *air-hunger.* Cyanosis may or may not be present. If it is, the pulse becomes rapid and weak and the patient gradually sinks into coma; the attack lasting from one to five days. There may be a very heavy sweetish odor of the breath, due to the presence of acetone. (γ) Cases in which, without any previous dyspnœa or distress, the patient is attacked with headache and a feeling of intoxication, and rapidly falls into a deep and fatal coma. There are atypical cases in which the coma is due to uræmia, to apoplexy, or to meningitis.

There has been much dispute as to the nature of these symptoms, but clinical laboratory investigations have practically afforded a satisfactory explanation. For years the coma symptoms were ascribed to the toxic effects of acetone and later to those of diacetic acid. Experimental work, however, showed that these views were incorrect. The almost universal opinion now is that the coma is due to an acid intoxication, or, as Naunyn terms it, an acidosis. The offending agent is believed to be β-oxybutyric acid, which accumulates in the tissues and circulating blood in enormous quantities, and is eliminated in the urine in combination with various base-forming elements, but never free. In 1884 Stadelmann, Külz, and Minkowski almost simultaneously found this acid in the urine of patients with diabetic coma. Subsequent researches, particularly those published from Naunyn's clinic, have fully confirmed these results, and it is now almost universally accepted that β-oxybutyric acid is the cause of diabetic coma. The amount of the acid excreted in the twenty-four hours may be enormous. Külz found in 3 cases 67, 100, and 226 grammes respectively. Magnus-Levy has estimated that from 100 to 200 grammes are often contained in the tissues of fatal cases. This author is of the belief that the β-oxybutyric acid is derived from the fats of the body, whereas most observers, including Naunyn, trace it to the disintegration of the tissue albumins. Acetone and diacetic acid are derivative products of the β-oxybutyric acid.

Saunders and Hamilton have described cases in which the lung capillaries were blocked with fat. They attributed the symptoms to fat embolism, but there are many cases on record in which this condition was not found, though lipæmia is by no means infrequent in diabetes.

Albuminuria frequently precedes or accompanies the attack, and numerous small, short, hyaline, and finely granular casts are demonstrable.

(2) *Peripheral Neuritis.*—The *neuralgias,* numbness, and tingling, which are not uncommon symptoms in diabetes, are probably minor neuritic manifestations. The involvement may be general of the upper and lower extremities. Sometimes it is unilateral, or the neuritis may be in a single nerve— the sciatic or the third nerve. Herpes zoster may occur. Perforating ulcer of the foot may develop.

Diabetic Tabes (so-called).—This is a peripheral neuritis, characterized by lightning pains in the legs, loss of knee-jerk—which may occur without the other symptoms—and a loss of power in the extensors of the feet. The gait is the characteristic *steppage,* as in arsenical, alcoholic, and other forms of neuritic paralysis. Charcot states that there may be atrophy of the optic nerves. Changes in the posterior columns of the cord have been found by Williamson and others.

Diabetic Paraplegia.—This is also in all probability due to neuritis. There are cases in which power has been lost in both arms and legs.

189

(3) *Mental Symptoms.*—The patients are often morose, and there is a strong tendency to become hypochondriacal. General paralysis has been met with. Some patients display an extraordinary degree of restlessness and anxiety.

(4) *Special Senses.*—Cataract is liable to occur, and with rapidity in young persons. Diabetic retinitis closely resembles the albuminuric form. Hæmorrhages are common. Sudden amaurosis, similar to that which occurs in uræmia, may occur. Paralysis of the muscles of accommodation may be present; and lastly, atrophy of the optic nerves. Aural symptoms may come on with great rapidity, either an otitis media, or in some instances inflammation of the mastoid cells.

(5) *Sexual Function.*—Impotence is common, and may be an early symptom. Conception is rare; if it occurs, abortion is apt to follow. A diabetic mother may bear a healthy child; there is no known instance of a diabetic mother bearing a diabetic child. The course of the disease is usually aggravated after delivery.

Course.—In children the disease is rapidly progressive, and may prove fatal in a few days. In young persons death almost invariably results from diabetic coma. It may be stated, as a general rule, that the older the patient at the time of onset the slower the course. Cases without hereditary influences are the most favorable. In stout, elderly men diabetes is a much more hopeful disease than it is in thin persons. Middle-aged patients may live for many years, and persons are met with who have had the disease for ten, twelve, or even fifteen years.

Diagnosis.—As stated in the definition, for a case to be considered diabetes the sugar eliminated in the urine must be grape sugar, it should be present for weeks, months, or years, and the excretion of sugar must take place after the ingestion of moderate amounts of carbohydrates. Alimentary or dietetic glycosuria must not be confused with true diabetes. As a rule, there is no difficulty in determining the presence of diabetes. The diagnosis must be made chiefly by the urine tests already given. More than one test must be used, and where there is any doubt the fermentation test, the most reliable single test, must be made. One must always exclude the possibility of the copper sulphate reduction being due to glycuronic acid compounds and to homogentisic acid, the latter the cause of alcaptonuria. Bremer showed that the red cells in diabetic blood fail to take the red stain as normal reds do. The test may be of some service when a patient is first seen in coma, which may be thought to be diabetic, and where urine is not at once available. Williamson found that diabetic blood possesses the power of decolorizing weak alkaline solutions of methylene blue to a yellowish-green or yellow color.

Occasionally intermittent glycosuria occurs. It is advisable in these cases to determine the assimilation limit for carbohydrates. According to Naunyn, 100 grammes of glucose given in solution two hours after a breakfast of a roll and butter with coffee ought not to cause a glycosuria. If it does, the individual's power of warehousing carbohydrates is lowered and a permanent glycosuria—true diabetes—may eventually ensue.

Deception may be practised. A young girl under my care had urine with a specific gravity of 1.065. The reactions were for cane sugar. There is one

190

case in the literature in which, after the cane-sugar fraud was detected, the woman bought grape sugar and put it into her bladder!

Prognosis.—In true diabetes instances of cure are rare. On the other hand, the transient or intermittent glycosuria, met with in stout overfeeders, or in persons who have undergone a severe mental strain, is very amenable to treatment. Not a few of the cases of reputed cures belong to this division. Practically, in cases under forty years of age the outlook is bad; in older persons the disease is less serious and much more amenable to treatment. It is a good plan at the outset to determine whether the urine of a patient contains sugar or not on a diet absolutely free from carbohydrates. If the sugar disappears the case may be regarded as a mild one. If, on the other hand, sugar continues to be excreted, it is a severe one, and the patient is manufacturing sugar from his body proteids. The presence of β-oxybutyric or diacetic acids in the urine is usually of serious import, and should warn the physician of the possible occurrence of coma. Occasionally diacetic acid may be present for months, apparently without serious consequences.

Treatment.—In families with a marked predisposition to the disease the use of starchy and saccharine articles of diet should be restricted.

The personal hygiene of a diabetic patient is of the first importance. Sources of worry should be avoided, and he should lead an even, quiet life, if possible in an equable climate. Flannel or silk should be worn next to the skin, and the greatest care should be taken to promote its action. A lukewarm, or, if tolerably robust, a cold bath, should be taken every day. An occasional Turkish bath is useful. Systematic, moderate exercise should be taken. When this is not feasible, massage should be given. It is well to study accurately the dietetic capabilities of each case. No two cases can be treated alike. The weight should be recorded weekly. A patient who is glycosuric and losing weight on a non-carbohydrate diet must be regarded as doing badly. By the addition of a certain amount of starchy food the same person may excrete a moderate amount of sugar and hold or even gain in weight.

DIET.—Our injunctions to-day are those of Sydenham: " Let the patient eat food of easy digestion, such as veal, mutton, and the like, and abstain from all sorts of fruit and garden stuff."

When a diabetic patient, in private or hospital practice, comes under treatment, it is well to keep him for three or four days on the ordinary diet, which contains moderate amounts of carbohydrates, in order to ascertain the amount of sugar excretion. For two days more the starches are gradually cut off. He is then placed on the following non-carbohydrate diet, modified in each case according to the patient's age and weight, and arranged from a list recommended by von Noorden:

Breakfast: 7.30, 200 cc. (℥ vi) of tea or coffee: 150 grammes (℥ iv) of beefsteak, mutton-chops without bone, or boiled ham; one or two eggs.

Lunch: 12.30, 200 grammes (℥ vi) cold roast beef; 60 grammes (℥ ij) celery, fresh cucumbers or tomatoes with vinegar, olive oil, pepper and salt to taste; 20 cc. (℥ v) whisky with 400 cc. (℥ xiij) water; 60 cc. (℥ ij) coffee, without milk or sugar.

Dinner: 6 P.M., 200 cc. clear bouillon; 250 grammes (℥ viiss) roast beef; 10 grammes (℥ iiss) butter; 80 grammes (℥ ij) green salad, with 10 grammes

(5 iiss) vinegar and 20 grammes (5 v) olive oil, or three tablespoonfuls of some well-cooked green vegetable; three sardines à l'huile; 20 cc. (5 v) whisky, with 400 cc. (℥ xiij) water.

Supper: 9 P. M., two eggs (raw or cooked); 400 cc. (℥ xiij) water.

This diet contains about 200 grammes of albumin and about 135 grammes of fat. The effect of the diet on the sugar excretion is remarkable. In many cases there is an entire disappearance of the sugar from the urine in three or four days. Chart XV shows very graphically the remarkable drop in the sugar excretion for the first twenty-four hours. In cases in which the urine becomes free from sugar, gradually increasing quantities of starch up to 20, 50, and 100 grammes are added daily. White bread contains fifty-five per cent of starch. The effect of the non-carbohydrate diet, according to von Noorden, is to improve the metabolic functions so that the system can ware-house considerable quantities of carbohydrates without sugar appearing in the urine. Naunyn emphasizes the importance of removing the hyperglycæmia and making the patient aglycosuric. In patients on a strict diet who continue to excrete from 0.1 to 0.5 per cent of glucose, he advises a " hunger-day," during which all food is cut off for twenty-four hours. In many such instances aglycosuria occurs, and the patient's power of assimilating carbohydrates is thought to be increased.

In cases in which a standard diet is not ordered it is well to begin cutting off article by article until the sugar disappears from the urine. Within a month or two the patient may be allowed a more liberal diet, testing the different kinds of food.

The *oatmeal diet*, introduced by von Noorden, is most excellent, particularly in the severer forms. Two hundred and fifty grammes of oatmeal, the same amount of butter and the whites of six or eight eggs constitute the day's food. The oatmeal is cooked for two hours, and the butter and albumin stirred in. It may be taken in four portions during the day. Coffee, tea, or whisky and water may be taken with it.

The following is a list of articles which diabetic patients may take:

Liquids: Soups—ox-tail, turtle, bouillon, and other clear soups. Lemonade, coffee, tea, chocolate, and cocoa; these to be taken without sugar, but they may be sweetened with saccharin. Potash or soda water, and Apollinaris, or the Saratoga-Vichy, and milk in moderation, may be used.

Of animal food: Fish of all sorts, including crabs, lobsters, and oysters; salt and fresh butcher's meat (with the exception of liver), poultry, and game. Eggs, butter, buttermilk, curds, and cream cheese.

Of bread: Gluten and bran bread, and almond and cocoanut biscuits. Aleuronat and roborat flours are made from wheat and contain large quantities of albumin and but little starch. They may be used in making bread or biscuits, and are highly recommended by Ebstein.

Of vegetables: Lettuce, tomatoes, spinach, chicory, sorrel, radishes, asparagus, water-cress, cucumbers, celery, endives, mustard and various pickles.

Fruits: Lemons and oranges. Currants, plums, cherries, pears, apples (tart), melons, raspberries, and strawberries may be taken in moderation. Nuts are, as a rule, allowable.

Among *prohibited articles* are the following: Thick soups and liver.

Ordinary bread of all sorts (in quantity), rye, wheaten, brown, or white.

192

All farinaceous preparations, such as hominy, rice, tapioca, semolina, arrow-root, sago, and vermicelli.

Of vegetables: Potatoes, turnips, parsnips, squashes, vegetable-marrows of all kinds, beets, corn, artichokes.

Of liquids: Beer, sparkling wine of all sorts, and the sweet aërated drinks.

In feeding a diabetic patient one of the greatest difficulties is in arranging a substitute for bread. Of the gluten foods, many are very unpalatable; others are frauds.

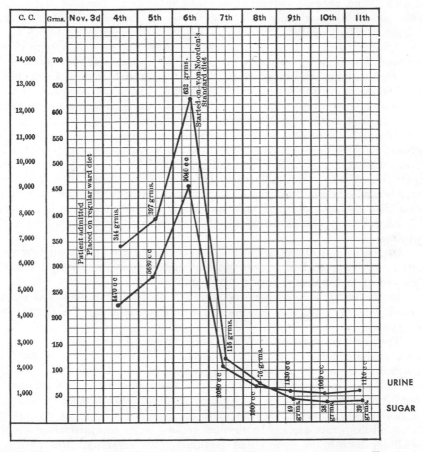

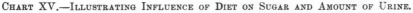

CHART XV.—ILLUSTRATING INFLUENCE OF DIET ON SUGAR AND AMOUNT OF URINE.

Other substitutes are the almond food, the Aleuronat bread, and soya bread, but these and other substitutes are not satisfactory as a rule. For sweetening purposes saccharin may be used, of which tablets are prepared. Mossé has shown that potato starch is more easily assimilated than wheat starch, and this view has been on the whole confirmed by comparative tests in my wards. He allows as much as a kilo (2¼ pounds) of potatoes, weighed fresh, to a diabetic daily. They are best baked.

193

MEDICINAL TREATMENT.—This is most unsatisfactory, and no one drug appears to have a directly curative influence. Opium alone stands the test of experience as a remedy capable of limiting the progress of the disease. Diabetic patients seem to have a special tolerance for this drug. Codeia is preferred by Pavy, and has the advantage of being less constipating than morphia. A patient may begin with half a grain three times a day, which may be gradually increased to 6 or 8 grains in the twenty-four hours. Not much effect is noticed unless the patient is on a rigid diet. When the sugar is reduced to a minimum, or is absent, the opium should be gradually withdrawn. The patients not only bear well these large doses of the drug, but they stand its gradual reduction. Potassium bromide is often a useful adjunct. The arsenite of bromine, a solution of arsenious acid with bromine in glycerin (dose, 3 to 5 minims after meals), has been very highly recommended, but it is by no means so certain as opium. Arsenic alone may be used. Antipyrin may be given in doses of 10 grains three times a day, and in cases with a marked neurotic constitution is sometimes satisfactory. The salicylates, iodoform, nitroglycerin, jambul, the lithium salts, strychnine, creasote, and lactic acid have been employed.

Preparations of the pancreas (glycerin extracts of the dried and fresh gland) have been used in the hope that they would supply the internal secretion necessary to normal sugar metabolism. The success has not, however, been in any way comparable with that obtained with the thyroid extract in myxœdema. Lépine has isolated a glycolytic ferment from the pancreas and also from the malt diastase, and has used it with some success in 4 cases.

As yet no practical therapeutic results have followed Cohnheim's observations.

Of the complications, the *pruritus* and *eczema* are best treated by cooling lotions of boric acid or hyposulphite of soda (1 ounce; water, 1 quart), or the use of ichthyol and lanolin ointment.

In the thin, nervous cases the bowels should be kept open and the urine tested at short intervals for acetone and diacetic acid—the derivatives of β-oxybutyric acid.

The *coma* is an almost hopeless complication. Inhalations of oxygen have been recommended. The use of bicarbonate of soda in very large doses is recommended to neutralize the acid intoxication. It may be used intravenously; as much as 80 grammes have been injected. The solution used for intravenous injection is a 1 to 2 per cent solution of sodium bicarbonate in normal salt solution. A litre may be injected slowly into a vein every six hours in desperate cases. In the less serious cases administration should be made by mouth, or mouth and rectum. This treatment was first recommended by Stadelmann, and has undoubtedly given the best results. Naunyn and Magnus-Levy report cases of recovery from coma by its use. I have had one recovery. The sodium bicarbonate should be pushed until the urine is alkaline. As much as 100 grammes should be given daily. All diabetics with a marked diacetic acid reaction in the urine should be placed on sodium bicarbonate. Next to the antacid treatment, subcutaneous or intravenous injections of normal salt solution have given the best results. The improvement, unfortunately, is only temporary with this line of treatment. Reynolds published 2 cases of recovery after the administration of a dose of castor oil, followed by 30 to 60 grains of citrate of potassium every hour in copious draughts of water. The bowels of a diabetic patient should be kept acting freely, as constipation is believed to predispose to the development of coma.

VI. DIABETES INSIPIDUS.

Definition.—A chronic affection characterized by the passage of large quantities of normal urine of low specific gravity.

The condition is to be distinguished from diuresis or polyuria, which is a frequent symptom in hysteria, in Bright's disease, and occasionally in cerebral or other affections. Willis, in 1674, first recognized the distinction between a saccharine and non-saccharine form of diabetes.

Etiology.—The disease is most common in young persons. Of the 85 cases collected by Strauss, 9 were under five years; 12 between five and ten years; 36 between ten and twenty-five years. Males are more frequently attacked than females. The affection may be congenital. A hereditary tendency has been noted in many instances, the most extraordinary of which has been reported by Weil. Of 91 members in four generations, 23 had persistent polyuria without any deterioration in health.

CLINICAL CLASSIFICATION.—There are two forms: primary or idiopathic, in which there is no evident organic basis, and secondary or symptomatic, in which there is evidence of disease in the brain or elsewhere. Of 9 cases reported from my clinic by Futcher, 4 belonged to the former and 5 to the latter group. Trousseau stated that the parents of children with diabetes insipidus frequently have glycosuria or albuminuria. Ralfe claimed that malnutrition is an important predisposing factor in children. The disease has followed rapidly the copious drinking of cold water, or a drinking bout, or has set in during the convalescence from an acute disease.

The secondary or symptomatic form is almost always associated with injury or disease of the nervous system, traumatism to the head, or, in some cases, to the trunk. It occurs in 30 per cent of the cases, according to Stoermer. Tumors of the brain, lesions of the medulla, cerebral hæmorrhage, have been met with in some cases. There is a remarkable association between diabetes insipidus and brain syphilis; 5 of the 9 cases reported by Futcher were in syphilitics. The lesion is usually at the base, and meningitic. Hemianopsia is present in a number of these cases; it occurred in 2 of Futcher's series. It is not necessary that the lesion should involve the medulla. It has been met with in spinal cord lesions. In tumors and aneurisms in the abdomen, in tuberculous peritonitis, and in carcinoma there may be polyuria of an extreme grade.

The most reasonable view of the production of the polyuria is that it results from a vaso-motor disturbance of the renal vessels, due either to local irritation, as in a case of abdominal tumor, to central disturbance in cases of brain-lesion, or to functional irritation of the centre in the medulla, giving rise to continuous renal congestion.

Morbid Anatomy.—There are no constant anatomical lesions. The *kidneys* have been found enlarged and congested. The *bladder* has been found hypertrophied. Dilatation of the ureters and of the pelves of the kidneys has

diabetes mellitus

Osler's chapter on diabetes might well evoke the paradoxical exclamation: "How much is still true; how much has been added!" The strength of Osler's approach is seen in the headings and subheadings, most of which continue to be the framework of modern texts. Thus, the incidence, heredity, relation to sex, age, race, and obesity continue to claim our attention. In these areas the modern reader notes the vastly increased knowledge of the disease, which has resulted from the greater use of epidemiological methods. Statistics on the worldwide occurrence of diabetes ("race") and prevalence based on better diagnostic procedures, screening tests of populations, and so on mark progress in knowledge which is sometimes obscured in our preoccupation with laboratory discovery. There is now a greater known prevalence of diabetes in children due to better diagnosis. In general, most of Osler's statements of this sort remain true but are much better documented.

The discovery of insulin is the dramatic addition to this chapter. Insulin has led to the prolonged survival of diabetic patients and to a new emphasis on the disease as modified by such treatment. It has also been a major stimulus to the study of the biochemistry and physiology of metabolism. "Our ignorance of the metabolic disturbances in diabetes has been largely due to the fact that we have not known how the carbohydrates are eventually disposed of in the body in health." In ultimate detail this is still true, but sections on biochemistry and summaries of the known reactions of carbohydrate and fat metabolism are now part of every chapter on diabetes. The reading of Osler drives home the magnitude of basic research in the last 58 years.

Laboratory tests have all been revised and improved. Thus, Fehling's solution has been replaced by Benedict's solution and that, in turn, by the glucose oxidase papers which are now used by the patient as well as by the physician. The glucose oxidase methods also take care of Osler's requirement: "For a case to be considered one of diabetes mellitus it is necessary that the form of sugar eliminated in the urine be grape sugar." If one recalls that Bang in 1909 first developed a practical method for the determination of blood sugar and that its hospital use really began about 1913, Osler was ahead of his time in referring to hyperglycemia, briefly as this is done. He mentions a glucose tolerance test based on the production of glycosuria but says nothing of the blood sugar curves used today and, of course, nothing of steroid-enforced tolerance tests. In connection with acidosis, there is no mention of CO_2, pH, blood urea nitrogen, or electrolytes. The tests for ketone bodies in blood and urine have been improved. At the

196

same time, one may regret the modern neglect of quantitative urinary glucose determination in the diagnosis and management of this condition. Only such medical history will remind us that the diabetic can excrete more than 200 grams a day of β-oxybutyric acid or 632 grams of sugar in 12 liters of urine (Chart XV of the 7th edition; see page 193).

Under morbid anatomy, one sees several remarkable statements. "R. T. Williamson has found changes in the posterior columns of the cord similar to those which occur in pernicious anaemia," is as up-to-date as Greenbaum and colleagues. Pathology of the islands is recognized. After 50 years of study, many investigators agree with Ogilvie that "every pancreas from established diabetic subjects will show detectable changes of one order or another." Finally, "a hyaline change occurs in the tubal epithelium . . . and *also in the capillary vessels of the tufts.*" The italics are added to this quotation of Osler whose informal observation antedates Kimmelstiel and Wilson by 25 years.

Under complications, infections and coma were more conspicuous than they are today. However, the definite recognition of retinopathy, albuminuria, neuropathy, and gangrene is noteworthy. In 1909 the diabetic vascular complications were not the result of immune reactions to exogenous insulin, and the severity of neuropathy was striking.

The treatment was the best of that era. The *measured* von Noorden diet (P = 176; F = 155; C = 15 grams by current evaluation) and the reduction of glycosuria which it might produce (Chart XV of the 7th edition; see page 193) are still instructive. But five years before the "Allen era" (1914–1922) caloric restriction was not featured as it now is. The statement, "It is well to study accurately the dietetic capabilities of each case," is advice which is all too neglected today. Medicinal treatment "is most unsatisfactory," and this judgment has been confirmed many times with great waste of time and money on empirical remedies since 1909. The use of sodium bicarbonate in coma still stands as an adjunct to treatment with insulin.

It is clear that Osler craved insulin and a better knowledge of metabolism. Fifty-eight years later, endowed with insulin and refined blood chemistry, we too are groping for better objectives and clearer criteria in the care of diabetes. It is evident that no single blood chemical determination now available measures the fully effective action of insulin, which is probably the desideratum of treatment. Modern methods and the ancient wisdom of Osler should be a good combination with which to face the future.

Francis D. W. Lukens

197

Diabetes mellitus

REFERENCES

Greenbaum, D., Richardson, P.C., Salmon, M.V., and Urich, H. Pathological observations on six cases of diabetic neuropathy. Brain, 87:201, 1964.

Joslin, E.P., Root, H.F., White, P., and Marble, A. The Treatment of Diabetes Mellitus, 10th ed. Philadelphia, Lea & Febiger, 1959.

Kimmelstiel, P., and Wilson, C. Intercapillary lesions in the glomeruli of the kidney. Amer. J. Path., 12:83, 1936.

Ogilvie, R.F. *In* Aetiology of Diabetes Mellitus and Its Complications, Ciba Foundation Colloquia on Endocrinology, Boston, Little, Brown and Company, 1964, Vol. 15, p. 67.

Peters, J.P., and Van Slyke, D.D. Quantitative Clinical Chemistry. Interpretations, Baltimore, The Williams & Wilkins Co., 1946, Vol. 1, p. 159.

Williams, R.H. Recent advances relative to diabetes mellitus. Ann. Intern. Med. 63:512, 1965.

There is an instance on record of a congenital malformation of the thoracic duct, in which the receptaculum formed a flattened cyst which discharged into the peritonæum, and a chylous ascitic fluid was withdrawn on several occasions. Homans, of Boston, reports an extraordinary case of a girl, who from the third to the thirteenth year had an enlarged abdomen. Laparotomy showed a series of cysts containing clear fluid. They were supposed to be dilated lymph vessels connected with the intestines.

(5) **Cysts of the Mesentery.**—Much attention has been directed of late years to the occurrence of mesenteric cysts, and the literature which is fully given by Dowd (Annals of Surgery, vol. xxxii) is already extensive. They may be either dermoid, hydatid, serous, sanguineous, or chylous. They occur at any portion of the mesentery, and range from a few inches in diameter to large masses occupying the entire abdomen. They are frequently adherent to the neighboring organs, to the liver, spleen, uterus, and sigmoid flexure.

The symptoms usually are those of a progressively enlarging tumor in the abdomen. Sometimes a mass develops rapidly, particularly in the hæmorrhagic forms. Colic and constipation are present in some cases. The general health, as a rule, is well maintained in spite of the progressive enlargement of the abdomen, which is most prominent in the umbilical region. Mesenteric cysts may persist for many years, even ten or twenty.

The diagnosis is extremely uncertain, and no single feature is in any way distinctive. Augagneur gives three important signs: the great mobility, the situation in the middle line, and the zone of tympany in front of the tumor. Of these, the second is the only one which is at all constant, as when the tumors are large the mobility disappears, and at this stage the intestines, too, are pushed to one side. It is most frequently mistaken for ovarian tumor. Movable kidney, hydronephrosis, and cysts of the omentum have also been confused with it. In certain instances puncture may be made for diagnostic purposes, but it is better to advise laparotomy for the purpose of drainage, or, if possible, enucleation may be practised.

H. DISEASES OF THE LIVER.

I. JAUNDICE (Icterus).

Definition.—Jaundice or icterus is a condition characterized by coloration of the skin, mucous membranes, and fluids of the body by the bile-pigment.

Like albuminuria, jaundice is a symptom and not a disease, and is met with in a variety of conditions.

For a full consideration of the theories of jaundice the reader is referred to William Hunter's article in Allbutt's System of Medicine. The cases with icterus may be divided into three great groups.

1. OBSTRUCTIVE JAUNDICE.

The following classification of the causes of obstructive jaundice is given by Murchison: (1) Obstruction by foreign bodies within the ducts, as gall-stones and parasites; (2) by inflammatory tumefaction of the duodenum or of the lining membrane of the duct; (3) by stricture or obliteration of the duct; (4) by tumors closing the orifice of the duct or growing in its interior; (5) by pressure on the duct from without, as by tumors of the liver itself, of the stomach, pancreas, kidney, or omentum; by pressure of enlarged glands in the fissures of the liver, and, more rarely, of abdominal aneurism, fæcal accumulation, or the pregnant uterus.

According to Rolleston, in these cases of extra-hepatic or obstructive jaundice the pressure within the biliary capillaries, usually low, becomes increased and the bile is absorbed by the lymphatics of the liver and not by the blood capillaries.

To these causes some add lowering of the blood pressure in the portal system so that the tension in the smaller bile-ducts is greater than in the bloodvessels. For this view, however, there is no positive evidence. In this class may perhaps be placed the cases of jaundice from mental shock or depressed emotions, which "may conceivably cause spasm and reversed peristalsis of the bile-duct" (W. Hunter).

GENERAL SYMPTOMS OF OBSTRUCTIVE JAUNDICE.—(1) *Icterus, or tinting of the skin and conjunctivæ.* The color ranges from a lemon-yellow in catarrhal jaundice to a deep olive-green or bronzed hue in permanent obstruction. In some instances the color of the skin is greenish black, the so-called "black jaundice." Except the central nervous system, the tissues are all stained.

(2) In the more chronic forms *pruritus* is a most distressing symptom. There is a curious preicteric itching, which Riessman thinks is suggestive of cancer, but I have seen it most marked in gall-stone cases. Sweating is common, and may be curiously localized to the abdomen or to the palms of the hands. Lichen, urticaria, and boils may occur. *Xanthoma multiplex* is rare. Only two cases have occurred under my observation. Usually in the flat form, rarely nodular, they are most common in the eyelids and on the hands and feet. They may be very numerous over the whole body. Occasionally the tumors are found in the bile duct. After persisting for years they may disappear. In very chronic cases telangiectases develop in the skin, sometimes in large numbers over the body and face, occasionally on the mucous membrane of the tongue and lips, forming patches of a bright red color from 1 to 2 cm. in breadth.

(3) The *secretions* are colored with bile-pigment. The sweat tinges the linen; the tears and saliva and milk are rarely stained. The expectoration is not often tinted unless there is inflammation, as when pneumonia coexists with jaundice. The urine may contain the pigment before it is apparent in the skin or conjunctiva. The color varies from light greenish yellow to a deep black-green. Gmelin's test is made by allowing five or six drops of urine and a similar amount of common nitric acid to flow together slowly on the flat surface of a white plate. A play of colors is produced—various shades of green, yellow, violet, and red. In cases of jaundice of long standing or great intensity the urine usually contains albumin and always bile-stained tube-casts.

(4) *No bile passes into the intestine.* The stools therefore are of a pale drab or slate-gray color, and usually very fetid and pasty. The "clay-color" of the stools is also in part due to the presence of undigested fat which,

according to Müller, may be increased from 7 to 10 per cent, which is normal, to 55 or 78.5 per cent. There may be constipation; in many instances, owing to decomposition, there is diarrhœa.

(5) *Slow pulse.* The heart's action may fall to 40, 30, or even to 20 per minute. It is particularly noticeable in the cases of catarrhal and recent jaundice, and is not as a rule an unfavorable symptom. This bradycardia has been ascribed to the inhibitory action of the bile salts on the cardiac ganglia. It occurs only in the early stages of jaundice. At this time bile acids pass into the blood, but are produced in very small quantities when jaundice is established. The respirations may fall to 10 or even to 7 per minute. Xanthopsia, or yellow vision, may occur.

(6) *Hæmorrhage.* The tendency to bleeding in chronic icterus is a serious feature in some cases. It has been shown that the blood-coagulation time may be much retarded, and instead of from three minutes and a half to four minutes and a half we have found it in some cases as late as eleven or twelve minutes. This is a point which should be taken account of by surgeons, inasmuch as incontrollable hæmorrhage is a well-recognized accident in operating upon patients with chronic obstructive jaundice. Purpura, large subcutaneous extravasations, more rarely hæmorrhages from the mucous membranes, occur in protracted jaundice, and in the more severe forms.

(7) *Cerebral symptoms.* Irritability, great depression of spirits, or even melancholia may be present. In any case of persistent jaundice special nervous phenomena may develop and rapidly prove fatal—such as sudden coma, acute delirium, or convulsions. Usually the patient has a rapid pulse, slight fever, and a dry tongue, and he passes into the so-called "typhoid state." These features are not nearly so common in obstructive as in febrile jaundice, but they not infrequently terminate a chronic icterus in whatever way produced. The group of symptoms has been termed *cholæmia* or, on the supposition that cholesterin is the poison, *cholesteræmia;* but its true nature has not yet been determined. In some of the cases the symptoms may be due to uræmia.

2. Toxæmic and Hæmolytic Jaundice.

The term hæmatogenous jaundice was formerly applied to this group in contradistinction to the hepatogenous jaundice, associated with manifest obstructive changes in the bile-passages. The toxic jaundice cases are essentially obstructive in origin, and it is doubtful whether there are any true non-obstructive cases. The manner in which the jaundice is produced in these cases has been experimentally worked out by Stadelmann and Afanassiew. The obstruction is due to the extreme viscidity of the bile associated with a mild angiocolitis. The sequence of events is as follows: Destruction of blood by hæmolysis; liberation of hæmoglobin with increased formation and excretion of bile pigments (polychromia); increased viscidity of the bile, which, at the low pressure at which the bile is excreted, causes a temporary obstruction, with reabsorption of the bile and jaundice; finally, as the drug exhausts itself, the bile loses its viscid character, the flow is re-established, and the jaundice disappears. Stadelmann found that a similar explanation applies to other varieties of jaundice associated with increased blood destruction. To show that the blood and liver both play a part in the production of the jaundice, Afanassiew has suggested the name " hæmohepatogenous " jaundice. Rolleston refers to them as cases of " intrahepatic " jaundice. Hunter groups the causes as follows: 1. Jaundice produced by the action of poisons, such as toluylendiamin, phosphorus, arsenic, snake-venom. 2. Jaundice met with in various specific fevers and conditions, such as yellow fever, malaria (remittent and intermittent), pyæmia, relapsing fever, typhus, enteric fever, scarlatina. 3. Jaundice met with in various conditions of unknown but more or less obscure infective nature, and variously designated as epidemic, infectious, febrile, malignant jaundice, icterus gravis, Weil's disease, acute yellow atrophy.

The symptoms are not nearly so striking as in the obstructive variety. The bile is present in the stools. The skin has in many cases only a light lemon tint. The urine may contain no bile-pigment, but the urinary pigments are considerably increased. In the severer forms, as in acute yellow atrophy, the color may be more intense, but in malaria and pernicious anæmia the tint is usually light. The constitutional disturbance may be very profound, with high fever, delirium, convulsions, suppression of urine, black vomit, and cutaneous hæmorrhages. In certain cases of hæmolytic jaundice the fragility of the red corpuscles is greatly increased and they may be smaller than normal (Widal, Chauffard) and show granular degeneration. This is particularly the case in the group of congenital icterus with enlarged spleen.

3. Hereditary Icterus.

A family form of icterus has long been known. We must recognize, indeed, several groups. First, icterus neonatorum, the remarkable instance described by Glaister (Lancet, March, 1879), in which a woman had eight children, six of whom died of jaundice shortly after birth; one of the cases had stenosis of the common duct, which, as John Thomson has shown, is, with angiocholitis, a common lesion in this affection. Still more remarkable is it that the mother of the woman had twelve children, all of whom were icteric after birth, but the jaundice gradually disappeared. A brother of the woman had several children who also were jaundiced at birth. Glaister states that all of the children of Morgagni, fifteen in number, had icterus neonatorum. Secondly, the congenital acholuric icterus. Minkowski reported eight cases in three generations. The jaundice is slight, the stools are not clay colored, the urine has no bile pigment but contains urobilin, the general health is little if at all disturbed. Splenic enlargement is a marked feature. Many cases have now been reported of this Minkowski type, nearly all in family groups, but Chauffard has met with a case without hereditary basis and I have seen at least one case of the kind. In the only autopsy so far reported no special changes were found in the liver or bile passages. Thirdly, a group of cases with enlargement of the spleen and liver and marked constitutional disturbances, dwarfing of stature, infantilism, slight jaundice, cases which have been described as Hanot's cirrhosis, have occurred in two or three members of a family, and the jaundice has dated from early childhood.

In connection with the various fevers, malaria, yellow fever, and Weil's disease jaundice has been described. Two special affections may here receive consideration, the icterus of the new-born and acute yellow atrophy.

202

II. ICTERUS NEONATORUM.

New-born infants are liable to jaundice, which in some instances rapidly proves fatal.   A mild and a severe form may be recognized.

The *mild or physiological icterus* of the new-born is a common disease in foundling hospitals, and is not very infrequent in private practice.   In 900 consecutive births at the Sloane Maternity, icterus was noted in 300 cases (Holt).   The discoloration appears early, usually on the first or second day, and is of moderate intensity.   The urine may be bile-stained and the fæces colorless.   The nutrition of the child is not usually disturbed, and in the majority of cases the jaundice disappears within two weeks.   This form is never fatal.   The cause of this jaundice is not at all clear.   Some have attributed it to stasis in the smaller bile-ducts, which are compressed by the distended radicals of the portal vein.   Others hold that the jaundice is due to the destruction of a large number of red blood-corpuscles during the first few days after birth.

The *severe form* of icterus in the new-born may depend upon (*a*) congenital absence of the common or hepatic duct, of which there are several instances on record; (*b*) congenital syphilitic hepatitis; and (*c*) septic poisoning, associated with phlebitis of the umbilical vein.   This is a severe and fatal form, in which also hæmorrhage from the cord may occur.

Curiously enough, in contradistinction to other forms, the brain and cord may be stained yellow in icterus neonatorum, sometimes diffusely, more rarely in definite foci corresponding to the ganglion cells which have become deeply stained (Schmorl).

III. ACUTE YELLOW ATROPHY.

(Malignant Jaundice; Icterus Gravis.)

Definition.—Jaundice associated with marked cerebral symptoms and characterized anatomically by extensive necrosis of the liver-cells with reduction in volume of the organ.

Etiology.—This is a rare disease.   The first authentic description of a case was by Ballonius, who died in 1616.   Bright in 1836 described the condition, and gave a good colored drawing of the liver.   Of 18,000 medical patients admitted to the Johns Hopkins Hospital in nearly sixteen years there were only 2 cases, one white and one colored.   Hunter has collected only 50 cases between 1880 and 1894 (inclusive), which brings up the total number of recorded cases to about 250.   On the other hand, a physician may see several cases within a few years, or even within a few months, as happened to Reiss, who saw five cases within three months at the Charité, in Berlin.   The disease seems to be rare in the United States.   It is more common in women than in men.   Of the 100 cases collected by Legg, 69 were in females; and of Thierfelder's 143 cases, 88 were in women.   There is a remarkable association between the disease and pregnancy, which was present in 25 of the 69 women in Legg's statistics, and in 33 of the 88 women in Thierfelder's collection.   This fact probably explains its prevalence in women.   It is most common between the ages of twenty and thirty, but has been met with as early as the fourth day and the tenth month. Rolleston has collected 22 cases occurring in the first decade. It has followed fright or profound mental emotion. In hypertrophic cirrhosis the symptoms of a profound icterus gravis may develop, with all the clinical features of acute yellow atrophy, including the presence of leucin and tyrosin in the urine, and convulsions. Though the symptoms produced by phosphorus poisoning closely simulate those of acute yellow atrophy, the two conditions are not identical. Acute yellow atrophy occasionally occurs in syphilis. This happens oftener in women than in men. The disease has followed a drinking bout. Various organisms, most frequently the colon bacillus, have been found in the liver, but possess no causal relationship to the disease.

Morbid Anatomy.—The liver is greatly reduced in size, looks thin and flattened, and sometimes does not reach more than one-half or even one-third of its normal weight. It is flabby and the capsule is wrinkled. Externally the organ has a greenish-yellow color. On section the color may be yellowish-brown, yellowish-red, or mottled, and the outlines of the lobules are indistinct. The yellow and dark-red portions represent different stages of the same process—the yellow an earlier, the red a more advanced stage. The organ may cut with considerable firmness. Microscopically the liver-cells are seen in all stages of necrosis, and in spots appear to have undergone complete destruction, leaving a fatty, granular *débris* with pigment grains and crystals of leucin and tyrosin. Hæmorrhages occur between the liver-cells. There is a cholangitis of the smaller bile-ducts. Marchand, MacCallum, and others have described regenerative changes in the cases which do not run an acute course. Regeneration occurs in two ways: (1) From hyperplasia of pre-existing liver-cells. Mitotic figures may be seen and the regeneration of the liver-cells leads to the production of hyperplastic or " œdematous " nodules in the liver, which project above the surface of the surrounding parts. (2) From hyperplasia of the interlobular bile-ducts by means of which cells approaching liver-cells are produced. The bile-ducts and gall-bladder are empty. Hunter concludes that it is a toxæmic catarrh of the finer bile-ducts, similar to that which is found after poisoning by toluylendiamin or phosphorus.

The other organs show extensive bile-staining, and there are numerous hæmorrhages. The kidneys may show marked granular degeneration of the epithelium, and usually there is fatty degeneration of the heart. In a majority of the cases the spleen is enlarged.

Symptoms.—In the initial stage there is a gastro-duodenal catarrh, and at first the jaundice is thought to be of a simple nature. In some instances this lasts only a few days, in others two or three weeks. Then severe symptoms set in—headache, delirium, trembling of the muscles, and, in some instances, convulsions. Vomiting is a constant symptom, and blood may be brought up. Hæmorrhages occur into the skin or from the mucous surfaces; in pregnant women abortion may occur. With the development of the head symptoms the jaundice usually increases. Coma sets in and gradually deepens until death. The body temperature is variable; in a majority of the cases the disease runs an afebrile course, though sometimes just before death there is an elevation. In some instances, however, there has been marked pyrexia. The pulse is usually rapid, the tongue coated and dry, and the patient is in a " typhoid state." There may be an entire obliteration of the liver dulness.

This is due to the flabby organ falling away from the abdominal walls and allowing the intestinal coils to take its place.

The urine is bile-stained and often contains tube-casts. Frequently albuminuria and occasionally albumosuria occur. Urea is markedly diminished. There is a corresponding increase in the percentage of nitrogen present as ammonia. Herter finds it may be increased from the normal 2 to 5 per cent up to 17 per cent. The diminution in urea is probably partly due to the liver-cells failing to manufacture urea from ammonia, but it may also be in part due to organic acids seizing on the ammonia, and thus preventing the formation of urea out of the basic ammonia. Leucin and tyrosin are not constantly present; of 23 cases collected by Hunter, in 9 neither was found; in 10 both were present; in 3 tyrosin only; in 1 leucin only. The leucin occurs as rounded disks, the tyrosin in needle-shaped crystals, arranged either in bundles or in groups. The tyrosin may sometimes be seen in the urine sediment, but it is best first to evaporate a few drops of urine on a cover-glass. The present view is that the leucin and tyrosin are derived from the liver-cells themselves as a result of their extensive destruction. In the majority of cases no bile enters the intestines, and the stools are clay-colored. The disease is almost invariably fatal. In a few instances recovery has been noted. I saw in Leube's clinic, at Würzburg, a case which was convalescent. In 1897 Legg gave a list of 28 cases of reputed recoveries.

Diagnosis.—Jaundice with vomiting, diminution of the liver volume, delirium, and the presence of leucin and tyrosin in the urine, form a characteristic and unmistakable group of symptoms. Leucin and tyrosin are not, however, distinctive. They may be present in cases of afebrile jaundice with slight enlargement of the liver.

It is not to be forgotten that any severe jaundice may be associated with intense cerebral symptoms. The clinical features in certain cases of hypertrophic cirrhosis are almost identical, but the enlargement of the liver, the more constant occurrence of fever, and the absence of leucin and tyrosin are distinguishing signs. Phosphorus poisoning may closely simulate acute yellow atrophy, particularly in the hæmorrhages, jaundice, and the diminution in the liver volume, but the gastric symptoms are usually more marked, and leucin and tyrosin are stated not to occur in the urine.

Treatment.—No known remedies have any influence on the course of the disease. Theoretically, efforts should be made to eliminate the toxins before they produce their degenerative effects by free purgation and the use of subcutaneous and intravenous saline injections. Gastric sedatives may be used to allay the distressing vomiting.

IV. AFFECTIONS OF THE BLOOD-VESSELS OF THE LIVER.

(1) **Anæmia.**—On the post-mortem table, when the liver looks anæmic, as in the fatty or amyloid organ, the blood-vessels, which during life were probably well filled, can be readily injected. There are no symptoms indicative of this condition.

(2) **Hyperæmia.**—This occurs in two forms. (a) ACTIVE HYPERÆMIA. After each meal the rapid absorption by the portal vessels induces transient

congestion of the organ, which, however, is entirely physiological; but it is quite possible that in persons who persistently eat and drink too much this active hyperæmia may lead to functional disturbance or, in the case of drinking too freely of alcohol, to organic change. In the acute fevers an acute hyperæmia may be present.

The *symptoms* of active hyperæmia are indefinite. Possibly the sense of distress or fulness in the right hypochondrium, so often mentioned by dyspeptics and by those who eat and drink freely, may be due to this cause. There are probably diurnal variations in the volume of the liver. In cirrhosis with enlargement the rapid reduction in volume after a copious hæmorrhage indicates the important part which hyperæmia plays even in organic troubles. It is stated that suppression of the menses or suppression of a hæmorrhoidal flow is followed by hyperæmia of the liver. Andrew H. Smith has described a case of periodical enlargement of the liver.

(*b*) PASSIVE CONGESTION.—This is much more common and results from an increase of pressure in the efferent vessels or sub-lobular branches of the hepatic veins. Every condition leading to venous stasis in the right heart at once affects these veins.

In chronic valvular disease, in emphysema, cirrhosis of the lung, and in intrathoracic tumors mechanical congestion occurs and finally leads to very definite changes. The liver is enlarged, firm, and of a deep-red color; the hepatic vessels are greatly engorged, particularly the central vein in each lobule and its adjacent capillaries. On section the organ presents a peculiar mottled appearance, owing to the deeply congested hepatic and the anæmic portal territories; hence the term *nutmeg* which has been given to this condition. Gradually the distention of the central capillaries reaches such a grade that atrophy of the intervening liver-cells is induced. Brown pigment is deposited about the centre of the lobules and the connective tissue is greatly increased. In this cyanotic induration or cardiac liver the organ is large in the early stage, but later it may become contracted. Occasionally in this form the connective tissue is increased about the lobules as well, but the process usually extends from the sub-lobular and central veins.

The symptoms of this form are not always to be separated from those of the associated conditions. Gastro-intestinal catarrh is usually present and hæmatemesis may occur. The portal obstruction in advanced cases leads to ascites, which may precede the development of general dropsy. There is often slight jaundice, the stools may be clay-colored, and the urine contains bile-pigment.

On examination the organ is found to be increased in size. It may be a full hand's breadth below the costal margin and tender on pressure. It is in this condition particularly that we meet with pulsation of the liver. We must distinguish the communicated throbbing of the heart, which is very common, from the heaving, diffuse impulse due to regurgitation into the hepatic veins, in which, when one hand is upon the ensiform cartilage and the other upon the right side at the margin of the ribs, the whole liver can be felt to dilate with each impulse.

The indications for *treatment* in passive hyperæmia are to restore the balance of the circulation and to unload the engorged portal vessels. In cases of intense hyperæmia 18 or 20 ounces of blood may be directly aspirated from the liver, as advised by George Harley and practised by many Anglo-Indian physicians.   Good results sometimes follow this hepato-phlebotomy.   The prompt relief and marked reduction in the volume of the organ which follow an attack of hæmatemesis or bleeding from piles suggests this practice.   Salts administered by Matthew Hay's method deplete the portal system freely and thoroughly.   As a rule, the treatment must be that of the condition with which it is associated.

(3) **Diseases of the Portal Vein.**—(*a*) THROMBOSIS; ADHESIVE PYLE-PHLEBITIS.—Coagulation of blood in the portal vein is met with in cirrhosis, in syphilis of the liver, invasion of the vein by cancer, proliferative perito-nitis involving the gastro-hepatic omentum, perforation of the vein by gall-stones, and occasionally follows sclerosis of the walls of the portal vein or of its branches (Borrmann).   In rare instances a complete collateral circula-tion is established, the thrombus undergoes the usual changes, and ultimately the vein is represented by a fibrous cord, a condition which has been called *pylephlebitis adhesiva.*   In a case of this kind which I dissected the portal vein was represented by a narrow fibrous cord; the collateral circulation, which must have been completely established for years, ultimately failed, ascites and hæmatemesis supervened and rapidly proved fatal.   The diagnosis of obstruc-tion of the portal vein can rarely be made.   A suggestive symptom, however, is a *sudden* onset of the most intense engorgement of the branches of the portal system, leading to hæmatemesis, melæna, ascites, and swelling of the spleen.

Infarcts are not common in the liver and may be either anæmic or hæmor-rhagic.   They are met with in obstruction of the portal vessels, or of the portal and hepatic veins at the same time, occasionally in disease of the hepatic artery.

(*b*) SUPPURATIVE PYLEPHLEBITIS will be considered in the section on abscess.

(4) **Affections of the hepatic vein** are extremely rare.   Dilatation occurs in cases of chronic enlargement of the right heart, from whatever cause pro-duced.   Emboli occasionally pass from the right auricle into the hepatic veins. A rare and unusual event is stenosis of the orifices of the hepatic veins, which I met in a case of fibroid obliteration of the inferior vena cava and which was associated with a greatly enlarged and indurated liver.

(5) **Hepatic Artery.**—Enlargement of this vessel is seen in cases of cir-rhosis of the liver.   It may be the seat of extensive sclerosis.   Aneurism of the hepatic artery is rare, but instances are on record, and will be referred to in the section on arteries.

V. DISEASES OF THE BILE-PASSAGES AND GALL-BLADDER.

I. ACUTE CATARRH OF THE BILE-DUCTS (*Catarrhal Jaundice*).

Definition.—Jaundice due to swelling and obstruction of the terminal por-tion of the common duct.

Etiology.—General catarrhal inflammation of the bile-ducts is usually asso-ciated with gall-stones.   The catarrhal process now under consideration is probably always an extension of a gastro-duodenal catarrh, and the process is most intense in the *pars intestinalis* of the duct, which projects into the duodenum. The mucous membrane is swollen, and a plug of inspissated mucus fills the diverticulum of Vater, and the narrower portion just at the orifice, completely obstructing the outflow of bile. It is not known how wide-spread this catarrh is in the bile-passages, and whether it really passes up the ducts. It would, of course, be possible to have a catarrh of the finer ducts within the liver, which some French writers think may initiate the attack, but the evidence for this is not strong, and it seems more likely that the terminal portion of the duct is always first involved. In the only instance which I have had an opportunity to examine post mortem the orifice was plugged with inspissated mucus, the common and hepatic ducts were slightly distended and contained a bile-tinged, not a clear, mucus, and there were no observable changes in the mucosa of the ducts.

This catarrhal or simple jaundice results from the following causes: (1) Duodenal catarrh, in whatever way produced, most commonly following an attack of indigestion. It is most frequently met with in young persons, but may occur at any age, and may follow not only errors in diet, but also cold, exposure, and malaria, as well as the conditions associated with portal obstruction, chronic heart-disease, and Bright's disease. (2) Emotional disturbances may be followed by jaundice, which is believed to be due to catarrhal swelling. Cases of this kind are rare and the anatomical condition is unknown. (3) Simple or catarrhal jaundice may occur in epidemic form. (4) Catarrhal jaundice is occasionally seen in the infectious fevers, such as pneumonia, and typhoid fever. The nature of acute catarrhal jaundice is still unknown. It may possibly be an acute infection. In favor of this view are the occurrence in epidemic form and the presence of slight fever. The spleen, however, is not often enlarged. In only 4 out of 23 cases was it palpable.

Symptoms.—There may be neither pain nor distress, and the patient's friends may first notice the yellow tint, or the patient himself may observe it in the looking-glass. In other instances there are dyspeptic symptoms and uneasy sensations in the hepatic region or pains in the back and limbs. In the epidemic form, the onset may be more severe, with headache, chill, and vomiting. Fever is rarely present, though the temperature may reach 101°, sometimes 02°. All the signs of obstructive jaundice already mentioned are present, the stools are clay-colored, and the urine contains bile-pigment. The skin has a bright-yellow tint; the greenish, bronzed color is never seen in the simple form. I have once seen spider angiomata on the face in catarrhal jaundice. They disappeared in a few months. The pulse may be normal, but occasionally it is remarkably slow, and may fall to 40 or 30 beats in the minute, and the respirations to as low as 8 per minute. Sleepiness, too, may be present. The liver may be normal in size, but is usually slightly enlarged, and the edge can be felt below the costal margin. Occasionally the enlargement is more marked. As a rule the gall-bladder can not be felt. The spleen may be increased in size. The duration of the disease is from four to eight weeks. There are mild cases in which the jaundice disappears within two weeks; on the other hand, it may persist for three months or even longer. The stools should be carefully watched, for they give the first intimation of removal of the obstruction.

208

Diagnosis.—The diagnosis is rarely difficult. The onset in young, comparatively healthy persons, the moderate grade of icterus, the absence of emaciation or of evidences of cirrhosis or cancer, usually make the diagnosis easy. Cases which persist for two or three months cause uneasiness, as the suspicion is aroused that it may be more than simple catarrh. The absence of pain, the negative character of the physical examination, and the maintenance of the general nutrition are the points in favor of simple jaundice. There are instances in which time alone can determine the true nature of the case. The possibility of Weil's disease must be borne in mind in anomalous types.

Treatment.—As a rule the patient can keep on his feet from the outset. Measures should be used to allay the gastric catarrh, if it is present. A dose of calomel may be given, and the bowels kept open subsequently by salines. The patient should not be violently purged. Bismuth and bicarbonate of soda may be given, and the patient should drink freely of the alkaline mineral waters, of which Vichy is the best. Irrigation of the large bowel with cold water may be practised. The cold is supposed to excite peristalsis of the gall-bladder and ducts, and thus aid in the expulsion of the mucus.

II. Chronic Catarrhal Angiocholitis.

This may possibly occur also as a sequel of the acute catarrh. I have never met with an instance, however, in which a chronic, persistent jaundice could be attributed to this cause. A chronic catarrh always accompanies obstruction in the common duct, whether by gall-stones, malignant disease, stricture, or external pressure. There are two groups of cases:

(1) With Complete Obstruction of the Common Duct.—In this form the bile-passages are greatly dilated, the common duct may reach the size of the thumb or larger, there is usually dilatation of the gall-bladder and of the ducts within the liver. The contents of the ducts and of the gall-bladder are a clear, colorless mucus. The mucosa may be everywhere smooth and not swollen. The clear mucus is usually sterile. The patients are the subjects of chronic jaundice, usually without fever.

(2) With Incomplete Obstruction of the Duct.—There is pressure on the duct or there are gall-stones, single or multiple, in the common duct or in the diverticulum of Vater. The bile-passages are not so much dilated, and the contents are a bile-stained, turbid mucus. The gall-bladder is rarely much dilated. In a majority of all cases stones are found in it.

The symptoms of this type of catarrhal angiocholitis are sometimes very distinctive. With it is associated most frequently the so-called hepatic intermittent fever, recurring attacks of chills, fever, and sweats. We need still further information about the bacteriology of these cases. In all probability the febrile attacks are due distinctly to infection. I can not too strongly emphasize the point that the recurring attacks of intermittent fever do not necessarily mean suppurative angiocholitis. The question will be referred to again under gall-stones.

III. Suppurative and Ulcerative Angiocholitis.

The condition is a diffuse, purulent angiocholitis involving the larger and smaller ducts. In a large proportion of all cases there is associated suppurative disease of the gall-bladder.

209

Etiology.—It is the most serious of the sequels of gall-stones. Occasionally a diffuse suppurative angiocholitis follows the acute infectious cholecystitis; this, however, is rare, since fortunately in the latter condition the cystic duct is usually occluded. Cancer of the duct, foreign bodies, such as lumbricoids or fish bones, are occasional causes. There may be extension from a suppurative pylephlebitis. In rare instances suppurative cholangitis occurs in the acute infections, as pneumonia and influenza.

The common duct is greatly dilated and may reach the size of the index finger or the thumb; the walls are thickened, and there may be fistulous communications with the stomach, colon, or duodenum. The hepatic ducts and their extensions in the liver are dilated and contain pus mixed with bile. On section of the liver small abscesses are seen, which correspond to the dilated suppurating ducts. The gall-bladder is usually distended, full of pus, and with adhesions to the neighboring parts, or it may have perforated.

Symptoms.—The symptoms of suppurative cholangitis are usually very severe. A previous history of gall-stones, the development of a septic fever, the swelling and tenderness of the liver, the enlargement of the gall-bladder, and the leucocytosis are suggestive features. Jaundice is always present, but is variable. In some cases it is very intense, in others it is slight. There may be very little pain. There is progressive emaciation and loss of strength. In a recent case parotitis developed on the left side, which subsided without suppuration.

Ulceration, stricture, perforation, and fistulæ of the bile-passages will be considered with gall-stones.

IV. Acute Infectious Cholecystitis.

Etiology.—Acute inflammation of the gall-bladder is usually due to bacterial invasion, with or without the presence of gall-stones. Three varieties or grades may be recognized: The catarrhal, the suppurative, and the phlegmonous. The condition is very serious, difficult to diagnose, often fatal, and may require for its relief prompt surgical intervention. The cases associated with gall-stones have of course long been recognized, but we now know that an acute infection of the gall-bladder leading to suppuration, gangrene, or perforation is by no means infrequent.

Acute non-calculous cholecystitis is a result of bacterial invasion. The colon bacillus, the typhoid bacillus, the pneumococcus and staphylococci and streptococci have been the organisms most often found. The frequency of gall-bladder infection in the fevers is a point already referred to, particularly in typhoid fever.

Condition of the Gall-bladder.—The organ is usually distended and the walls tense. Adhesions may have formed with the colon or the omentum. In other instances perforation has taken place and there is a localized abscess, or in the more fulminant forms general peritonitis. The contents of the organ are usually dark in color, muco-purulent, purulent, or hæmorrhagic. In the cases with acute phlegmonous inflammation there may be a very foul odor. As Richardson remarks, the cystic duct is often found closed even when no stone is impacted. It should be borne in mind that in the acutely distended gall-bladder the elongation and enlargement may take place chiefly upward and inward, toward the foramen of Winslow.

210

Symptoms.—Severe paroxysmal pain is, as a rule, the first indication, most commonly in the right side of the abdomen in the region of the liver. It may be in the epigastrium or low down in the region of the appendix. "Nausea, vomiting, rise of pulse and temperature, prostration, distention of the abdomen, rigidity, general tenderness becoming localized" usually follow (Richardson). In this form, without gall-stones, jaundice is not often present. The local tenderness is extreme, but it may be deceptive in its situation. Associated probably with the adhesion and inflammatory processes between the gall-bladder and the bowel are the intestinal symptoms, and there may be complete stoppage of gas and fæces; indeed, the operation for acute obstruction has been performed in several cases. The distended gall-bladder may sometimes be felt. As sequels there may be serious distention or empyema.

Diagnosis.—The diagnosis is by no means easy. The symptoms may not indicate the section of the abdomen involved. In two of our cases and in three of Richardson's appendicitis was diagnosed; in two of his cases acute intestinal obstruction was suspected. This was the diagnosis in a case of acute phlegmonous cholecystitis which I reported in 1881. The history of the cases is often a valuable guide. Occurring during the convalescence from typhoid fever, after pneumonia, or in a patient with previous cholecystitis, such a group of symptoms as mentioned would be highly suggestive. The differentiation of the variety of the cholecystitis can not be made. In the acute suppurative and phlegmonous forms the symptoms are usually more severe, perforation is very apt to occur, with local or general peritonitis, and unless operative measures are undertaken death ensues.

There is an acute cholecystitis, probably an infective form, in which the patient has recurring attacks of pain in the region of the gall-bladder. The diagnosis of gall-stones is made, but an operation shows simply an enlarged gall-bladder filled with mucus and bile, and the mucous membrane perhaps swollen and inflamed. In some of these cases gall-stones may have been present and have passed before the operation.

V. Cancer of the Bile-passages.

Females suffer in the proportion of 3 to 1 (Musser), or 4 to 1 (Ames). In cases of primary cancer of the bile-duct, on the other hand, men and women appear to be about equally affected. In Musser's series 65 per cent of the cases occurred between the ages of forty and seventy. The association of malignant disease of the gall-bladder with gall-stones has long been recognized. The fact is well put by Kelynack as follows: "While gall-stones are found in from 6 to 12 per cent of all general cases (that is, coming to autopsy), they occur in association with cancer of the gall-bladder in from 90 to 100 per cent." In Futterer's series calculi were present in 70 per cent.

The exact nature of the association is not very clear, but it is usually regarded as an effect of the chronic irritation. On the other hand, it is urged that the presence of the malignant disease may itself favor the production of gall-stones. Histologically, "carcinoma of the gall-bladder varies much, both in the form of the cells and in their structural arrangement; it may be either columnar or spheroidal-celled" (Rolleston). The fundus is usually first involved in the gall-bladder, and in the ducts the ductus communis choledochus.

211

When the disease involves the *gall-bladder,* a tumor can be detected extending diagonally downward and inward toward the navel, variable in size, occasionally very large, due either to great distention of the gall-bladder or to involvement of contiguous parts. It is usually very firm and hard.

Among the important symptoms are jaundice, which was present in 69 per cent of Musser's cases; pain, often of great severity and paroxysmal in character. The pain and tenderness on pressure persist in the intervals between the paroxysmal attacks. In one of my three cases, which Ames reported, there was a very profound anæmia, but an absence of jaundice throughout. Gall-stones were present in two of the cases, and a history of gall-stone attacks was obtained from the third. When the liver becomes involved the picture is that of carcinoma of the organ.

Primary malignant disease in the *bile-ducts* is less common, and rarely forms tumors that can be felt externally. The tumor is usually in the common duct, 57 of 80 cases collected by Rolleston. Kelynack gives very fully a number of important points in the differential diagnosis between tumors in the duct and tumors in the gall-bladder. There is usually an early, intense, and persistent jaundice. The dilated gall-bladder may rupture. At best the diagnosis is very doubtful, unless cleared up by an exploratory operation. A very interesting form of malignant disease of the ducts is that which involves the diverticulum of Vater. Rolleston has collected 16 cases. An elderly woman was admitted under my care with jaundice of some months' duration, without pain, with progressive emaciation, and a greatly enlarged gall-bladder. My colleague, Halsted, operated and found obstruction at the orifice of the common duct. He opened the duodenum, removed a cylindrical-celled epithelioma of the ampulla of Vater, and stitched the common duct to another portion of the duodenum. The patient made an uninterrupted recovery, and, fourteen weeks after the operation, had gained twenty-five pounds in weight and passed bile with the fæces. A year later death occurred from secondary disease of the head of the pancreas.

VI. Stenosis and Obstruction of the Bile-ducts.

Stenosis.—Stenosis or complete occlusion may follow ulceration, most commonly after the passage of a gall-stone. In these instances the obstruction is usually situated low down in the common duct. Instances are extremely rare. Foreign bodies, such as the seeds of various fruits, may enter the duct, and occasionally round worms crawl into it. Liver-flukes and echinococci are rare causes of obstruction in man.

Obstruction.—Obstruction by *pressure* from without is more frequent. Cancer of the head of the pancreas, less often a chronic interstitial inflammation, may compress the terminal portion of the duct; rarely, cancer of the pylorus. Secondary involvement of the lymph-glands of the liver is a common cause of occlusion of the duct, and is met with in many cases of cancer of the stomach and other abdominal organs. Rare causes of obstruction are aneurism of a branch of the cœliac axis of the aorta, and pressure of very large abdominal tumors.

Symptoms.—The symptoms produced are those of chronic obstructive jaundice. At first, the liver is usually enlarged, but in chronic cases it may be reduced in size, and be found of a deeply bronzed color. The hepatic intermittent fever is not often associated with complete occlusion of the duct from any cause, but it is most frequently met with in chronic obstruction by gall-stones. Permanent occlusion of the duct terminates in death. In a majority of the cases the conditions which lead to the obstruction are in themselves fatal. The liver, which is not necessarily enlarged, presents a moderate grade of cirrhosis. Cases of cicatricial occlusion may last for years. A patient under my care, who was permanently jaundiced for nearly three years, had a fibroid occlusion of the duct.

Diagnosis.—The diagnosis of the nature of the occlusion is often very difficult. A history of colic, jaundice of varying intensity, paroxysms of pain, and intermittent fever points to gall-stones. In cancerous obstruction the tumor mass can sometimes be felt in the epigastric region. In cases in which the lymph-glands in the transverse fissure are cancerous, the primary disease may be in the pelvic organs or the rectum, or there may be a limited cancer of the stomach, which has not given any symptoms. In these cases the examination of the other lymphatic glands may be of value. In a man who came under observation with a jaundice of seven weeks' duration, believed to be catarrhal (as the patient's general condition was good and he was not said to have lost flesh), a small nodular mass was detected at the navel, which on removal proved to be scirrhus. Involvement of the clavicular groups of lymph-glands may also be serviceable in diagnosis. The gall-bladder is usually enlarged in obstruction of the common duct, except in the cases of gall-stones (Courvoisier's law). Great and progressive enlargement of the liver with jaundice and moderate continued fever is more commonly met with in cancer.

Congenital obliteration of the ducts is an interesting condition, of which there are some 60 or 70 cases on record. It may occur in several members of one family. Spontaneous hæmorrhages are frequent, particularly from the navel. The subjects may live for three or even eight weeks. The liver is usually cirrhotic and the spleen is enlarged. Rolleston suggests that the disease is primarily a congenital cirrhosis with consecutive involvement of the ducts. For a recent careful consideration of the subject, see John Thomson's article in Allbutt's System of Medicine.

VI. CHOLELITHIASIS.

No chapter in medicine is more interesting than that which deals with the question of gall-stones. Few affections present so many points for study—chemical, bacteriological, pathological, and clinical. The past few years have seen a great advance in our knowledge in two directions: First, as to the mode of formation of the stones, and, secondly, as to the surgical treatment of the cases. The recent study of the origin of stones dates from Naunyn's work in 1891. Marion Sims's suggestion that gall-stones came within the sphere of the surgeon has been most fruitful.

Origin of Gall-stones.—Two important points with reference to the formation of calculi in the bile-passages were brought out by Naunyn: (*a*) The origin of the cholesterin of the bile, as well as of the lime salts from the mucous membrane of the biliary passages, particularly when inflamed; and (*b*) the remarkable association of micro-organisms with gall-stones. It is stated that Bristowe first noticed the origin of cholesterin in the gall-bladder itself, but Naunyn's observations showed that both the cholesterin and the lime were in great part a production of the mucosa of the gall-bladder and of the bile-ducts, particularly when in a condition of catarrhal inflammation excited by the presence of microbes. According to the views of this author, the lithogenous catarrh (which, by the way, is quite an old idea) modifies materially the chemical constitution of the bile and favors the deposition about epithelial *débris* and bacteria of the insoluble salts of lime in combination with the bilirubin. Welch and others have demonstrated the presence of micro-organisms in the centre of gall-stones. Three additional points of interest may be referred to:

First, the demonstration that the gall-bladder is a peculiarly favorable habitat for micro-organisms. The colon bacilli, staphylococci, streptococci, pneumococci, and the typhoid bacilli have all been found here under varying conditions of the bile. A remarkable fact is the length of time that they may live in the gall-bladder, as was first demonstrated by Blachstein in Welch's laboratory. The typhoid bacillus has been isolated in pure culture seven years after an attack.

Secondly, the experimental production of gall-stones has been successfully accomplished by Gilbert and Fournier by injecting micro-organisms into the gall-bladder of animals.

Thirdly, the association of gall-stones with the specific fevers. Bernheim, in 1889, first called attention to the frequency of gall-stone attacks after typhoid. Since that time Dufort has collected a series of cases, and Chiari, Mason, and Camac have called attention to the great frequency of gall-bladder complications during and after this disease.

While it is probable that a lithogenous catarrh, induced by micro-organisms, is the most important single factor, there are other accessory causes of great moment.

Country.—Gall-stones are less frequent in the United States than in Germany, 6.94 to 12 per cent (Mosher). They are less common in England than on the Continent. Cholelithiasis is found in India.

Age.—Nearly 50 per cent of all the cases occur in persons above forty years of age. They are rare under twenty-five. They have been met with in the new-born, and in infants (John Thomson).

Sex.—Three-fourths of the cases occur in women. Pregnancy has an important influence. Naunyn states that 90 per cent of women with gall-stones have borne children.

All conditions which favor *stagnation of bile* in the gall-bladder predispose to the formation of stones. Among these may be mentioned corset-wearing, enteroptosis, nephroptosis, and occupations requiring a "leaning forward" position. Lack of exercise, sedentary occupations, particularly when combined with over-indulgence in food, constipation, depressing mental emotions are also to be regarded as favoring circumstances. The belief prevailed formerly that there was a lithiac diathesis closely allied to that of gout.

Physical Characters of Gall-stones.—They may be single, in which case the stone is usually ovoid and may attain a very large size. Instances are on record of gall-stones measuring more than 5 inches in length. They may be extremely numerous, ranging from a score to several hundreds or even several

214

thousands, in which case the stones are very small. When moderately numerous, they show signs of mutual pressure and have a polygonal form, with smooth facets; occasionally, however, five or six gall-stones of medium size are met with in the bladder which are round or ovoid and without facets. They are sometimes mulberry-shaped and very dark, consisting largely of bile-pigments. Again there are small, black calculi, rough and irregular in shape, and varying in size from grains of sand to small shot. These are sometimes known as gall-sand. On section, a calculus contains a nucleus, which consists of bile-pigment, rarely a foreign body. The greater portion of the stone is made up of cholesterin, which may form the entire calculus and is arranged in concentric laminæ showing also radiating lines. Salts of lime and magnesia, bile acids, fatty acids, and traces of iron and copper are also found in them. Most gall-stones consist of from 70 to 80 per cent of cholesterin, in either the amorphous or the crystalline form. As above stated, it is sometimes pure, but more commonly it is mixed with the bile-pigment. The outer layer of the stone is usually harder and brownish in color.

The Seat of Formation.—Within the liver itself calculi are occasionally found, but are here usually small and not abundant, and in the form of ovoid, greenish-black grains. A large majority of all calculi are formed within the gall-bladder. The stones in the larger ducts have usually had their origin in the gall-bladder.

Symptoms.—In a majority of the cases, gall-stones cause no symptoms. The gall-bladder will tolerate the presence of large numbers for an indefinite period of time, and post-mortem examinations show that they are present in 25 per cent of all women over sixty years of age (Naunyn). Moynihan claims that in most cases there are early symptoms—a sense of fulness, weight, and oppression in the epigastrium; a catch in the breath, a feeling of faintness or nausea, and a chilliness after eating. Attacks of indigestion are common. I have seen two cases with obstinate attacks of urticaria. I have had many cases in which the most careful inquiry failed to elicit the existence of any symptoms prior to the attack of colic.

The French writers have suggested a useful division, dealing with the main symptoms of cholelithiasis, into (1) the aseptic, mechanical accidents in consequence of migration of the stone or of obstruction, either in the ducts or in the intestines; (2) the septic, infectious accidents, either local (the angiocholitis and cholecystitis with empyema of the gall-bladder, and the fistulæ and abscess of the liver and infection of the neighboring parts) or general, the biliary fever and the secondary visceral lesions.

1. BILIARY COLIC.—Gall-stones may become engaged in the cystic or the common duct without producing pain or severe symptoms. More commonly the passage of a stone excites the violent symptoms known as biliary colic. The attack sets in abruptly with agonizing pain in the right hypochondriac region, which radiates to the shoulder, or is very intense in the epigastric and in the lower thoracic regions. It is often associated with a rigor and a rise in temperature from 102° to 103°. The pain is usually so intense that the patient rolls about in agony. There are vomiting, profuse sweating, and great depression of the circulation. There may be marked tenderness in the region of the liver, which may be enlarged, and the gall-bladder may become palpable and very tender. In other cases the fever is more marked. The spleen is enlarged

215

(Naunyn) and the urine contains albumin with red blood-corpuscles. Ortner holds that *cholecystitis acuta*, occurring in connection with gall-stones, is a septic (bacterial) infection of the bile-passages. The symptoms of acute infectious cholecystitis and those of what we call gall-stone colic are very similar, and surgeons have frequently performed cholecystotomy for the former condition, believing calculi were present. In a large number of the cases jaundice occurs, but it is not a necessary symptom. Of course it does not happen during the passage of the stone through the cystic duct, but only when it becomes lodged in the common duct. The pain is due (*a*) to the slow progress in the cystic duct, in which the stone takes a rotary course owing to the arrangement of the Heisterian valve; the cystic duct is poor in muscle fibres but rich in nerves and ganglia; (*b*) to the acute inflammation which usually accompanies an attack; (*c*) to the stretching and distention of the gall-bladder by retained secretions.

The attack varies in duration. It may last for a few hours, several days, or even a week or more. If the stone becomes impacted in the orifice of the common duct, the jaundice becomes intense; much more commonly it is a slight transient icterus. The attack of colic may be repeated at intervals for some time, but finally the stone passes and the symptoms disappear.

Occasionally accidents occur, such as rupture of the duct with fatal peritonitis. Fatal syncope during an attack, and the occurrence of repeated convulsive seizures have come under my observation. These are, however, rare events. Palpitation and distress about the heart may be present, and occasionally a mitral murmur occurs during the paroxysm, but the cardiac conditions described by some writers as coming on acutely in biliary colic are possibly pre-existent in these patients.

The *diagnosis* of acute hepatic colic is generally easy. The pain is in the upper abdominal and thoracic regions, whereas the pain in nephritic colic is in the lower abdomen. A chill, with fever, is much more frequent in biliary colic than in gastralgia, with which it is liable, at times, to be confounded. A history of previous attacks is an important guide, and the occurrence of jaundice, however slight, determines the diagnosis. To look for the gall-stones, the stools should be thoroughly mixed with water and carefully filtered through a narrow-meshed sieve. Pseudo-biliary colic is not infrequently met with in nervous women, and the diagnosis of gall-stones made. This nervous hepatic colic may be periodical; the pain may be in the right side and radiating; sometimes associated with other nervous phenomena, often excited by emotion, tire, or excesses. The liver may be tender, but there are neither icterus nor inflammatory conditions. The combination of colic and jaundice, so distinctive of gall-stones, is not always present. The pains may be not colicky, but more constant and dragging in character. Of 50 cases operated upon by Riedel, 10 had not had colic, only 14 presented a gall-bladder tumor, while a majority had not had jaundice. A remarkable xanthoma of the bile-passages has been found in association with hepatic colic. I have already spoken of the diagnosis of acute cholecystitis from appendicitis and obstruction of the bowels. Recurring attacks of pain in the region of the liver may follow adhesions between the gall-bladder and adjacent parts.

2. OBSTRUCTION OF THE CYSTIC DUCT.—The effects may be thus enumerated:

216

(*a*) *Dilatation* of the gall-bladder—hydrops vesicæ felleæ. In acute obstruction the contents are bile mixed with much mucus or muco-purulent material. In chronic obstruction the bile is replaced by a clear fluid mucus. This is an important point in diagnosis, particularly as a dropsical gall-bladder may form a very large tumor. The reaction is not always constant. It is either alkaline or neutral; the consistence is thin and mucoid. Albumin is usually present. A dilated gall-bladder may reach an enormous size, and in one instance Tait found it occupying the greater part of the abdomen. In such cases, as is not unnatural, it has been mistaken for an ovarian tumor. I have described a case in which it was attached to the right broad ligament. The dilated gall-bladder can usually be felt below the edge of the liver, and in many instances it has a characteristic outline like a gourd. An enlarged and relaxed organ may not be palpable, and in acute cases the distention may be upward toward the hilus of the liver. The dilated gall-bladder usually projects directly downward, rarely to one side or the other, though occasionally toward the middle line. It may reach below the navel, and in persons with thin walls the outline can be accurately defined. Riedel has called attention to a tongue-like projection of the anterior margin of the right lobe in connection with enlarged gall-bladder. It is to be remembered that distention of the gall-bladder may occur without jaundice; indeed, the greatest enlargement has been met with in such cases.

Gall-stone crepitus may be felt when the bladder is very full of stones and its walls not very tense. It is rarely well felt unless the abdominal walls are much relaxed. It may be found in patients who have never had any symptoms of cholelithiasis.

(*b*) *Acute cholecystitis.* The simple form is common, and to it are due probably very many of the symptoms of the gall-stone attack. Phlegmonous cholecystitis is rare; only seven instances are found in the enormous statistics of Courvoisier. It is, however, much more common than these figures indicate. Perforation may occur with fatal peritonitis.

(*c*) *Suppurative cholecystitis*, empyema of the gall-bladder, is much more common, and in the great majority of cases is associated with gall-stones—41 in 55 cases (Courvoisier). There may be enormous dilatation, and over a litre of pus has been found. Perforation and the formation of abscesses in the neighborhood are not uncommon.

(*d*) *Calcification* of the gall-bladder is commonly a termination of the previous condition. There are two separate forms: incrustation of the mucosa with lime salts and the true infiltration of the wall with lime, the so-called ossification.

(*e*) *Atrophy* of the gall-bladder. This is by no means uncommon. The organ shrinks into a small fibroid mass, not larger, perhaps, than a good-sized pea or walnut, or even has the form of a narrow fibrous string; more commonly the gall-bladder tightly embraces a stone. This condition is usually preceded by hydrops of the bladder.

Occasionally the gall-bladder presents diverticula, which may be cut off from the main portion, and usually contain calculi.

(3) OBSTRUCTION OF THE COMMON DUCT.—There may be a single stone tightly wedged in the duct in any part of its course, or a series of stones, sometimes extending into both hepatic and cystic ducts, or a stone lies in

217

the diverticulum of Vater. There are three groups of cases: (*a*) In rare instances a stone tightly corks the common duct, causing *permanent occlusion;* or it may partly rest in the cystic duct, and may have caused thickening of the junction of the ducts; or a big stone may compress the hepatic or upper part of the common duct. The jaundice is deep and enduring, and there are no septic features. The pains, the previous attacks of colic, and the absence of enlarged gall-bladder help to separate the condition from obstruction by new growths, although it can not be differentiated with certainty. The ducts are usually much dilated and everywhere contain a clear mucoid fluid.

(*b*) *Incomplete obstruction, with infective cholangitis.* There may be a series of stones in the common duct, a single stone which is freely movable, or a stone (ball-valve stone) in the diverticulum of Vater. These conditions may be met with at autopsy, without the subjects having had symptoms pointing to gall-stones; but in a majority of cases there are very characteristic features.

The common duct may be as large as the thumb; the hepatic duct and its branches through the liver may be greatly dilated, and the distention may be even apparent beneath the liver capsule. Great enlargement of the gall-bladder is rarer. The mucous membrane of the ducts is usually smooth and clear, and the contents consist of a thin, slightly turbid bile-stained mucus.

Naunyn has given the following as the distinguishing signs of stone in the common duct: " (1) The continuous or occasional presence of bile in the fæces; (2) distinct variations in the intensity of the jaundice; (3) normal size or only slight enlargement of the liver; (4) absence of distention of the gall-bladder; (5) enlargement of the spleen; (6) absence of ascites; (7) presence of febrile disturbance; and (8) duration of the jaundice for more than a year."

In connection with the ball-valve stone, which is most commonly found in the diverticulum of Vater, though it may be in the common duct itself, there is a special symptom group: (*a*) Ague-like paroxysms, chills, fever, and sweating; the *hepatic intermittent fever* of Charcot; (*b*) jaundice of varying intensity, which persists for months or even years, and deepens after each paroxysm; (*c*) at the time of the paroxysm, pains in the region of the liver with gastric disturbance. These symptoms may continue on and off for three or four years, without the development of suppurative cholangitis. In one of my cases the jaundice and recurring hepatic intermittent fever existed from July, 1879, until August, 1882; the patient recovered and still lives. The condition has lasted from eight months to three years. The rigors are of intense severity, and the temperature rises to 103° or 105°. The chills may recur daily for weeks, and present a tertian or quartan type, so that they are often attributed to malaria, with which, however, they have no connection. The jaundice is variable, and deepens after each paroxysm. The itching may be most intense. Pain, which is sometimes severe and colicky, does not always occur. There may be marked vomiting and nausea. As a rule there is no progressive deterioration of health. In the intervals between the attacks the temperature is normal.

The clinical history and the post-mortem examinations in my cases show conclusively that this condition may persist for years without a trace of suppuration within the ducts. There must, however, be an infection, such as may exist for years in the gall-bladder, without causing suppuration. It is probable that the toxic symptoms develop only when a certain grade of tension is reached.

An interesting and valuable diagnostic point is the absence of dilatation of the gall-bladder in cases of obstruction from stone—Courvoisier's rule. Ecklin, who has recently reviewed this point, finds that of 172 cases of obstruction of the common duct by calculus in 34 the gall-bladder was normal, in 110 it was contracted, and in 28 it was dilated. Of 139 cases of occlusion of the common duct from other causes the gall-bladder was normal in 9, shrunken in 9, and dilated in 121.

(*c*) *Incomplete obstruction, with suppurative cholangitis.* When suppurative cholangitis exists the mucosa is thickened, often eroded or ulcerated; there may be extensive suppuration in the ducts throughout the liver, and even empyema of the gall-bladder. Occasionally the suppuration extends beyond the ducts, and there is localized liver abscess, or there is perforation of the gall-bladder with the formation of abscess between the liver and stomach.

Clinically it is characterized by a fever which may be intermittent, but more commonly is remittent and without prolonged intervals of apyrexia. The jaundice is rarely so intense, nor do we see the deepening of the color after the paroxysms. There is usually greater enlargement of the liver, and tenderness and more definite signs of septicæmia. The cases run a shorter course, and recovery never takes place.

(4) THE MORE REMOTE EFFECTS OF GALL-STONES.—(*a*) *Biliary Fistulæ.* These are not uncommon. There may, for instance, be abnormal communication between the gall-bladder and the hepatic duct or the gall-bladder and a cavity in the liver itself. More rarely perforation occurs between the common duct and the portal vein. Of this there are at least four instances on record, among them the celebrated case of Ignatius Loyola. Perforation into the abdominal cavity is not uncommon; 119 cases exist in the literature (Courvoisier), in 70 of which the rupture occurred directly into the peritoneal cavity; in 49 there was an encapsulated abscess. Perforation may take place from an intrahepatic branch or from the hepatic, common, or cystic ducts. Perforation from the gall-bladder is the most common.

Fistulous communications between the bile-passages and the gastro-intestinal canal are frequent. Openings into the stomach are rare. Between the duodenum and bile-passages they are much more common. Courvoisier has collected 10 instances of communication between the ductus communis and the duodenum, and 73 cases between the gall-bladder and the duodenum. Communication with the ileum and jejunum is extremely rare. Of fistulous opening into the colon 39 cases are on record. These communications can rarely be diagnosed; they may be present without any symptoms whatever. It is probably by ulceration into the duodenum or colon that the large gall-stones escape.

Occasionally the urinary passages may be opened into and the stones may be found in the bladder. Many instances are on record of fistulæ between the bile-passages and the lungs. Courvoisier has collected 24 cases, to which list J. E. Graham has added 10, including 2 cases of his own. (Trans. of Assoc. of Am. Physicians, xiii.) Bile may be coughed up with the expectoration, sometimes in considerable quantities.

Of all fistulous communications the external or cutaneous is the most common. Courvoisier's statistics number 184 cases, in 50 per cent of which the perforation took place in the right hypochondrium; in 29 per cent in the region of the navel. The number of stones discharged varied from one or two to many hundreds. Recovery took place in 78 cases; some with, some without operation.

(*b*) *Obstruction of the Bowel by Gall-stones.*—Reference has already been made to this; its frequency appears from the fact that of 295 cases of obstruction, occurring during eight years, analyzed by Fitz, 23 were by gall-stone. Courvoisier's statistics give a total number of 131 cases, in 6 of which the calculi had a peculiar situation, as in a diverticulum or in the appendix. Of the remaining 125 cases, in 70 the stone was spontaneously passed, usually with severe symptoms. The post-mortem reports show that in some of these cases even very large stones have passed *per viam naturalem*, as the gall-duct has been enormously distended, its orifice admitting the finger freely. This, however, is extremely rare. The stones have been found most commonly in the ileum.

Treatment of Gall-stones and their Effects.—In an attack of biliary colic the patient should be kept under morphia, given hypodermically, in quarter-grain doses. In an agonizing paroxysm it is well to give a whiff or two of chloroform until the morphia has had time to act. Great relief is experienced from the hot bath and from fomentations in the region of the liver. The patient should be given laxatives and should drink copiously of alkaline mineral waters. Olive oil has proved useless in my hands. When taken in large quantities, fatty concretions are passed with the stools, which have been regarded as calculi; and concretions due to eating pears have been also mistaken, particularly when associated with colic attacks. Since the days of Durande, whose mixture of ether and turpentine is still largely used in France, various remedies have been advised to dissolve the stones within the gall-bladder, none of which are efficacious.

The diet should be regulated, the patient should take regular exercise and avoid, as much as possible, the starchy and saccharine foods. The soda salts recommended by Prout are believed to prevent the concentration of the bile and the formation of gall-stones. Either the sulphate or the phosphate may be taken in doses of from 1 to 2 drachms daily. For the intolerable itching McCall Anderson's dusting powder may be used: starch, an ounce; camphor, a drachm and a half; and oxide of zinc, half an ounce. Some of this should be finely dusted over the skin with a powder-puff. Powdering with starch, strong alkaline baths (hot), pilocarpin hypodermically (gr. $\frac{1}{8}$–$\frac{1}{6}$), and antipyrin (gr. viij), may be tried. Ichthyol and lanolin ointment sometimes gives relief.

Exploratory puncture, as practised by the elder Pepper, in 1857, in a case of empyema of the gall-bladder, and by Bartholow in 1878 is not now often done. Aspiration is usually a safe procedure, though a fatal result has followed.

The surgical treatment of gall-stones has of late years made rapid progress. The operation of cholecystotomy, or opening the gall-bladder and removing the stones, which was advised by Sims, has been remarkably successful. The removal of the gall-bladder, cholecystectomy, has also been practised with success. The indications for operation are: (*a*) Repeated attacks of gall-stone

220

colic. The operation is now attended with such slight risk that the patient is much safer in the hands of a surgeon than when left to Nature, with the feeble assistance of drugs and mineral waters. (*b*) The presence of a distended gall-bladder, associated with attacks of pain or with fever. (*c*) When a gall-stone is permanently lodged in the common duct, and the group of symptoms above described are present, the question, then, of advising operation depends largely upon the personal methods and success of the surgeon who is available.

In 1,000 consecutive operations for gall-stone disease the brothers Mayo, of Rochester, Minn., had 50 deaths, 5 per cent. In 673 cases of cholecystotomy the mortality was only 2.4 per cent. In 186 cholecystectomies the mortality was 4.3 per cent. In 137 operations for stone in the common duct the mortality was 11 per cent.

VII. THE CIRRHOSES OF THE LIVER.

General Considerations.—The many forms of cirrhoses of the liver have one feature in common—an increase in the connective tissue of the organ. In fact, we use the term cirrhosis (by which Laennec characterized the tawny, yellow color of the common atrophic form) to indicate similar changes in other organs.

The cirrhoses may be classified, etiologically, according to the supposed causation; anatomically, according to the structure primarily involved; or clinically, according to certain special symptoms.

Etiological Classification.—1. *Toxic Cirrhosis.*—Alcohol is the chief cause of cirrhosis of the liver. Other poisons, such as lead and the toxic products of faulty metabolism in gout, diabetes, rickets, and indigestion, play a minor *rôle.*

2. *Infectious Cirrhoses.*—With many of the specific fevers necrotic changes occur in the liver which, when wide-spread, may be followed by cirrhosis. Possibly the hypertrophic cirrhosis of Hanot and other forms met with in early life are due to infection. The malarial cirrhosis is a well-recognized variety. The syphilitic poison produces a very characteristic form.

3. *Cirrhosis from chronic congestion of the blood-vessels* in heart-disease —the cardiac liver.

4. *Cirrhosis from chronic obstruction of the bile-ducts,* a form of very slight clinical interest. In anthracosis the carbon pigment may reach the liver in large quantities and be deposited in the connective tissue about the portal canal, leading to cirrhosis (Welch).

Anatomical Classification.—1. *Vascular cirrhoses,* in which the new growth of connective tissue has its starting point about the finer branches of the portal or hepatic veins.

2. *Biliary cirrhoses,* in which the process is supposed to begin about the finer bile-ducts, as in the hypertrophic cirrhosis of Hanot and in the form from obstruction of the larger ducts.

3. *Capsular cirrhoses,* a perihepatitis leading to great thickening of the capsule and reduction in the volume of the liver.

Clinical Classification.—For practical purposes we may recognize the following varieties of cirrhosis of the liver:

1. The alcoholic cirrhosis of Laennec, including with this the fatty cirrhotic liver.

2. The hypertrophic cirrhosis of Hanot.

3. Syphilitic cirrhosis.

4. Capsular cirrhosis—chronic perihepatitis.

Other forms, of slight clinical interest, are considered elsewhere under diabetes, malaria, tuberculosis, and heart-disease. The cirrhosis from malaria, upon which the French writers lay so much stress (one describes thirteen varieties!), is excessively rare. In our large experience with malaria during the past fifteen years not a single case of advanced cirrhosis due to this cause has been seen in the wards or autopsy-room of the Johns Hopkins Hospital.

I. Alcoholic Cirrhosis.

Etiology.—The disease occurs most frequently in middle-aged males who have been addicted to drink. Whisky, gin, and brandy are more potent to cause cirrhosis than beer. It is more common in countries in which strong spirits are used than in those in which malt liquors are taken. Among 1,000 autopsies in my colleague Welch's department of the Johns Hopkins Hospital there were 63 cases of small atrophic liver, and 8 cases of the fatty cirrhotic organ. Lancereaux claims that the *vin ordinaire* of France is a common cause of cirrhosis. Of 210 cases, excess in wine alone was present in 68 cases. He thinks it is the sulphate of potash in the plaster of Paris used to give the " dry " flavor which damages the liver.

Cirrhosis of the liver in young children is not very rare. Palmer Howard collected 63 cases, to which Hatfield added 93 and Musser 529. In a certain number of the cases there is an alcoholic history, in others syphilis has been present, while a third group, due to the poisons of the infectious diseases, embraces a certain number of the cases of Hanot's hypertrophic cirrhosis.

Morbid Anatomy.—Practically on the post-mortem table we see alcoholic cirrhosis in two well-characterized forms:

The Atrophic Cirrhosis of Laennec.—The organ is greatly reduced in size and may be deformed. The weight is sometimes not more than a pound or a pound and a half. It presents numerous granulations on the surface; is firm, hard, and cuts with great resistance. The substance is seen to be made up of greenish-yellow islands, surrounded by grayish-white connective tissue. W. G. MacCallum has shown that regenerative changes in the cells are almost constantly present. This yellow appearance of the liver induced Laennec to give to the condition the name of cirrhosis. Apart from the fatty liver there may be enlargement as pointed out by Foxwell and Rolleston.

The Fatty Cirrhotic Liver.—Even in the atrophic form the fat is increased, but in typical examples of this variety the organ is not reduced in size, but is enlarged, smooth or very slightly granular, anæmic, yellowish-white in color, and resembles an ordinary fatty liver. It is, however, firm, cuts with resistance, and microscopically shows a great increase in the connective tissue. This form occurs most frequently in beer-drinkers.

The two essential elements in cirrhosis are destruction of liver-cells and obstruction to the portal circulation.

In an autopsy on a case of atrophic cirrhosis the peritonæum is usually found to contain a large quantity of fluid, the membrane is opaque, and there is chronic catarrh of the stomach and of the small intestines. The spleen is enlarged, in part, at least, from the chronic congestion, possibly due in part to a " vital reaction," to a toxic influence (Parkes Weber). The pancreas frequently shows chronic interstitial changes. The kidneys are sometimes cirrhotic, the bases of the lungs may be much compressed by the ascitic fluid, the heart often shows marked degeneration, and arterio-sclerosis is usually present. A remarkable feature is the association of acute tuberculosis with cirrhosis. In seven cases of my series the patients died with either acute tuberculous peritonitis or acute tuberculous pleurisy. Rolleston has found that tuberculosis was present in 28 per cent of 706 fatal cases of cirrhosis. Peritoneal tuberculosis was found in 9 per cent of a series of 584 cases.

The compensatory circulation is usually readily demonstrated. It is carried out by the following set of vessels: (1) The accessory portal system of Sappey, of which important branches pass in the round and suspensory ligaments and unite with the epigastric and mammary systems. These vessels are numerous and small. Occasionally a large single vein, which may attain the size of the little finger, passes from the hilus of the liver, follows the round ligament, and joins the epigastric veins at the navel. Although this has the position of the umbilical vein, it is usually, as Sappey showed, a para-umbilical vein—that is, an enlarged vein by the side of the obliterated umbilical vessel. There may be produced about the navel a large bunch of varices, the so-called caput Medusæ. Other branches of this system occur in the gastro-epiploic omentum, about the gall-bladder, and, most important of all, in the suspensory ligament. These latter form large branches, which anastomose freely with the diaphragmatic veins, and so unite with the vena azygos. (2) By the anastomosis between the œsophageal and gastric veins. The veins at the lower end of the œsophagus may be enormously enlarged, producing varices which project on the mucous membrane. (3) The communications between the hæmorrhoidal and the inferior mesenteric veins. The freedom of communication in this direction is very variable, and in some instances the hæmorrhoidal veins are not much enlarged. (4) The veins of Retzius, which unite the radicles of the portal branches in the intestines and mesentery with the inferior vena cava and its branches. To this system belong the whole group of retroperitoneal veins, which are in most instances enormously enlarged, particularly about the kidneys, and which serve to carry off a considerable proportion of the portal blood.

Symptoms.—The most extreme grade of atrophic cirrhosis may exist without symptoms. *So long as the compensatory circulation is maintained* the patient may suffer little or no inconvenience. The remarkable efficiency of this collateral circulation is well seen in those rare instances of permanent obliteration of the portal vein. The symptoms may be divided into two groups —obstructive and toxic.

OBSTRUCTIVE.—The overfilling of the blood-vessels of the stomach and intestine lead to chronic catarrh, and the patients suffer with nausea and vomiting, particularly in the morning; the tongue is furred and the bowels are irregular. Hæmorrhage from the stomach may be an early symptom; it is often profuse and liable to recur. It seldom proves fatal. The amount vomited may be remarkable, as in a case already referred to, in which ten pounds were ejected in seven days. Following the hæmatemesis melæna is common;

but hæmorrhages from the bowels may occur for several years without hæmatemesis. The bleeding very often comes from the œsophageal varices already described (p. 459). Very frequently epistaxis occurs. Enlargement of the spleen may, as Parkes Weber suggests, be due to a toxemia. The organ can usually be felt. Evidences of the establishment of the collateral circulation are seen in the enlarged epigastric and mammary veins, more rarely in the presence of the caput Medusæ and in the development of hæmorrhoids. The distended venules in the lower thoracic zone along the line of attachment of the diaphragm are not specially marked in cirrhosis. The most striking feature of failure in the compensatory circulation is ascites, the effusion of serous fluid into the peritoneal cavity, which may appear suddenly. The conditions under which this occurs are still obscure. In some cases it is due more to chronic peritonitis than to the cirrhosis. The abdomen gradually distends, may reach a large size, and contain as much as 15 or 20 litres. Œdema of the feet may precede or develop with the ascites. The dropsy is rarely general.

Jaundice is usually slight, and was present in 107 of 293 cases of cirrhosis collected by Rolleston. The skin has frequently a sallow, slightly icteroid tint. The urine is often reduced in amount, contains urates in abundance, often a slight amount of albumin, and, if jaundice is intense, tube-casts. The disease may be afebrile throughout, but in many cases, as shown by Carrington, there is slight fever, from 100° to 102.5°.

Examination at any early stage of the disease may show an enlarged and painful liver. Dreschfeld, Foxwell, and Rolleston have of late years called particular attention to the fact that in very many of the cases of alcoholic cirrhosis the organ is "enlarged at all stages of the disease, and that whether enlarged or contracted the clinical symptoms and course are much the same" (Foxwell). The patient may first come under observation for dyspepsia, hæmatemesis, slight jaundice, or nervous symptoms. Later in the disease, the patient has an unmistakable hepatic facies; he is thin, the eyes are sunken, the conjunctivæ watery, the nose and cheeks show distended venules, and the complexion is muddy or icteroid. On the enlarged abdomen the vessels are distended, and a bunch of dilated veins may surround the navel. Nævi of a remarkable character may appear on the skin, either localized stellate varices— spider angiomata—usually on the face, neck, and back, and also "mat" nævi, as I have called them—areas of skin of a reddish or purplish color due to the uniform distention of small venules. When much fluid is in the peritonæum it is impossible to make a satisfactory examination, but after withdrawal the area of liver dulness is found to be diminished, particularly in the middle line, and on deep pressure the edge of the liver can be detected, and occasionally the hard, firm, and even granular surface. The spleen can be felt in the left hypochondriac region. Examination of the anus may reveal the presence of hæmorrhoids.

TOXIC SYMPTOMS.—At any stage of atrophic cirrhosis the patient may have cerebral symptoms, either a noisy, joyous delirium, or stupor, coma, or even convulsions. The condition is not infrequently mistaken for uræmia. The nature of the toxic agent is not yet settled. Without jaundice, and not attributable to cholæmia, the symptoms may come on in hospital when the patient has not had alcohol for weeks.

224

The fatty cirrhotic liver may produce symptoms similar to those of the atrophic form, but more frequently it is latent and is found accidentally in topers who have died from various diseases. The greater number of the cases clinically diagnosed as cirrhosis with enlargement come in this division.

Diagnosis.—With ascites, a well-marked history of alcoholism, the hepatic facies, and hæmorrhage from the stomach or bowels, the diagnosis is rarely doubtful. If, after withdrawal of the fluid, the spleen is found to be enlarged and the liver either not palpable or, if it is enlarged, hard and regular, the probabilities in favor of cirrhosis are very great. In the early stages of the disease, when the liver is increased in size, it may be impossible to say whether it is a cirrhotic or a fatty liver. The differential diagnosis between common and syphilitic cirrhosis can sometimes be made. A marked history of syphilis or the existence of other syphilitic lesions, with great irregularity in the surface or at the edge of the liver, are the points in favor of the latter. Thrombosis or obliteration of the portal vein can rarely be differentiated. In a case of fibroid transformation of the portal vein which came under my observation, the collateral circulation had been established for years, and the symptoms were simply those of extreme portal obstruction, such as occur in cirrhosis. Thrombosis of the portal vein may occur in cirrhosis and be characterized by a rapidly developing ascites.

Prognosis.—The prognosis is bad. When the collateral circulation is fully established the patient may have no symptoms whatever. Three cases of advanced atrophic cirrhosis have died under my observation of other affections without presenting during life any symptoms pointing to disease of the liver. There are instances, too, of enlargement of the liver, slight jaundice, cerebral symptoms, and even hæmatemesis, in which the liver becomes reduced in size, the symptoms disappear, and the patient may live in comparative comfort for many years. There are cases, too, possibly syphilitic, in which, after one or two tappings, the symptoms have disappeared and the patients have apparently recovered. Ascites is a very serious event, especially if due to the cirrhosis and not to an associated peritonitis. Of 34 cases with ascites 10 died before tapping was necessary; 14 were tapped, and the average duration of life after the swelling was first noticed was only eight weeks; of 10 cases the diagnosis was wrong in 4, and in the remaining 6, who were tapped oftener than once, chronic peritonitis and perihepatitis were present (Hale White).

II. Hypertrophic Cirrhosis (*Hanot*).

This well-characterized form was first described by Requin in 1846, but our accurate knowledge of the condition dates from the work of the lamented Hanot (1875), whose name in France it bears—*maladie de Hanot.*

Cirrhosis with enlargement occurs in the early stage of atrophic cirrhosis; there is an enlarged fatty and cirrhotic liver of alcoholics, a pigmentary form in diabetes has been described, and in association with syphilis the organ is often very large. The hypertrophic cirrhosis of Hanot is easily distinguished from these forms.

Etiology.—Males are more often affected than females—in 22 of Schachmann's 26 cases. The subjects are young; some of the cases in children probably belong to this form. Of four recent cases under my care the ages were from twenty to thirty-five. Two were brothers. Alcohol plays a minor part. Not one of the four cases referred to had been a heavy drinker. The absence of all known etiological factors is a remarkable feature in a majority of the cases.

Morbid Anatomy.—The organ is enlarged, weighing from 2,000 to 4,000 grammes. The form is maintained, the surface is smooth, or presents small granulations; the color in advanced cases is of a dark olive green; the consistence is greatly increased. The section is uniform, greenish-yellow in color, and the liver nodules may be seen separated by connective tissue. The bile-passages present nothing abnormal. In a case without much jaundice exploratory operation showed a very large red organ, with a slightly roughened surface. Microscopically the following characteristics are described by French writers: The cirrhosis is mono- or multilobular, with a connective tissue rich in round cells. The bile-vessels are the seat of an angiocholitis, catarrhal and productive, and there is an extraordinary development of new biliary canaliculi. The liver-cells are neither fatty nor pigmented, and may be increased in size and show karyokinetic figures. From the supposed origin about the bile-vessels it has been called biliary cirrhosis, but the histological details have not yet been worked out fully, and the separation of this as a distinct form should, for the present at least, rest upon clinical rather than anatomical grounds. The spleen is greatly enlarged and may weigh 600 or more grammes.

Symptoms.—Hanot's hypertrophic cirrhosis presents the following very characteristic group of symptoms. As previously stated, the cases occur in young persons; there is not, as a rule, an alcoholic history, and males are usually affected: (*a*) A remarkably chronic course of from four to six, or even ten years. (*b*) Jaundice, usually slight, often not more than a lemon tint, or a tinging of the conjunctivæ. At any time during the course an *icterus gravis*, with high fever and delirium, may develop. There is bile in the urine; the stools are not clay-colored as in obstructive jaundice, but may be very dark and " bilious." (*c*) Attacks of pain in the region of the liver, which may be severe and associated with nausea and vomiting. The pain may be slight and dragging, and in some cases is not at all a prominent symptom. The jaundice may deepen after attacks of pain. (*d*) Enlarged liver. A fulness in the upper abdominal zone may be the first complaint. On inspection the enlargement may be very marked. In one of my cases the left lobe was unusually prominent and stood out almost like a tumor. An exploratory operation showed only an enlarged, smooth organ without adhesions. On palpation the hypertrophy is uniform, the consistence is increased, and the edge distinct and hard. The gall-bladder is not enlarged. The vertical flatness is much increased and may extend from the sixth rib to the level of the navel. (*e*) The spleen is enlarged, easily palpable, and very hard. (*f*) Certain negative features are of moment—the usual absence of ascites and of dilatation of the subcutaneous veins of the abdomen. Among other symptoms may be mentioned hæmorrhages. One of my cases had bleeding at the gums for a year; another had had for years most remarkable attacks of purpura with urticaria. Pruritus, xanthoma, lichen, and telangiectasis may be present in the skin. In one of my cases the skin became very bronzed, almost as deeply as in Addison's disease. Slight fever may be present, which increases during the crises of pain. There may be a marked leucocytosis. A curious attitude of the body has been seen, in which the right shoulder and right side look dragged down. The patients die with the symptoms of icterus gravis, from hæmorrhage, from an intercurrent infection, or in a profound cachexia. Certain of the cases of cirrhosis of the liver in children are of this type; the enlargement of the spleen may be very pronounced.

III. SYPHILITIC CIRRHOSIS.

This has already been considered in the section on syphilis (p. 275). I refer to it again to emphasize (1) its frequency; (2) the great importance of its differentiation from the alcoholic form; (3) its curability in many cases; and (4) the tumor formations in connection with it.

IV. CAPSULAR CIRRHOSIS—PERIHEPATITIS.

Local capsulitis is common in many conditions of the liver. The form of disease here described is characterized by an enormous thickening of the entire capsule, with great contraction of the liver, but not necessarily with special increase in the connective tissue of the organ itself. Our chief knowledge of the disease we owe to the Guy's Hospital physicians, particularly to Hilton Fagge and to Hale White, who has collected from the records 22 cases. The liver substance itself was " never markedly cirrhotic; its tissue was nearly always soft." Chronic capsulitis of the spleen and a chronic proliferative peritonitis are almost invariably present. In 19 of the 22 cases the kidneys were granular. Hale White regards it as a sequel of interstitial nephritis. The youngest case in his series was twenty-nine. The symptoms are those of atrophic cirrhosis—ascites, often recurring and requiring many tappings. Jaundice is not often present. I have met with two groups of cases—the one in adults usually with ascites and regarded as ordinary cirrhosis. I have never made a diagnosis in such a case. Signs of interstitial nephritis, recurring ascites, and absence of jaundice are regarded by Hale White as important diagnostic points. In the second group of cases the perihepatitis, perisplenitis, and proliferative peritonitis are associated with adherent pericardium and chronic mediastinitis. In one such case the diagnosis of capsular hepatitis was very clear, as the liver could be grasped in the hand and formed a rounded, smooth organ resembling the spleen. The child was tapped 121 times (Archives of Pædiatrics, 1896).

Treatment of the Cirrhoses.—The portal function of the liver may be put out of action without much damage to the body. There may be an extreme grade of cirrhotic atrophy without symptoms; the portal vein may be obliterated, or, experimentally the portal vein may be anastomosed with the cava. So long as there is an active compensatory circulation a patient with atrophic cirrhosis may remain well. In the hypertrophic form toxæmia is the special danger. In the hypertrophic cirrhosis we have no means of arresting the progress of the disease. In the alcoholic form it is too late, as a rule, to do much after symptoms have occurred. In a few cases an attack of jaundice or hæmatemesis may prove the salvation of the patient, who may afterward take to a temperate life and a bland diet. An occasional course of potassium iodide may be given. With the advent of ascites the critical stage is reached. A dry diet, without salt, and free purgation may relieve a small exudate, rarely a large one, and it is best to tap early, or to advise Talma's operation. In the syphilitic cirrhosis much more can be done, and a majority of the cases of cure after ascites are of this variety. Iodide of potassium in moderate doses, 15 to 30 drops of the saturated solution, and the Addison pill save a number of cases even after repeated tapping. The diagnosis may be reached only after removal of the fluid, but in every case with a history of syphilis or with irregularity of the liver this treatment should be tried.

SURGICAL TREATMENT.—(*a*) *Tapping.*—When the ascites increases it is better to tap early. As Hale White remarks, a case of cirrhosis of the liver which is tapped rarely recovers, but there are instances in which early and repeated paracentesis is followed by cure. Accidents are rare; hæmorrhage occasionally follows; acute peritonitis; erysipelas at the point of puncture; collapse during the operation, to guard against which Mead advised the use of the abdominal binder. Continuous drainage with Southey's tubes is not often practicable and has no special advantages. (*b*) *Laparotomy*, with complete removal of the fluid, and freshening or rubbing the peritoneal surfaces, to stimulate the formation of adhesions. (*c*) *Omentopexy*, the stitching of the omentum to the abdominal wall, and the establishment of collateral circulation in this way between the portal and the systemic vessels. This operation is sometimes very successful, and may be recommended. In 224 cases there were 84 deaths and 129 recoveries; 11 cases doubtful. Among the 129 successful cases, in 25 the ascites recurred; 70 appeared to have completely recovered. (*d*) *Fistula of Eck.* The porto-caval anastomosis has been performed once in man in cirrhosis of the liver by Widal (*La Semaine Médicale*, 1903). The patient lived for three months.

VIII. ABSCESS OF THE LIVER.

Etiology.—Suppuration within the liver, either in the parenchyma or in the blood or bile passages, occurs under the following conditions:

(1) The *tropical abscess*, also called the *solitary*, commonly follows amœbic dysentery. It frequently occurs among Europeans in India, particularly those who drink alcohol freely and are exposed to great heat. The relation of this form of abscess to dysentery is still under discussion, and Anglo-Indian practitioners are by no means unanimous on the subject. Certainly cases may occur without a history of previous dysentery, and there have been fatal cases without any affection of the large bowel. In the United States the large solitary abscess is not very infrequent. The relation of this form of abscess to the *Amœba dysenteriæ* has been considered.

(2) *Traumatism* is an occasional cause. The injury is generally in the hepatic region. Two instances of it have come under my notice in brakemen who were injured while coupling cars. Injury to the head is not infrequently followed by liver abscess.

(3) *Embolic* or *pyæmic abscesses* are the most numerous, occurring in a general pyæmia or following foci of suppuration in the territory of the portal vessels. The infective agents may reach the liver through the hepatic artery, as in those cases in which the original focus of infection is in the area of the systemic circulation; though it may happen occasionally that the infective agent, instead of passing through the lungs, reaches the liver through the infe-

rior vena cava and the hepatic veins. A remarkable instance of multiple abscesses of arterial origin was afforded by the case of aneurism of the hepatic artery reported by Ross and myself. Infection through the portal vein is much more common. It results from dysentery and other ulcerative affections of the bowels, appendicitis, occasionally after typhoid fever, in rectal affections, and in abscesses in the pelvis. In these cases the abscesses are multiple and, as a rule, within the branches of the portal vein—suppurative pylephlebitis.

(4) A not uncommon cause of suppuration is *inflammation of the bile-passages* caused by gall-stones, more rarely by parasites—suppurative cholangitis.

In some instances of tuberculosis of the liver the affection is chiefly of the bile-ducts, with the formation of multiple tuberculous abscesses containing a bile-stained pus.

(5) *Foreign bodies and parasites.* In rare instances foreign bodies, such as a needle, may pass from the stomach or gullet, lodge in the liver, and excite an abscess, or, as in several instances which have been reported, a foreign body, such as a needle or a fish-bone, has perforated a branch or the portal vein itself and induced pylephlebitis. Echinococcus cysts frequently cause suppuration, the penetration of round worms into the liver less commonly, and most rarely of all the liver-fluke.

Morbid Anatomy.—(*a*) OF THE SOLITARY OR TROPICAL ABSCESS.—This has been described under amœbic dysentery (p. 4).

(*b*) OF SEPTIC AND PYÆMIC ABSCESSES.—These are usually multiple, though occasionally, following injury, there may be a large solitary collection of pus.

In suppurative pylephlebitis the liver is uniformly enlarged. The capsule may be smooth and the external surface of the organ of normal appearance. In other instances, numerous yellowish-white points appear beneath the capsule. On section there are isolated pockets of pus, either having a round outline or in some places distinctly dendritic, and from these the pus may be squeezed. They look like small, solitary abscesses, but, on probing, are found to communicate with the portal vein and to represent its branches, distended and suppurating. The entire portal system within the liver may be involved; sometimes territories are cut off by thrombi. The suppuration may extend into the main branch or even into the mesenteric and gastric veins. The pus may be fetid and is often bile-stained; it may, however, be thick, tenacious, and laudable. In suppurative cholangitis there is usually obstruction by gall-stones, the ducts are greatly distended, the gall-bladder enlarged and full of pus, and the branches within the liver are extremely distended, so that on section there is an appearance not unlike that described in pylephlebitis.

Suppuration about the echinococcus cysts may be very extensive, forming enormous abscesses, the characters of which are at once recognized by the remnants of the cysts.

Symptoms.—(*a*) OF THE LARGE SOLITARY ABSCESS.—The abscess may be latent and run a course without definite symptoms; death may occur suddenly from rupture.

Fever, pain, enlargement of the liver, and a septic condition are the important symptoms of hepatic abscess. The temperature is elevated at the outset and is of an intermittent or septic type. It is irregular, and may remain normal or even subnormal for a few days; then the patient has a rigor and the temperature rises to 103° or higher. Owing to this intermittent character of the fever the disease is often mistaken for malaria. The fever may rise every afternoon without a rigor. Profuse sweating is common, particularly when the patient falls asleep. In chronic cases there may be little or no fever. One of my patients, with a liver abscess which had perforated the lung, coughed up pus after his temperature had been normal for weeks. The pain is variable, and is usually referred to the back or shoulder; or there is a dull aching sensation in the right hypochondrium. When turned on the left side, the patient often complains of a heavy, dragging sensation, so that he usually prefers to lie on the right side; at least, this has been the case in a majority of the instances which have come under my observation. Pain on pressure over the liver is usually present, particularly on deep pressure at the costal margin in the nipple line.

The enlargement of the liver is most marked in the right lobe, and, as the abscess cavity is usually situated more toward the upper than the under surface, the increase in volume is upward and to the right, not downward, as in cancer and the other affections producing enlargement. Percussion in the mid-sternal and parasternal lines may show a normal limit. At the nipple-line the curve of liver dulness begins to rise, and in the mid-axillary it may reach the fifth rib, while behind, near the spine, the area of dulness may be almost on a level with the angle of the scapula. Of course there are instances in which this characteristic feature is not present, as when the abscess occupies the left lobe. The enlargement of the liver may be so great as to cause bulging of the right side, and the edge may project a hand's-breadth or more below the costal margin. In such instances the surface is smooth. Palpation is painful, and there may be fremitus on deep inspiration. In some instances fluctuation may be detected. Adhesions may form to the abdominal wall and the abscess may point below the margin of the ribs, or even in the epigastric region. In many cases the appearance of the patient is suggestive. The skin has a sallow, slightly icteroid tint, the face is pale, the complexion muddy, the conjunctivæ are infiltrated, and often slightly bile-tinged. There is in the facies and in the general appearance of the patient a strong suggestion of the existence of abscess. There is no internal affection associated with suppuration which gives, I think, just the same hue as certain instances of abscess of the liver. Marked jaundice is rare. Diarrhœa may be present and may give an important clew to the nature of the case, particularly if amœbæ are found in the stools. Constipation may occur.

Perforation of the lung occurred in 9 of the 27 cases in my series. The symptoms are most characteristic. The extension may occur through the diaphragm, without actual rupture, and with the production of a purulent pleurisy and invasion of the lung. With cough of an aggravated and convulsive character, there are signs of involvement at the base of the right lung, defective resonance, feeble tubular breathing, and increase in the tactile fremitus; but the most characteristic feature is the presence of a reddish-brown expectoration of a brick-dust color, resembling anchovy sauce. This, which was noted originally by Budd, was present in our cases, and in addition Reese and Lafleur found the *amœbæ coli* identical with those which exist in the liver abscess and

230

in the stools. They are present in variable numbers and display active amœboid movements. The brownish tint of the expectoration is due to blood-pigment and blood-corpuscles, and there may be orange-red crystals of hæmatoidin.

The abscess may perforate externally, as mentioned already, or into the stomach or bowel; occasionally into the pericardium. The duration of this form is very variable. It may run its course and prove fatal in six or eight weeks or may persist for several years.

The prognosis is serious, as the mortality is more than 50 per cent. The death-rate has been lowered of late years, owing to the great fearlessness with which the surgeons now attack these cases.

(*b*) Of the Pyæmic Abscess and Suppurative Pylephlebitis.—Clinically these conditions can not be separated. Occurring in a general pyæmia, no special features may be added to the case. When there is suppuration within the portal vein the liver is uniformly enlarged and tender, though pain may not be a marked feature. There is an irregular, septic fever, and the complexion is muddy, sometimes distinctly icteroid. The features are indeed those of pyæmia, plus a slight icteroid tinge, and an enlarged and painful liver. The latter features alone are peculiar. The sweats, chills, prostration, and fever have nothing distinctive.

Diagnosis.—Abscess of the liver may be confounded with intermittent fever, a common mistake in malarial regions. Practically an intermittent fever which resists quinine is not malarial. Laveran's organisms are also absent from the blood. When the abscess bursts into the pleura a right-sided empyema is produced and perforation of the lung usually follows. When the liver abscess has been latent and dysenteric symptoms have not been marked, the condition may be considered empyema or abscess of the lung. In such cases the anchovy-sauce-like color of the pus and the presence of the amœbæ will enable one to make a definite diagnosis. Perforation externally is readily recognized, and yet in an abscess cavity in the epigastric region it may be difficult to say whether it has proceeded from the liver or is in the abdominal wall. When the abscess is large, and the adhesions are so firm that the liver does not descend during inspiration, the exploratory needle does not make an up-and-down movement during aspiration. The diagnosis of suppurating echinococcus cyst is rarely possible, except in Australia and Iceland, where hydatids are so common.

Perhaps the most important affection from which suppuration within the liver is to be separated is the intermittent hepatic fever associated with gall-stones. Of the cases reported a majority have been considered due to suppuration, and in two of my cases the liver had been repeatedly aspirated. Post-mortem examinations have shown conclusively that the high fever and chills may recur at intervals for years without suppuration in the ducts. The distinctive features of this condition are paroxysms of fever with rigors and sweats—which may occur with great regularity, but which more often are separated by long intervals—the deepening of the jaundice after the paroxysms, the entire apyrexia in the intervals, and the maintenance of the general nutrition. The time element also is important, as in some of these cases the disease has lasted for several years. Finally, it is to be remembered that abscess of the liver, in temperate climates at least, is invariably secondary, and the primary source must be carefully sought for, either in dysentery, slight ulceration of the rectum, suppurating hæmorrhoids, ulcer of the stomach, or in suppurative disease of other parts of the body, particularly within the skull or in the bones.

Leucocytosis may be absent in the amœbic abscess of the liver; in septic cases it may be very high.

In suspected cases, whether the liver is enlarged or not, exploratory aspiration may be performed without risk. The needle may be entered in the anterior axillary line in the lowest interspace, or in the seventh interspace in the mid-axillary line, or over the centre of the area of dulness behind. The patient should be placed under ether, for it may be necessary to make several deep punctures. It is not well to use too small an aspirator. No ill effects follow this procedure, even though blood may leak into the peritoneal cavity. Extensive suppuration may exist, and yet be missed in the aspiration, particularly when the branches of the portal vein are distended with pus.

Treatment.—Pyæmic abscess and suppurative pylephlebitis are invariably fatal. Treves, however, reports a case of pyæmic abscess following appendicitis in which the patient recovered after an exploratory operation. Surgical measures are not justified in these cases, unless an abscess shows signs of pointing. As the abscesses associated with dysentery are often single, they afford a reasonable hope of benefit from operation. If, however, the patient is expectorating the pus, if the general condition is good and the hectic fever not marked, it is best to defer operation, as many of these instances recover spontaneously. The large single abscesses are the most favorable for operation. The general medical treatment of the cases is that of ordinary septicæmia.

IX. NEW GROWTHS IN THE LIVER.

These may be cancer, either primary or secondary, sarcoma, or angioma.

Etiology.—Cancer of the liver is third in order of frequency of internal cancer. It is rarely primary, usually secondary to cancer in other organs. It is a disease of late adult life. According to Leichtenstern, over 50 per cent of the cases occur between the fortieth and the sixtieth years. It occasionally occurs in children. Women are attacked less frequently than men. It is stated by some authors that secondary cancer is more common in women, owing to the frequency of cancer of the uterus. Heredity is believed to have an influence in from 15 to 20 per cent.

In many cases trauma is an antecedent, and cancer of the bile-passages is associated in many instances with gall-stones. Cancer is stated to be less common in the tropics.

Morbid Anatomy.—The following forms of new growths occur in the liver and have a clinical importance:

CANCER.—(1) *Primary cancer*, of which three forms may be recognized.

(*a*) The *massive cancer*, which causes great enlargement and on section shows a uniform mass of new growth, which occupies a large portion of the organ. It is grayish-white, usually not softened, and is abruptly outlined from the contiguous liver substance.

(*b*) *Nodular cancer*, in which the liver is occupied by nodular masses, some large, some small, irregularly scattered throughout the organ. Usu-

232

ally in one region there is a larger, perhaps firmer, older-looking mass, which indicates the primary seat, and the numerous nodules are secondary to it. This form is much like the secondary cancerous involvement, except that it seldom reaches a large size.

(c) *Adeno-carcinoma with cirrhosis.* The liver varies in size, small as a rule, but in a few cases enlarged. The surface is usually mottled dark green, with elevated yellowish nodules beneath the capsule, or even large globular masses projecting. On section the tissue is bile-stained, and there are innumerable tumor masses, varying in size, separated from each other by strands of connective tissue, which may be 5 to 10 mm. across. The growths may be unevenly distributed. The connection between the adenoma and the cirrhosis is not known, nor is it known which is primary. There is, as a rule, extensive vicarious hypertrophy of the liver tissue. Of the two cases which have been under my care, in one I diagnosed cirrhosis, and the clinical picture was that of the ordinary atrophic form; the other I thought to be carcinoma (C. H. Travis, J. H. H. Bull., 1902). The latter patient died of hæmorrhage into the peritoneal cavity, a similar ending to that in the case reported by Peabody.

Histologically, the primary cancers are epitheliomata—alveolar and trabecular. The character of the cells varies greatly. In some varieties they are polymorphous; in others small polyhedral; in others, again, giant cells are found. In rare instances, as in one described by Greenfield, the cells are cylindrical. The trabecular form of epithelioma is also known as adenoma or adenocarcinoma.

(2) *Secondary Cancer.*—The organ may reach an enormous size, $30\frac{1}{2}$ pounds (Osler), 33 pounds (Christian). The cancerous nodules project beneath the capsule, and can be felt during life or even seen through the thin abdominal walls. They are usually disseminated equally, though in rare instances they may be confined to one lobe. The consistence of the nodules varies; in some cases they are firm and hard and those on the surface show a distinct umbilication, due to the shrinking of the fibrous tissue in the centre. These superficial cancerous masses are still sometimes spoken of as " Farre's tubercles." More frequently the masses are on section grayish-white in color, or hæmorrhagic. Rupture of blood-vessels is not uncommon in these cases. In one specimen there was an enormous clot beneath the capsule of the liver, together with hæmorrhage into the gall-bladder and into the peritonæum. The secondary cancer shows the same structure as the initial lesion, and is usually either an alveolar or cylindrical carcinoma. Degeneration is common in these secondary growths; thus the hyaline transformation may convert large areas into a dense, dry, grayish-yellow mass. Extensive areas of fatty degeneration may occur, sclerosis is not uncommon, and hæmorrhages are frequent. Suppuration sometimes follows.

(3) *Cancer of the bile-passages* which has been already considered.

SARCOMA.—Of primary sarcoma of the liver very few cases have been reported. Secondary sarcoma is more frequent, and many examples of lympho-sarcoma and myxo-sarcoma are on record, less frequently glio-sarcoma or the smooth or striped myoma.

The most important form is the melano-sarcoma, secondary to sarcoma of the eye or of the skin. Very rarely melano-sarcoma occurs primarily in the liver. Of the reported cases Hanot excludes all but one. In this form the liver is greatly enlarged, is either uniformly infiltrated with the growth which gives the cut surface the appearance of dark granite, or there are large nodular masses of a deep black or marbled color. There are usually extensive metastases, and in some instances every organ of the body is involved. Nodules of melano-sarcoma of the skin may give a clew to the diagnosis.

OTHER FORMS OF LIVER TUMOR.—One of the commonest tumors in the liver is the angioma, which occurs as a small, reddish body the size of a walnut, and consists simply of a series of dilated vessels. Occasionally in children angiomata grow and produce large tumors.

Cysts are occasionally found in the liver, either single, which is not very uncommon, or multiple, when they usually coexist with congenital cystic kidneys.

Symptoms.—It is often impossible to differentiate primary and secondary cancer of the liver unless the primary seat of the disease is evident, as in the case of scirrhus of the breast, or cancer of the rectum, or of a tumor in the stomach, which can be felt. As a rule, cancer of the liver is associated with progressive enlargement; but in some cases of primary nodular cancer, and in the cancer with cirrhosis the organ may not be enlarged. Gastric disturbance, loss of appetite, nausea, and vomiting are frequent. Progressive loss of flesh and strength may be the first symptoms. Pain or a sensation of uneasiness in the right hypochondriac region may be present, but enormous enlargement of the liver may occur without the slightest pain. Jaundice, which is present in at least one-half of the cases, is usually of moderate extent, unless the common duct is occluded. Ascites is rare, except in the form of cancer with cirrhosis, in which the clinical picture is that of the atrophic form. Pressure by nodules on the portal vein or extension of the cancer to the peritonæum may also induce ascites.

Inspection shows the abdomen to be distended, particularly in the upper zone. In late stages of the disease, when emaciation is marked, the cancerous nodules can be plainly seen beneath the skin, and in rare instances even the umbilications. The superficial veins are enlarged. On palpation the liver is felt, a hand's-breadth or more below the costal margin, descending with each inspiration. The surface is usually irregular, and may present large masses or smaller nodular bodies, either rounded or with central depressions. In instances of diffuse infiltration the liver may be greatly enlarged and present a perfectly smooth surface. The growth is progressive, and the edge of the liver may ultimately extend below the level of the navel. Although generally uniform and producing enlargement of the whole organ, occasionally the tumor in the left lobe forms a solid mass occupying the epigastric region. By percussion the outline can be accurately limited and the progressive growth of the tumor estimated. The spleen is rarely enlarged. Pyrexia is present in many cases, usually a continuous fever, ranging from 100° to 102°; it may be intermittent, with rigors. This may be associated with the cancer alone, or, as in one of my cases, with suppuration. Œdema of the feet, from anæmia, usually supervenes. Cancer of the liver kills in from three to fifteen months. One of my patients lived for more than two years.

Diagnosis.—The diagnosis is easy when the liver is greatly enlarged and the surface nodular. The smoother forms of diffuse carcinoma may at first be mistaken for fatty or amyloid liver, but the presence of jaundice, the rapid

234

enlargement, and the more marked cachexia will usually suffice to differentiate it. Perhaps the most puzzling conditions occur in the rare cases of enlarged amyloid liver with irregular gummata. The large echinococcus liver may present a striking similarity to carcinoma, but the projecting nodules are usually softer, the disease lasts much longer, and the cachexia is not marked.

Hypertrophic cirrhosis may at first be mistaken for carcinoma, as the jaundice is usually deep and the liver very large; but the absence of a marked cachexia and wasting, and the painless, smooth character of the enlargement are points against cancer. When in doubt in these cases, aspiration may be safely performed, and positive indication may be gained from the materials so obtained. In large, rapidly growing secondary cancers the superficial rounded masses may almost fluctuate and these soft tumor-like projections may contain blood. The form of cancer with cirrhosis can scarcely be separated from atrophic cirrhosis itself. Perhaps the wasting is more extreme and more rapid, but the jaundice and the ascites are identical. Melano-sarcoma causes great enlargement of the organ. There are frequently symptoms of involvement of other viscera, as the lungs, kidneys, or spleen. Secondary tumors may occur in the skin. A very important symptom, not present in all cases, is melanuria, the passage of a very dark-colored urine, which may, however, when first voided, be quite normal in color. The existence of a melano-sarcoma of the eye, or the history of blindness in one eye, with subsequent extirpation, may indicate at once the true nature of the hepatic enlargement. The secondary tumors may arise some time after the extirpation of the eye, as in a case under the care of J. C. Wilson, at the Philadelphia Hospital, or, as in a case under Tyson at the same institution, the patient may have a sarcoma of the choroid which had never caused any symptoms.

The *treatment* must be entirely symptomatic. The question of surgical interference may be discussed. Keen has collected reports of 76 cases of resection of tumors of the liver, 63 of which recovered.

X. FATTY LIVER.

Two different forms of this condition are recognized—the fatty infiltration and fatty degeneration.

Fatty infiltration occurs, to a certain extent, in normal livers, since the cells always contain minute globules of oil.

In fatty degeneration, which is a much less common condition, the protoplasm of the liver-cells is destroyed and the fat takes its place, as seen in cases of malignant jaundice and in phosphorus poisoning.

Fatty liver occurs under the following conditions: (*a*) In association with general obesity, in which case the liver appears to be one of the storehouses of the excessive fat. (*b*) In conditions in which the oxidation processes are interfered with, as in cachexia, profound anæmia, and in phthisis. The fatty infiltration of the liver in heavy drinkers is to be attributed to the excessive demand made by the alcohol upon the oxygen. (*c*) Certain poisons, of which phosphorus is the most characteristic, produce an intense fatty degeneration with necrosis of the liver-cells. The poison of acute yellow atrophy, whatever its nature, acts in the same way.

The fatty liver is uniformly increased in size. The edge may reach below the level of the navel. It is smooth, looks pale and bloodless; on section it is dry, and renders the surface of the knife greasy. The liver may weigh many pounds, and yet the specific gravity is so low that the entire organ floats in water.

The symptoms of fatty liver are not definite. Jaundice is never present; the stools may be light-colored, but even in the most advanced grades the bile is still formed. Signs of portal obstruction are rare. Hæmorrhoids are not very infrequent. Altogether, the symptoms are ill-defined, and are chiefly those of the disease with which the degeneration is associated. In cases of great obesity, the physical examination is uncertain; but in phthisis and cachectic conditions, the organ can be felt to be greatly enlarged, though smooth and painless. Fatty livers are among the largest met with at the bedside.

XI. AMYLOID LIVER.

The waxy, lardaceous, or amyloid liver occurs as part of a general degeneration, associated with cachexias, particularly when the result of long-standing suppuration.

In practice, it is found oftenest in the prolonged suppuration of tuberculous disease, either of the lungs or of the bones. Next in order of frequency are the cases associated with syphilis. Here there may be ulceration of the rectum, with which it is often connected, or chronic disease of the bone, or it may be present when there are no suppurative changes. It is found occasionally in rickets, in prolonged convalescence from the infectious fevers, and in the cachexia of cancer.

The amyloid liver is large, and may attain dimensions equalled only by those of the cancerous organ. Wilks speaks of a liver weighing fourteen pounds. It is solid, firm, resistant, on section anæmic, and has a semitranslucent, infiltrated appearance. Stained with a dilute solution of iodine, the areas infiltrated with the amyloid matter assume a rich mahogany-brown color. The precise nature of this change is still in question. It first attacks the capillaries, usually of the median zone of the lobules, and subsequently the interlobular vessels and the connective tissue. The cells are but little if at all affected.

There are no characteristic *symptoms* of this condition. Jaundice does not occur; the stools may be light-colored, but the secretion of bile persists. The physical examination shows the organ to be uniformly enlarged and painless, the surface smooth, the edge rounded, and the consistence greatly increased. Sometimes the edge, even in very great enlargement, is sharp and hard. The spleen also may be involved, but there are no evidences of portal obstruction.

The *diagnosis* of the condition is, as a rule, easy. Progressive and great enlargement in connection with suppuration of long standing or with syphilis, is almost always of this nature. In rare instances, however, the amyloid liver is reduced in size.

In *leukæmia* the liver may attain considerable size and be smooth and uniform, resembling, on physical examination, the fatty organ. The blood condition at once indicates the true nature of the case.

236

XII. ANOMALIES IN FORM AND POSITION OF THE LIVER.

In transposition of the viscera the right lobe of the organ may occupy the left side. A common and important anomaly is the tilting forward of the organ, so that the antero-posterior axis becomes vertical, not horizontal. Instead of the edge of the right lobe presenting just below the costal margin, a considerable portion of the surface of the lobe is in contact with the abdominal parietes, and the edge may be felt as low, perhaps, as the navel. This anteversion is apt to be mistaken for enlargement of the organ.

The "lacing" liver is met with in two chief types. In one the anterior portion, chiefly of the right lobe, is greatly prolonged, and may reach the transverse navel line, or even lower. A shallow transverse groove separates the thin extension from the main portion of the organ. The peritoneal coating of this groove may be fibroid, and in rare instances the deformed portion is connected with the organ by an almost tendinous membrane. The liver may be compressed laterally and have a pyramidal shape, and the extreme left border and the hinder margin of the left lobe may be much folded and incurved. The projecting portion of the liver, extending low in the right flank, may be mistaken for a tumor, or more frequently for a movable right kidney. Its continuity with the liver itself may not be evident on palpation or on percussion, as coils of intestine may lie in front. It descends, however, with inspiration, and usually the margin can be traced continuously with that of the left lobe of the liver. The greatest difficulty arises when this anomalous lappet of the liver is either naturally very thick and united to the liver by a very thin membrane, or when it is swollen in conditions of great congestion of the organ.

The other principal type of lacing liver is quite different in shape. It is thick, broader above than below, and lies almost entirely above the transverse line of the cartilages. There is a narrow groove just above the anterior border, which is placed more transversely than normal.

Movable Liver.—This rare condition has received much attention, and J. E. Graham collected 70 reported cases from the literature. In a very considerable number of these there has been a mistaken diagnosis. A slight grade of mobility of the organ is found in the pendulous abdomen of enteroptosis, and after repeated ascites.

The organ is so connected at its posterior margin with the inferior vena cava and diaphragm that any great mobility from this point is impossible, except on the theory of a meso-hepar or congenital ligamentous union between these structures. The ligaments, however, may show an extreme grade of relaxation (the suspensory 7.5 cm., and the triangular ligament 4 cm., in one of Leube's cases); and when the patient is in the erect posture the organ may drop down so far that its upper surface is entirely below the costal margin. The condition is rarely met with in men; 56 of the cases were in women.

diseases of the liver

It may be safely assumed that Osler's great interest in the liver was maintained throughout his career. One of his best known classic papers, "On Fever of Hepatic Origin," appeared in 1890 (Johns Hopkins Hospital Reports, Vol. II, No. 1), two years before the publication of *The Principles and Practice of Medicine.* In this he refers to many personal experiences with problems of jaundice and liver disease, studied at the bedside and the autopsy table.

In his textbook Osler devotes the first part of the section on liver disease to a discussion of jaundice. He recognized obstructive jaundice as we do now but placed hemolytic and hepatocellular (his "toxemic") jaundice in a single group. In 1909 Virchow's catarrhal jaundice (our viral hepatitis) was presented under "Diseases of the Bile Passages and Gallbladder." Only following the observations of Eppinger in 1920 was this disease clearly removed from one beginning in the bile ducts and proper emphasis placed on the parenchymal hepatocellular damage. This basic confusion led to partial merging, in Osler's discussion, of parenchymal and obstructive jaundice.

The penetration of Osler's clinical observations, without benefit of any of the laboratory methods which have come to be regarded as more or less the sine qua non in the differential diagnosis of jaundice, is truly impressive.

No mention is made, of course, of the serum bilirubin in terms either of amount or form in relation to the different types of jaundice. The great contributions of Hijmans van der Bergh, Snapper, and Mueller were a few years ahead, appearing first in definitive form just at the end of World War I. The impact of their observations on the clinical study of jaundice was strong, and it is not unlikely that Osler learned of these even in the short space of time between the publication of van den Bergh's monograph in 1918 and Osler's death in late 1919. Similarly, Osler would have been much interested in the basic classification of jaundice proposed by Arnold Rich in 1930, which depended in considerable part on the results of the van den Bergh test and on whether bilirubin was present in the urine. Rich observed two different kinds of jaundice — one characterized by accumulation of indirect or delayed-reacting bilirubin in the blood without bilirubinuria ("retention jaundice"), and one by the accumulation of direct-reacting bilirubin in both the bile and urine ("regurgitation jaundice") — as two highly different forms of jaundice. This concept has been further extended by the demonstration that direct-reacting bilirubin is almost entirely a glucuronide conjugate.

238

Diseases of the liver

In describing hereditary icterus, Osler first considered icterus neonatorum. He cited some remarkable examples of the familial type which, in the light of present knowledge, are probably erythroblastosis fetalis. He reports that the brain and cord may be stained yellow in fatal cases of icterus neonatorum, in contrast to adult cases of jaundice — a reflection of more permeable blood-brain barrier in the immature individual, together with much greater concentration of free bilirubin in the blood. He also recognized congenital absence of the common or hepatic duct, congenital syphilitic hepatitis, and septic poisoning associated with phlebitis of the umbilical vein. Osler discusses Minkowski's congenital acholuric icterus, now generally designated as hereditary spherocytosis. Current interest in familial jaundice has identified at least four forms of jaundice not referred to by Osler. In addition, jaundice is a feature of several types of nonspherocytic hemolytic anemia caused by a genetic defect of a red cell enzyme — glucose-6-phosphate dehydrogenase, pyruvate kinase, and triosephosphate isomerase — as discovered in the last few years.

In discussing vascular affection of the liver, Osler does not mention the Budd-Chiari syndrome, most vividly brought to clinical attention by Chiari in 1889. The omission of constrictive pericarditis as a disease closely mimicking cirrhosis with ascites and edema is also noteworthy.

Little can be added to Osler's description of obstructive and suppurative disease of the bile ducts, biliary colic, common duct stone, and suppurative cholangitis. His description of intermittent hepatic fever of Charcot is excellent. His entire discussion of the various aspects of the diseases of the gallbladder and bile ducts is clinical. The advent of cholecystography, cholangiograms, transhepatic cholangiography and laboratory studies of the blood have supplemented his observations. Osler ascribed all acute cholecystitis to bacterial infection. A few would still agree with this, but most hold that chemical factors are quite significant. Osler's views on the genesis of gallstones are modern. He recognized the importance of stasis of bile, bacterial inflammation, and change in the chemical constitution of the bile.

Osler discussed hepatic cirrhosis from clinical, etiological, and anatomical points of view. Thus, alcoholic cirrhosis was "toxic," syphilitic cirrhosis was "infectious." He clearly implicated alcohol in respect to the atrophic cirrhosis of Laennec and the fatty cirrhotic liver without mentioning dietary deficiency. A few years ago protein deficiency in the chronic alcoholic would be given the prime role in the etiology of Laennec's cirrhosis, but more recent concepts have come full cycle back to the view of Osler that alcohol is directly toxic. The large fatty cirrhotic liver was considered by Osler a milder form of the disease. Osler's description of the collateral circulation is up to date, except that he gives more emphasis to the relative frequency of "caput Medusae" and less emphasis on esophageal varices than would be given by most clinicians today. The statement on hemorrhage ("Haemorrhage from the stomach may be an early symptom; it is often profuse and liable to recur. It seldom proves fatal.") is certainly at variance with present-day experience which places bleeding from varices as the cause of death in about one third of patients with cirrhosis.

In speaking of ascites Osler observed: "The conditions under which this occurs are still obscure." While it cannot yet be said that the ascites of cirrhosis is fully understood, there is agreement that hormone-mediated renal retention of sodium is essential for its formation, probably of greater importance than portal hypertension or the often lowered oncotic pressure of the plasma. Ratnoff and Patek presented data in 1945 illustrating Osler's view: "Ascites is a very serious event, especially if due to the cirrhosis and not to an associated peritonitis." Although still regarded as a serious complication, the ascites of cirrhosis can now be managed with a far greater degree of optimism because of the newer information of the past two decades. Osler said, "With the advent of ascites, the critical stage is reached. A dry diet, without salt, and free purgation may relieve a small exudate, rarely a large one, and it is best to tap early or to advise Talma's operation:"* The reference to restriction of salt is highly interesting, as in recent years this has become the cornerstone of much more successful treatment of ascites. Presently, reduction in total body sodium is achieved in part by dietary restriction and in part by natriuretic agents. Osler used the much less effective purgation to deplete his patients of sodium.

The clinical description of the patient with advanced cirrhosis is truly on a par with any of the classical descriptions of disease. "Later in the disease, the patient has an unmistakable hepatic facies; he is thin, the eyes are sunken, the conjunctivae watery, the nose and cheeks show distended venules, and the complexion is muddy or icteroid."

Osler's description of the hypertrophic cirrhosis of Hanot corresponds closely with what today is generally termed primary biliary cirrhosis ("cholangiolitic" cirrhosis). He commented upon the pruritus and

*Omentopexy: suturing of omentum to abdominal wall to encourage portacaval anastomoses.

the pigmentation, but mentioned the xanthoma only casually. The lipid abnormalities have been a focal point of biochemists for the last two decades. The "pigmentary form of cirrhosis in diabetes" is alluded to but is not clearly discussed in the sections on cirrhosis. Apart from this, hemochromatosis is not considered.

Treatment has, of course, changed. Osler's treatment of hepatitis, emphasizing keeping the bowels open with calomel or saline, the use of Vichy water, and cold irrigations of the colon, would find little support today. In alcoholic cirrhosis "it is too late, as a rule, to do much after symptoms have occurred." Today the early precise diagnosis of cirrhosis at a stage when symptoms are mild and often lead to treatment in time for restoration to health, at least in individuals who will continue to abstain from alcohol. In the last two decades we have come to appreciate the great significance of protein, first its value and later its dangers. Protein is highly beneficial in defatting the liver and in promoting normal hepatic regeneration. Protein is dangerous from the standpoint of promoting encephalopathy. Although Osler recognized encephalopathy, he did not discern its cause.

Osler mentioned that portacaval anastomosis had been performed once in a man with cirrhosis of the liver (Widal, 1903). He would have been surprised to see the surge of interest in portacaval shunting for combating the problem of esophageal varices, a problem that he did not clearly recognize.

Osler devoted a large section to liver abscess. His clinical description of amebic abscess and its complications is excellent and is still complete except for modern chemotherapy.

Though our knowledge of jaundice and of the various forms of liver disease, their pathogenesis, and treatment has no doubt increased extensively since Osler wrote his great textbook, one can still read his lucid descriptions of these disorders with pleasure and often with profit.

Cecil J. Watson

Diseases of the liver

REFERENCES

Baggenstoss, A.H. The changing concepts of pathology in liver disease. Amer. J. Dig. Dis., 6:178, 1961.

Popper, H., and Schaffner, F. Progress in Liver Diseases. New York and London, Grune & Stratton, Inc., 1961, Vol. 1; 1965, Vol. 2.

Ratnoff, O.D., and Patek, A.J., Jr. The natural history of Laennec's cirrhosis of the liver. Medicine, 21:207, 1942.

Rich, A.R. The pathogenesis of the forms of jaundice. Bull. Hopkins Hosp., 47:338, 1930.

Schmid, R. Hyperbilirubinemia. Ch. 37 In The Metabolic Basis of Inherited Disease, 2nd ed. Stanbury J.B., Wyngaarden, J.B., and Frederickson, D.S., eds. New York, Blakiston Div. of McGraw-Hill Book Company, 1966, p. 871.

acute rheumatism, lead poisoning, and intestinal hæmorrhages. This pigment has been found very frequently after the administration of sulphonal, and sometimes imparts a very dark color to the urine.

V. URÆMIA.

Definition.—A toxæmia developing in the course of nephritis or in conditions associated with anuria. The nature of the poison or poisons is as yet unknown, whether they are the retained normal products or the products of an abnormal metabolism.

Theories of Uræmia.—The view most widely held is that uræmia is due to the accumulation in the blood of excrementitious material—body poisons— which should be thrown off by the kidneys. "If, however, from any cause, these organs make default, or if there be any prolonged obstruction to the outflow of urine, accumulation of some or of all the poisons takes place, and the characteristic symptoms are manifested, but the accumulation may be very slow and the earlier symptoms, corresponding to the comparatively small dose of poison, may be very slight; yet they are in kind, though not in degree, as indicative of uræmia as are the more alarming, which appear toward the end, and to which alone the name uræmia is often given" (Carter). Herter and others have shown that the toxicity of the blood-serum in uræmic states is increased. The part played by urea itself, by the salts, and by the nitrogenous extractives has not been determined.

Another view is that uræmia depends on the products of an abnormal metabolism. Brown-Séquard suggested that the kidney has an internal secretion, and it is urged that the symptoms of uræmia are due to its disturbance. Bradford's experiments show that the kidneys do influence profoundly the metabolism of the tissues of the body, particularly of the muscles. If more than two-thirds of the total kidney weight be removed, there is an extraordinary increase in the production of urea and of the nitrogenous bodies of the creatin class. He favors this view, but acknowledges that we are still ignorant of the nature of the poison. From a careful study of the question, Hughes and Carter concluded that the poison was an albuminous product quite different from anything in normal urine. In Bradford's Goulstonian Lectures (1898) will be found a full discussion of the question.

Traube believed that the symptoms of uræmia, particularly the coma and convulsions, were due to localized œdema of the brain.

Symptoms.—Clinically, we may recognize latent, acute, and chronic forms of uræmia. The latent form has been considered under the section on anuria. Acute uræmia may arise in any form of nephritis. It is more common in the post-febrile varieties. Bradford thinks that it is specially associated with a form of contracted white kidney in young subjects. Chronic forms of uræmia are more frequent in the arterio-sclerotic and granular kidney. For convenience the symptoms of uræmia may be described under cerebral, dyspnœic, and gastro-intestinal manifestations.

Among the CEREBRAL symptoms of uræmia may be described:

(*a*) *Mania.*—This may come on abruptly in an individual who has shown no previous indications of mental trouble, and who may not be known to have Bright's disease. In a remarkable case of this kind which came under my observation the patient became suddenly maniacal and died in six days. More commonly the delirium is less violent, but the patient is noisy, talkative, restless, and sleepless.

(*b*) *Delusional Insanity* (*Folie Brightique*).—Cases are by no means uncommon, and excellent clinical reports have been issued on the subject from several of the asylums, particularly by Bremer, Christian, and Alice Bennett. Delusions of persecution are common. One of my cases committed suicide by jumping out of a window. The condition is of interest medico-legally because of its bearing on testamentary capacity. Profound melancholia may also supervene.

(*c*) *Convulsions.*—These may come on unexpectedly or be preceded by pain in the head and restlessness. The attacks may be general and identical with those of ordinary epilepsy, though the initial cry may not be present. The fits may recur rapidly, and in the interval the patient is usually unconscious. Sometimes the temperature is elevated, but more frequently it is depressed, and may sink rapidly after the attack. Local or Jacksonian epilepsy may occur in most characteristic form in uræmia. A remarkable sequence of the convulsions is blindness—*uræmic amaurosis*—which may persist for several days. This, however, may occur apart from the convulsions. It usually passes off in a day or two. There are, as a rule, no ophthalmoscopic changes. Sometimes uræmic deafness supervenes, and is probably also a cerebral manifestation. It may also occur in connection with persistent headache, nausea, and other gastric symptoms.

(*d*) *Coma.*—Unconsciousness invariably accompanies the general convulsions, but a coma may develop gradually without any convulsive seizures. Frequently it is preceded by headache, and the patient gradually becomes dull and apathetic. In these cases there may have been no previous indications of renal disease, and unless the urine is examined the nature of the case may be overlooked. Twitchings of the muscles occur, particularly in the face and hands, but there are many cases of coma in which the muscles are not involved. In some of these cases a condition of torpor persists for weeks or even months. The tongue is usually furred and the breath very foul and heavy.

(*e*) *Local Palsies.*—In the course of chronic Bright's disease hemiplegia or monoplegia may come on spontaneously or follow a convulsion, and post mortem no gross lesions of the brain be found, but only a localized or diffused œdema. These cases, which are not very uncommon, may simulate almost every form of organic paralysis of cerebral origin.

(*f*) Of other cerebral symptoms, HEADACHE is important. It is most often occipital and extends to the neck. It may be an early feature and associated with giddiness. Other nervous symptoms of uræmia are intense itching of the skin, numbness and tingling in the fingers, and cramps in the muscles of the calves, particularly at night. An erythema may be present.

URÆMIC DYSPNŒA is classified by Palmer Howard as follows: (1) Continuous dyspnœa; (2) paroxysmal dyspnœa; (3) both types alternating; and (4) Cheyne-Stokes breathing. The attacks of dyspnœa are most commonly nocturnal; the patient may sit up, gasp for breath, and evince as much distress as in true asthma. Occasionally the breathing is noisy and stridulous. The Cheyne-Stokes type may persist for weeks, and is not necessarily associated with coma. I have seen it in a man who travelled over a hundred miles to consult a physician. In another instance a patient, up and about, could when at meals feed himself only in the apnœa period. Though usually of serious omen and occurring with coma and other symptoms, recovery may follow even after persistence for weeks or even months.

The GASTRO-INTESTINAL manifestations of uræmia often set in with abruptness. Uncontrollable vomiting may come on and its cause be quite unrecognizable. A young married woman was admitted to my wards in the Montreal General Hospital with persistent vomiting of four or five days' duration. The urine was slightly albuminous, but she had none of the usual signs of uræmia, and the case was not regarded as one of Bright's disease. The vomiting persisted and caused death. The post mortem showed extensive sclerosis of both kidneys. The attacks may be preceded by nausea and may be associated with diarrhœa. In some instances the diarrhœa may come on without the vomiting; sometimes it is profuse and associated with an intense catarrhal or even diphtheritic inflammation of the colon.

A special URÆMIC STOMATITIS has been described (Barie) in which the mucosa of the lips, gums, and tongue is swollen and erythematous. The saliva may be increased, and there is difficulty in swallowing and in mastication. The tongue is usually very foul and the breath heavy and fetid. A cutaneous erythema may occur and a remarkable urea " frost " on the skin.

FEVER is not uncommon in uræmic states, and may occur with the acute nephritis, with the complications, and as a manifestation of the uræmia itself (Stengel).

Very many patients with chronic uræmia succumb to what I have called terminal infections—acute peritonitis, pericarditis, pleurisy, meningitis, or endocarditis.

Diagnosis.—Herter calls attention to the value of the clinical determination of the urea in the blood (for which purpose only a few cubic centimetres are required) as an index of the degree of renal inadequacy. Cryoscopy, the electrical conductivity of blood and urine, also the methylene blue, potassium iodide, salicylic-acid tests have been employed in the hope of testing the functional ability of the kidneys. The result has been that while in some cases of uræmia one finds the expected accumulation of urea and ions in the blood, in others the kidneys are, judged by these tests, normal. In some cases of nephritis without any signs of uræmia the kidneys are apparently as insufficient as the worst uræmia cases. In but 2 of 96 cases could the urea determination have been of any value in predicting uræmia, and equal drops in the urea occurred without this symptom (Emerson).

It is still common to depend on the urea estimation as of service in foretelling an uræmia, but in the 96 cases of nephritis with uræmia in my wards in but 2 cases was it of any real value.

Uræmia may be confounded with:

(*a*) Cerebral lesions, such as hæmorrhage, meningitis, or even tumor. In apoplexy, which is so commonly associated with kidney disease and stiff arteries, the sudden loss of consciousness, particularly if with convulsions, may simulate a uræmic attack; but the mode of onset, the existence of complete hemiplegia, with conjugate deviation of the eyes, suggest hæmorrhage. As already noted, there are cases of uræmic hemiplegia or monoplegia which can not be separated from those of organic lesion and which post mortem show no trace of coarse disease of the brain. I know of an instance in which a consultation was held upon the propriety of operation in a case of hemiplegia believed to be due to subdural hæmorrhage which post mortem was shown to be uræmic. Indeed, in some of these cases it is quite impossible to distinguish between the two conditions. So, too, cases of meningitis, in a condition of deep coma, with perhaps slight fever, furred tongue, but without localizing symptoms, may readily be confounded with uræmia.

(*b*) With certain infectious diseases. Uræmia may persist for weeks or months and the patient lies in a condition of torpor or even unconsciousness, with a heavily coated, perhaps dry, tongue, muscular twitchings, a rapid feeble pulse, with slight fever. This state not unnaturally suggests the existence of one of the infectious diseases. Cases of the kind are not uncommon, and I have known them to be mistaken for typhoid fever and for miliary tuberculosis.

(*c*) Uræmic coma may be confounded with poisoning by alcohol or opium. In opium poisoning the pupils are contracted; in alcoholism they are more commonly dilated. In uræmia they are not constant; they may be either widely dilated or of medium size. The examination of the eye-ground should be made to determine the presence or absence of albuminuric retinitis. The urine should be drawn off and examined. The odor of the breath sometimes gives an important hint.

The condition of the heart and arteries should also be taken into account. Sudden uræmic coma is more common in the chronic interstitial nephritis. The character of the delirium in alcoholism is sometimes important, and the coma is not so deep as in uræmia or opium poisoning. It may for a time be impossible to determine whether the condition is due to uræmia, profound alcoholism, or hæmorrhage into the pons Varolii.

And lastly, in connection with sudden coma, it is to be remembered that insensibility may occur after prolonged muscular exertion, as after running a ten-mile race. In some instances unconsciousness has come on rapidly with stertorous breathing and dilated pupils. Cases have occurred under conditions in which sun-stroke could be excluded; and Poore, who reports a case in the Lancet (1894), considers that the condition is due to the too rapid accumulation of waste products in the blood, and to hyperpyrexia from suspension of sweating.

The treatment will be considered under Chronic Bright's Disease.

VI. ACUTE BRIGHT'S DISEASE.

Definition.—Acute diffuse nephritis, due to the action of cold or of toxic agents upon the kidneys.

In all instances changes exist in the epithelial, vascular, and intertubular tissues, which vary in intensity in different forms; hence writers have described a tubular, a glomerular, and an acute interstitial nephritis. Delafield recognizes *acute exudative* and *acute productive* forms, the latter characterized by proliferation of the connective-tissue stroma and of the cells of the Malpighian tufts.

Etiology.—The following are the principal causes of acute nephritis:

(1) Cold. Exposure to cold and wet is one of the most common causes. It is particularly prone to follow exposure after a drinking-bout.

246

(2) The poisons of the specific fevers, particularly scarlet fever, less commonly typhoid fever, measles, diphtheria, small-pox, chicken-pox, malaria, cholera, yellow fever, meningitis, and, very rarely, dysentery. Acute nephritis may be associated with syphilis and with acute tuberculosis, particularly the former, to which Bradford has recently called attention as an important cause. He suggests that many of the idiopathic cases and those ascribed to cold may be of syphilitic origin. It may also occur in septicæmia and in acute tonsillitis. In exudative erythema and the allied purpuric affections acute nephritis is not uncommon. Among 1,832 cases of malaria at the Johns Hopkins Hospital there were 26 of nephritis (Thayer).

(3) Toxic agents, such as turpentine, cantharides, potassium chlorate, and carbolic acid may cause an acute congestion which sometimes terminates in nephritis. Alcohol probably never excites an acute nephritis.

(4) Pregnancy, in which the condition is thought by some to result from compression of the renal veins, although this is not yet finally settled. The condition may in reality be due to toxic products as yet undetermined.

(5) Acute nephritis occurs occasionally in connection with extensive lesions of the skin, as in burns or in chronic skin-diseases, and also after trauma. It may follow operations on the kidney.

Morbid Anatomy.—The kidneys may present to the naked eye in mild cases no evident alterations. When seen early in more severe forms the organs are congested, swollen, dark, and on section may drip blood. Bright's original description is as follows:

" The kidneys . . . stripped easily out of their investing membrane, were large and less firm than they often are, of the darkest chocolate color, interspersed with a few white points, and a great number nearly black; and this, with a little tinge of red in parts, gave the appearance of a polished fine-grained porphyry or greenstone. . . . On (section) these colors were found to pervade the whole cortical part; but the natural striated appearance was not lost, and the external part of each mass of tubuli was particularly dark . . . a very considerable quantity of blood oozed from the kidney, showing a most unusual accumulation in the organ."

In other instances the surface is pale and mottled, the capsule strips off readily, and the cortex is swollen, turbid, and of a grayish-red color, while the pyramids have an intense beefy-red tint. The glomeruli in some instances stand out plainly, being deeply swollen and congested; in other instances they are pale.

Histology.—The histology may be thus summarized: (*a*) *Glomerular changes.* In a majority of the cases of nephritis due to toxic agents, which reach the kidney through the blood-vessels, the tufts suffer first, and there is either an acute intracapillary glomerulitis, in which the capillaries become filled with cells and thrombi, or involvement of the epithelium of the tuft and of Bowman's capsule, the cavity of which contains leucocytes and red blood-corpuscles. Hyaline degeneration of the contents and of the walls of the capillaries of the tuft is an extremely common event. These processes are perhaps best marked in scarlatinal nephritis. There may be proliferation about Bowman's capsule. These changes interfere with the circulation in the tufts and seriously influence the nutrition of the tubular structures beyond them.

(*b*) The *alterations in the tubular epithelium* consist in cloudy swelling, fatty change, and hyaline degeneration. In the convoluted tubules, the accumulation of altered cells with leucocytes and blood-corpuscles causes the enlargement and swelling of the organ. The epithelial cells lose their striation, the nuclei are obscured, and hyaline droplets often accumulate in them.

(*c*) *Interstitial changes.* In the milder forms a simple inflammatory exudate—serum mixed with leucocytes and red blood-corpuscles—exists between the tubules. In severer cases areas of small-celled infiltration occur about the capsules and between the convoluted tubes. These changes may be wide-spread and uniform throughout the organs or more intense in certain regions.

Councilman has described an *acute interstitial nephritis* occurring chiefly in children after fevers, characterized by the presence of cells similar to those described by Unna as plasma cells. He thinks that these cells are formed in other organs, chiefly the spleen and bone marrow, and are carried to the kidneys in the blood-current.

Symptoms.—The onset is usually sudden, and when the nephritis follows cold, dropsy may be noticed within twenty-four hours. After fevers the onset is less abrupt, but the patient gradually becomes pale and a puffiness of the face or swelling of the ankles is first noticed. In children there may at the outset be convulsions. Chilliness or rigors initiate the attack in a limited number of cases. Pain in the back, nausea, and vomiting may be present. The fever is variable. Many cases in adults have no rise in temperature. In young children with nephritis from cold or scarlet fever the temperature may, for a few days, range from 101° to 103°.

The most characteristic symptoms are the *urinary changes*. There may at first be suppression; more commonly the urine is scanty, highly colored, and contains blood, albumin, and tube-casts. The quantity is reduced and only 4 or 5 ounces may be passed in the twenty-four hours; the specific gravity is high—1.025, or even more; the color varies from a smoky to a deep porter color, but is seldom bright red. On standing there is a heavy deposit; microscopically there are blood-corpuscles, epithelium from the urinary passages, and hyaline, blood, and epithelial tube-casts. The albumin is abundant, forming a curdy, thick precipitate. The largest amounts of albumin are seen in the early acute nephritis of syphilis. In Hoffmann's case this reached 8.5 per cent. The total excretion of urea is reduced, though the percentage is high.

Anæmia is an early and marked symptom. In cases of extensive dropsy, effusion may take place into the pleuræ and peritonæum. There are cases of scarlatinal nephritis in which the dropsy of the extremities is trivial and effusion into the pleuræ extensive. The lungs may become œdematous. In rare cases there is œdema of the glottis. Epistaxis may occur or cutaneous ecchymoses may develop in the course of the disease.

The pulse may be hard, the tension increased, and the second sound in the aortic area accentuated. Occasionally dilatation of the heart comes on rapidly and may cause sudden death (Goodhart). The skin is dry and it may be difficult to induce sweating.

Uræmic symptoms occur in a limited number of cases, either at the onset

248

with suppression, more commonly later in the disease. Ocular changes are not so common in acute as in chronic Bright's disease, but hæmorrhagic retinitis may occur and occasionally papillitis.

The course of acute Bright's disease varies considerably. The description just given is of the form which most commonly follows cold or scarlet fever. In many of the febrile cases dropsy is not a prominent symptom, and the diagnosis rests rather with the examination of the urine. Moreover, the condition may be transient and less serious. In other cases, as in the acute nephritis of typhoid fever, there may be hæmaturia and pronounced signs of interference with the renal function. The most intense acute nephritis may exist without anasarca.

In scarlatinal nephritis, in which the glomeruli are most seriously affected, suppression of the urine may be an early symptom, the dropsy is apt to be extreme, and uræmic manifestations are common. Acute Bright's disease in children, however, may set in very insidiously and be associated with transient or slight œdema, and the symptoms may point rather to affection of the digestive system or to brain-disease.

Diagnosis.—It is very important to bear in mind that the most serious involvement of the kidneys may be manifested only by slight œdema of the feet or puffiness of the eyelids, without impairment of the general health. On the other hand from the urine alone a diagnosis can not be made with certainty since simple cloudy, swelling, and circulatory changes may cause a similar condition of urine. The first indication of trouble may be a uræmic convulsion. This is particularly the case in the acute nephritis of pregnancy, and it is a good rule for the practitioner, when engaged to attend a case, invariably to ask that during the seventh and eighth months the urine should occasionally be sent for examination.

In nephritis from cold and in scarlet fever the symptoms are usually marked and the diagnosis is rarely in doubt. As already mentioned, every case in which albumin is present must not be called acute Bright's disease, not even if tube-casts be present. Thus the common febrile albuminuria, although it represents the first link in the chain of events leading to acute Bright's disease, should not be placed in the same category.

There are occasional cases of acute Bright's disease with anasarca, in which albumin is either absent or present only as a trace. This is a rare condition. Tube-casts are usually found, and the absence of albumin is rarely permanent. The urine may be reduced in amount.

The character of the casts is of use in the diagnosis of the form of Bright's disease, but scarcely of such extreme value as has been stated. Thus, the hyaline and granular casts are common to all varieties. The blood and epithelial casts, particularly those made up of leucocytes, are most common in the acute cases.

Prognosis.—The outlook varies somewhat with the cause of the disease. Recoveries in the form following exposure to cold are much more frequent than after scarlatinal nephritis. In younger children the mortality is high, amounting to at least one-third of the cases. Serious symptoms are low arterial tension, the occurrence of uræmia, and effusion into the serous sacs. The persistence of the dropsy after the first month, intense pallor, and a large amount of albumin indicate the possibility of the disease becoming chronic.

For some months after the disappearance of the dropsy there may be traces of albumin and a few tube-casts.

In a case of scarlatinal nephritis, if the progress is favorable, the dropsy diminishes in a week or ten days, the urine increases, the albumin lessens, and by the end of a month the dropsy has disappeared and the urine is nearly free. In very young children the course may be rapid, and I have known the urine to be free from albumin in the fourth week. Other cases are more insidious, and though the dropsy may disappear, the albumin persists in the urine, the anæmia is marked, and the condition becomes chronic, or, after several recurrences of the dropsy, improves and complete recovery takes place.

Treatment.—The patient should be in bed and there remain until all traces of the disease have disappeared. As sweating plays such an important part in the treatment, it is well, if possible, to accustom the patient to blankets. He should also be clad in thin Canton flannel.

The diet should consist of milk or butter-milk, gruels made of arrow-root or oat-meal, barley water, and, if necessary, beef tea and chicken broth. It is better, if possible, to confine the patient to a strictly milk diet. As convalescence is established, bread and butter, lettuce, water-cress, grapes, oranges, and other fruits may be given. Meats should be used very sparingly. As there is marked retention of the chlorides, which seem to bear a relation to the dropsy, salt should be withheld.

The patient should drink freely of alkaline mineral waters, ordinary water, or lemonade. The fluids keep the kidneys flushed and wash out the *débris* from the tubes. A useful drink is a drachm of cream of tartar in a pint of boiling water, to which may be added the juice of half a lemon and a little sugar. Taken when cold, this is a pleasant and satisfactory diluent drink.

No remedies, so far as known, control directly the changes which are going on in the kidneys. The indications are: (1) To give the excretory function of the kidney rest by utilizing the skin and the bowels, in the hope that the natural processes may be sufficient to effect a cure; (2) to meet the symptoms as they arise.

In a case of scarlet fever it may occasionally be possible to avert an attack, the premonitory symptoms of which are marked increase in the arterial tension and the presence of blood coloring matter in the urine (Mahomed). An active saline cathartic may completely relieve this condition.

At the onset, when there is pain in the back or hæmaturia, the Paquelin cautery or the dry or wet cups give relief. The last should not be used in children. Warm poultices are often grateful. In cases which set in with suppression of urine, these measures should be adopted, and in addition the hot bath with subsequent pack, copious diluents, and a free purge. The dropsy is best treated by hydrotherapy—either the hot bath, the wet pack, or the hot-air bath. In children the wet pack is usually satisfactory. It is applied by wringing a blanket out of hot water, wrapping the child in it, covering this with a dry blanket, and then with a rubber cloth. In this the child may remain for an hour. It may be repeated daily. In the case of adults, the hot-air bath or the vapor bath may be conveniently given by allowing the vapor or air to pass from a funnel beneath the bed-clothes, which are raised on a low cradle. More efficient, as a rule, is a hot bath of from fifteen or twenty minutes, after which the patient is wrapped in blankets. The sweating produced by these measures is usually profuse, rarely exhausting, and in a majority of cases the dropsy can in this way be relieved. There are some cases, however, in which the skin does not respond to the baths, and if the symptoms are serious, particularly if uræmia supervenes, jaborandi or its active principle, pilocarpine, may be used. The latter may be given hypodermically, in doses of from a sixth to an eighth of a grain in adults, and from a twentieth to a twelfth of a grain in children of from two to ten years.

The bowels should be kept open by a morning saline purge; in children the fluid magnesia is readily taken; in adults the sulphate of magnesia may be given by Hay's method, in concentrated form, in the morning, before anything is taken into the stomach. In Bright's disease it not infrequently causes vomiting. The compound powder of jalap, in half-drachm doses, or, if necessary, elaterium may be used. If the dropsy is not extreme, the urine not very concentrated, and uræmic symptoms are not present, the bowels should be kept loose without active purgation. If these measures fail to reduce the dropsy and it has become extreme, the skin may be punctured with a lancet or drained by a small silver canula (Southey's tube), which is inserted beneath it. A fine aspirator needle may be used, and the fluid allowed to drain through a piece of long, narrow rubber tubing into a vessel beneath the bed. If the dyspnœa is marked, owing to pressure of fluid in the pleuræ, aspiration should be performed. In rare instances the ascites is extreme and may require paracentesis, or a Southey's tube may be inserted and the fluid gradually withdrawn. If uræmic convulsions occur, the intensity of the paroxysms may be limited by the use of chloroform; to an adult a pilocarpine injection should be at once given, and from a robust, strong man 20 ounces of blood may be withdrawn. In children the loins may be dry cupped, the wet pack used, and a brisk purgative given. Bromide of potassium and chloral sometimes prove useful.

Vomiting may be relieved by ice and by restricting the amount of food. Drop doses of creasote, iodine, and carbolic acid may be given. The dilute hydrocyanic acid with bismuth is often effectual.

The question of the use of diuretics in acute Bright's disease is not yet settled. The best diuretic, after all, is water, which may be taken freely with the citrate of potash or the benzoate of soda, salts which are held to favor the conversion of the urates into less irritating and more easily excreted compounds. Digitalis and strophanthus are useful diuretics, and may be employed without risk when the arterial tension is low and the cardiac impulse is not forcible. I have never seen any injurious effects from their employment after the early symptoms had lessened in intensity.

For the persistent albuminuria, I agree with Roberts and Rosenstein that we have no remedy of the slightest value. Nothing indicates more clearly our helplessness in controlling kidney metabolism than inability to meet this common symptom. Astringents, alkalies, nitroglycerin, and mercury have been recommended.

For the anæmia always associated with acute Bright's disease iron should be employed. It should not be given until the acute symptoms have subsided. In the adult it may be used in the form of the perchloride in increasing doses, as convalescence proceeds. In children, the syrup of the iodide of iron or the syrup of the phosphate of iron are better preparations. Tyson has recently urged caution in the too free use of iron in kidney disease. The dilatation of the heart is best treated with digitalis, strophanthus, and strychnia.

In the convalescence from acute Bright's disease, care should be taken to guard the patient against cold. The diet should still consist chiefly of milk and a return to mixed food should be gradual. A change of air is often beneficial, particularly a residence in a warm, equable climate.

VII. CHRONIC BRIGHT'S DISEASE.

Here, too, in all forms we deal with a diffuse process, involving epithelial, interstitial, and glomerular tissues. Clinically two groups are recognized— (*a*) the chronic parenchymatous nephritis, which follows the acute attack or comes on insidiously, is characterized by marked dropsy, and post mortem by the *large white kidney.* In the later stages of this process the kidney may be smaller—a condition known as the *small white kidney; (b)* chronic interstitial nephritis, in which dropsy is not common and the cardio-vascular changes are pronounced. Delafield recognizes a chronic diffuse nephritis with exudation and a chronic productive diffuse nephritis without exudation, the latter corresponding to the contracted kidney of authors.

The amyloid kidney is usually spoken of as a variety of Bright's disease, but in reality it is a degeneration which may accompany any form of nephritis.

1. CHRONIC PARENCHYMATOUS NEPHRITIS

(*Chronic Desquamative and Chronic Tubal Nephritis; Chronic Diffuse Nephritis with Exudation*).

Etiology.—In many cases the disease follows the acute nephritis of cold, scarlet fever, or pregnancy. More frequently than is usually stated the disease has an insidious onset and occurs independently of any acute attack. The fevers may play an important *rôle* in certain of these cases. Rosenstein, Bartels, and, in this country, I. E. Atkinson and Thayer have laid special stress upon malaria as a cause. The use of alcohol is believed to lead to this form of nephritis. In chronic suppuration, syphilis, and tuberculosis the diffuse parenchymatous nephritis is not uncommon, and is usually associated with amyloid disease. Males are rather more subject to the affection than females. It is met with most commonly in young adults, and is by no means infrequent in children as a sequence of scarlatinal nephritis.

Morbid Anatomy.—Several varieties of this form have been recognized. The *large white kidney* of Wilks, in which the organ is enlarged, the capsule is thin, and the surface white with the stellate veins injected is not very common in America. On section the cortex is swollen and yellowish-white in color, and often presents opaque areas. The pyramids may be deeply congested. On microscopical examination it is seen that the epithelium is granular and fatty, and the tubules of the cortex are distended, and contain tube-casts. Hyaline changes are also present in the epithelial cells. The glomeruli are large, the capsules thickened, the capillaries show hyaline changes, and the epithelium of the tuft and of the capsule is extensively altered. The interstitial tissue is everywhere increased, though not to an extreme degree. I have had in my wards but 30 such cases with autopsy. The average weight of both kidneys was 420 grammes, the heaviest 580 grammes.

The second variety of this form results from the gradual increase in the connective tissue and the subsequent shrinkage, forming what is called the *small white kidney* or the pale granular kidney. It is doubtful whether this is always preceded by the large white kidney. Some observers hold that it may be a primary independent form. The capsule is thickened and the surface is rough and granular. On section the resistance is greatly increased, the cortex is reduced and presents numerous opaque white or whitish-yellow foci, consisting of accumulations of fatty epithelium in the convoluted tubules. This combination of contracted kidney with the areas of marked fatty degeneration has given the name of small granular fatty kidney to this form. The interstitial changes are marked, many of the glomeruli are destroyed, the degeneration of epithelium in the convoluted tubules is wide-spread, and the arteries are greatly thickened.

Belonging to this chronic tubal nephritis is a variety known as the *chronic hæmorrhagic nephritis,* in which the organs are enlarged, yellowish-white in color, and in the cortex are many brownish-red areas, due to hæmorrhage into and about the tubes. In other respects the changes are identical with those in the large white kidney.

Of changes in the other organs the most marked are thickening of the blood-vessels and hypertrophy of the left heart.

Symptoms.—Following an acute nephritis, the disease may present, in a modified way, the symptoms of that affection. In many cases it sets in insidiously, and after an attack of dyspepsia or a period of failing health and loss of strength the patient becomes pale, and puffiness of the eyelids or swollen feet are noticed in the morning.

The symptoms are as follows: The urine is, as a rule, diminished in quantity, averaging 500 cc., often scanty. It has a dirty-yellow, sometimes smoky, color, and is turbid from the presence of urates. On standing, a heavy sediment falls, in which are found numerous tube-casts of various forms and sizes, hyaline, both large and small, epithelial, granular, and fatty casts. Leucocytes are abundant; red blood-corpuscles are frequently met with, and epithelium from the kidneys and pelves. The albumin is abundant and may be from 4 to 6 per cent. It is more abundant in the urine passed during the day. The specific gravity may be high in the early stages—from 1.020 to 1.025, even 1.040—though in the later stages it is lower. The urea is always reduced in quantity. As the case improves from 5 to 6 litres a day may be voided.

Dropsy is a marked and obstinate symptom of this form of Bright's disease. The face is pale and puffy, and in the morning the eyelids are œdematous. The anasarca is general, and there may be involvement of the serous sacs. In these chronic cases associated with large white kidney there is often a distinctive appearance in the face; the complexion is pasty, the pallor marked, and the eyelids are œdematous. The dropsy is peculiarly obstinate. Uræmic symptoms are common, though convulsions are perhaps less frequent than in the interstitial nephritis.

The tension of the pulse is usually increased; the vessels ultimately become stiff and the heart hypertrophied, though there are instances of this form of nephritis in which the heart is not enlarged. The aortic second sound is

253

accentuated. Retinal changes, though less frequent than in the chronic interstitial nephritis, occur in a considerable number of cases.

Gastro-intestinal symptoms are common. Vomiting is frequently a distressing and serious symptom, and diarrhœa may be profuse. Ulceration of the colon may occur and prove fatal.

It is sometimes impossible to determine, even by the most careful examination of the urine or by analysis of the symptoms, whether the condition of the kidney is that of the large white or of the small white form. In cases, however, which have lasted for several years, with the progressive increase in the renal connective tissue and the cardio-vascular changes, the clinical picture may approach, in certain respects, that of the contracted kidney. The urine is increased, with low specific gravity. It is often turbid, may contain traces of blood, the tube-casts are numerous and of every variety of form and size, and the albumin is abundant. Dropsy is usually present, though not so extensive as in the early stages.

Prognosis.—The prognosis is extremely grave. In a case which has persisted for more than a year recovery rarely takes place. Death is caused either by great effusion with œdema of the lungs, by uræmia, or by secondary inflammation of the serous membranes. Occasionally in children, even when the disease has persisted for two years, the symptoms disappear and recovery takes place.

Treatment.—Essentially the same treatment should be carried out as in acute Bright's disease. Milk or butter-milk should constitute for a time the chief article of food. Later more food may be allowed, oysters, fresh vegetables, and fruit. The dropsy should be treated by the hot baths, and a salt-free diet. Iron preparations should be given when there is marked anæmia. It is to be remembered that the pallor of the face may not be a good index of the blood condition. The acetate of potash, digitalis, and diuretin are useful in increasing the flow of urine. Basham's mixture given in plenty of water will be found beneficial.

2. Chronic Interstitial Nephritis

(Contracted Kidney; Granular Kidney; Cirrhosis of the Kidney; Gouty Kidney; Renal Sclerosis).

Sclerosis of the kidney is met with (*a*) as a sequence of the large white kidney, forming the so-called pale granular or secondary contracted kidney; (*b*) as an independent primary affection; (*c*) as a sequence of arterio-sclerosis.

Etiology.—The *primary form* is chronic from the outset, and is a slow, creeping degeneration of the kidney substance—in many respects only an anticipation of the gradual changes which take place in the organ in extreme old age. In many cases no satisfactory cause can be assigned. In others there are hereditary influences, as in the remarkable family studied by Dickinson, in which a pronounced tendency to chronic Bright's disease occurred in four generations. Families in which the arteries tend to degenerate early are more prone to interstitial nephritis. Syphilis is held by some to be a cause, and possibly in some cases the mercurial treatment. Alcohol probably plays an important part, particularly in conjunction with other factors. Among the better classes in America chronic Bright's disease is very common, and is, I believe, caused more frequently by overeating than by excesses in alcohol. Some believe excessive use of meat is injurious, since it increases the materials out of which uric acid is formed. By many a functional disorder of the liver, leading to lithæmia, is regarded as the most efficient factor. It is quite possible that in persons who habitually eat and drink too much the work thrown upon this organ is excessive, and the elaboration of certain materials is so defective that in their excretion from the general circulation they irritate the kidneys. Actual gout, which in England is a common cause of interstitial nephritis, is not an important factor here. Lead, as is well known, may produce renal sclerosis. For a full discussion on the etiology and varieties of renal cirrhosis the student is referred to the work of S. West.

Arterio-sclerotic Form.—By far the most common form in America is secondary to arterio-sclerosis. The kidneys are not much, if at all, contracted, very hard, red, and show patches of cortical atrophy. It is seen in men over forty who have worked hard, eaten freely, and taken alcohol to excess. They are conspicuous victims of the " strenuous life," the incessant tension of which is felt first in the arteries. After forty in men of this class nothing is more salutary than to experience the shock brought by the knowledge of the presence of albumin and tube-casts in the urine. The associated cardio-vascular changes are of varying degrees of intensity, and upon them, not upon the renal condition, does the outlook depend.

Morbid Anatomy.—The contracted kidneys are small, and together may weigh no more than an ounce and a half. Of 174 cases of chronic interstitial nephritis (white kidney) from my wards, with autopsy, in 79 cases the combined weight of kidneys was over 300 grammes; in 57 cases, 200–300 grammes; 30 cases, 150–200 grammes; and below 150 grammes, 8 cases. Of the arterio-sclerotic form 61 per cent weighed over 300 grammes and but 6 per cent below 200 grammes. Unilateral nephritis is excessively rare, not occurring once in the series, a striking contrast to Edebohl's figures, 9 of 72 cases in which the operation of stripping the capsule was performed. The capsule is thick and adherent; the surface of the organ irregular and covered with small nodules, which have given to it the name of granular kidney. In stripping off the capsule, portions of the kidney substance are removed. Small cysts are frequently seen on the surface. The color is usually reddish, often a very dark red. On section the substance is tough and resists cutting; the cortex is thin and may measure no more than a couple of millimetres. The pyramids are less wasted. The small arteries are greatly thickened and stand out prominently. The fat about the pelvis is greatly increased. Bright's original description is as follows:

" . . . The kidney is quite rough and scabrous to the touch externally, and is seen to rise in numerous projections not much exceeding a large pin's head, yellow, red, and purplish. The form of the kidney is often inclined to be lobulated, the feel is hard, and on making an incision the texture is found approaching to semi-cartilaginous firmness, giving great resistance to the knife. The tubular portions are observed to be drawn near to the surface of the organ, with less interstitial deposit than in the last variety . . . the kidney . . . (is usually) . . . of a purplish gray tinge."

Microscopically there is seen a marked increase in the connective tissue and degeneration and atrophy of the secreting structures, glomerular and tubal, the former predominating and giving the main characters to the lesion.   The following are the most important changes:

(*a*) An increase in the fibrous elements, widely distributed throughout the organ, but more advanced in the cortex, particularly in the tissue between the medullary rays.   In the pyramids the distribution of new growth is less patchy and more diffuse.   In the early stages of the process there is a small-celled infiltration between the tubes and around the glomeruli, and finally this becomes fibrillated and is seen encircling the tubules and Bowman's capsules, around the latter often forming concentric layers.

(*b*) The changes in the glomeruli are striking, and in advanced cases a very considerable number of them have undergone complete atrophy and are represented as densely encapsulated hyaline structures.   The atrophy is partly due to changes in the capillary walls and multiplication of cells between the loops, partly to extensive hyaline degeneration, and in part, no doubt, to the alterations in the afferent vessels.   The normal glomeruli usually show some thickening of the capsule and increase in the cells of the tufts.

(*c*) The tubules show changes in the epithelium, which vary a good deal in different localities.   Where the connective-tissue growth is most advanced they are greatly atrophied and the epithelium may be represented by small cubical cells.   In other instances the epithelium has entirely disappeared. On the other hand, in the regions represented by the projecting granules the tubules are usually dilated, and the epithelium shows hyaline, fatty, and granular changes.   Very many of them contain dark masses of epithelial *débris* and tube-casts.   In the interstitial tissue and in the tubules there may be pigmentary changes due to hæmorrhage.   The dilatation of the tubules may reach an extreme grade, forming definite cysts.

(*d*) The arteries show an advanced sclerosis.   The intima is greatly thickened and there are changes in the adventitia and in the media, consisting in increase in the thickness due to proliferation of the connective tissue, in the latter coat at the expense of the muscular elements.

The view most generally entertained at present is that the essential lesion is in the secreting tissues of the tubules and the glomeruli, and that the connective-tissue overgrowth is secondary to this.   Greenfield holds that the primary change is in most instances in the glomeruli, to which both the degeneration in the epithelium of the convoluted tubules and the increase in the intertubular connective tissue are secondary.

Associated with contracted kidney are general arterio-sclerosis and hypertrophy of the heart.   The changes in the arteries have already been described in the section on arterio-sclerosis.   The hypertrophy of the heart is constant, and the enlargement may reach an extreme grade.   Variations depend, no doubt, in part upon the extent of the diffuse arterial degeneration, but there are instances in which the term *cor bovinum* may be applied to the enlarged organ.   In such cases the hypertrophy is not confined to the left ventricle, but involves the entire heart.   The explanation of this has been much discussed. It was at first held to be due to the increased work thrown upon the organ in driving the impure blood through the capillary system.   Basing his opinion upon the supposed muscular increase in the smaller arteries, Johnson regarded it as an effort to overcome a sort of stop-cock action of these vessels, which, under the influence of the irritating ingredient in the blood, contracted and

256

increased greatly the peripheral resistance. Traube believed that the obliteration of a large number of capillary territories in the kidney materially raised the arterial pressure, and in this way led to the hypertrophy of the heart; an additional factor, he thought, was the diminished excretion of water, which also heightened the pressure within the blood-vessels.

With our present knowledge the most satisfactory explanation is that given by Cohnheim, which is thus clearly and succinctly put by Fagge: " He gives reasons for thinking that the activity of the circulation through the kidneys at any moment—in other words, the state of the smaller renal arteries as regards contraction or dilatation—depends not (as in the case of the tissues generally) upon the need of those organs for blood, but solely upon the amount of material for the urinary secretion that the circulatory fluid happens then to contain. This suggestion has bearings . . . upon the development of hypertrophy in one kidney when the other has been entirely destroyed. But another consequence deducible from it is that when parts of both kidneys have undergone atrophy, the blood-flow to the parts that remain must, *cæteris paribus,* be as great as it would have been to the whole of the organs if they had been intact. But in order that such a quantity of blood should pass through the restricted capillary area now open to it, an excessive pressure must obviously be necessary. This can be brought to bear only by the exertion of more than the normal degree of force on the part of the left ventricle, combined with the maintenance of a corresponding resistance in all other districts of the arterial system. And so one can account at once for the high arterial pressure and for the cardio-vascular changes that are secondary to it." W. P. Herringham in a recent study of the subject concludes that the cardiac hypertrophy depends upon degeneration and rigidity of the aorta and large arteries, changes which incapacitate them from acting as an elastic reservoir and transfer their functions to the smaller vessels, which naturally offer much more resistance and give the heart more work to do.

Symptoms.—Perhaps a majority of the cases are latent, and are not recognized until the occurrence of one of the serious or fatal complications. Even an advanced grade of contracted kidney may be compatible with great mental and bodily activity. There may have been no symptoms whatever to suggest to the patient the existence of a serious malady. In other cases the general health is disturbed. The patient complains of lassitude, is sleepless, has to get up at night to micturate; the digestion is disordered, the tongue is furred; there are complaints of headache, failing vision, and breathlessness on exertion.

So complex and varied is the clinical picture of chronic Bright's disease that it will be best to consider the symptoms under the various systems.

URINARY SYSTEM.—In the *small contracted kidney* polyuria is common. Frequently the patient has to get up two or three times during the night to empty the bladder, and there is increased thirst. It is for these symptoms occasionally that relief is sought. And yet in many cases with very small kidneys this feature has not been present. A careful study of the cases from my wards, of the urine and the anatomical condition, showed that almost no parallelism could be made between the weight of the kidney, its appearance, and the urine it secreted before death. Of the 174 cases with autopsy, in almost a third the renal changes were so slight that the nephritis was not mentioned as a part of the clinical diagnosis (Emerson). The color is a light yellow, and the specific gravity ranges from 1.005 to 1.012. Persistent low specific gravity is one of the most constant and important features of the disease. Traces of albumin are found, but may be absent at times, particularly in the early morning urine. It is often simply a slight cloudiness, and may be apparent only with the more delicate tests. The sediment is scanty, and in it a few hyaline or granular casts are found. The quantity of the solid constituents of the urine is, as a rule, diminished, though in some instances the urea may be excreted in full amount. In attacks of dyspepsia or bronchitis, or in the later stages when the heart fails, the quantity of albumin may be greatly increased and the urine diminished. Occasionally blood occurs in the urine, and there may even be hæmaturia (S. West). Slight leakage, represented by the constant presence of a few red cells, may be present early in the disease and persist for years. In the *arterio-sclerotic form* the quantity of urine is normal, or reduced rather than increased; the specific gravity is normal or high, the color of the urine is good, and there are hyaline and finely granular casts. The amount of albumin varies greatly with the food and exercise, and is usually much in excess of that seen with the contracted kidneys, and does not show so often the albumin-free intervals of that form, also it is more common to find albumin, no casts, while in the contracted kidney casts, no albumin, should one be absent.

CIRCULATORY SYSTEM.—The pulse is hard, the tension increased, and the vessel wall, as a rule, thickened. As already mentioned, a distinction must be made between increased tension and thickening of the arterial wall. The tension may be plus in a normal vessel, but in chronic Bright's disease it is more common to have increased tension in a stiff artery.

A pulse of increased tension has the following characters: It is hard and incompressible, requiring a good deal of force to overcome it; it is persistent, and in the intervals between the beats the vessel feels full and can be rolled beneath the finger. These characters may be present in a vessel the walls of which are little, if at all, increased in thickness. To estimate the latter the pulse wave should be obliterated in the radial, and the vessel wall felt beyond it. In a perfectly normal vessel the arterial coats, under these circumstances, can not be differentiated from the surrounding tissue; whereas, if thickened, the vessel can be rolled beneath the finger. Persistent high blood pressure is one of the earliest and most important symptoms of interstitial nephritis. During the disease the pressure may rise to 250 mm. or even 300 mm., but this is very rare. With dropsy and cardiac dilatation the pressure may fall, but not necessarily. The cardiac features are equally important, though often less obvious. Hypertrophy of the left ventricle occurs to overcome the resistance offered in the arteries. The enlargement of the heart ultimately becomes more general. The apex is displaced downward and to the left; the impulse is forcible and may be heaving. In elderly persons with emphysema, the displacement of the apex may not be evident. The first sound at the apex may be duplicated; more commonly the second sound at the aortic cartilage is accentuated, a very characteristic sign of increased tension. The sound in extreme cases may have a bell-like quality. In many cases a systolic murmur develops at the apex, probably as a result of relative insufficiency. It may be loud and transmitted to the axilla. Finally the hypertrophy fails, the heart becomes dilated, gallop rhythm is present, and the general condition is that of a chronic heart-lesion.

RESPIRATORY SYSTEM.—Sudden œdema of the glottis may occur. Effusion into the pleuræ or sudden œdema of the lungs may prove fatal. Acute pleurisy and pneumonia are not uncommon. Bronchitis is a frequent accompaniment, particularly in the winter. Sudden attacks of oppressed breathing, particularly at night, are not infrequent. This is often a uræmic symptom, but is sometimes cardiac. The patient may sit up in bed and gasp for breath, as in true asthma. Cheyne-Stokes breathing may be present, most commonly toward the close, but the patient may be walking about and even attending to his occupation.

DIGESTIVE SYSTEM.—Dyspepsia and loss of appetitie are common. Severe and uncontrollable vomiting may be the first symptom. This is usually regarded as a manifestation of uræmia, but it may occur without any other indications, and I have known it to prove fatal without any suspicion that chronic Bright's disease was present. Severe and even fatal diarrhœa may develop. The tongue may be coated and the breath heavy and urinous.

NERVOUS SYSTEM.—Various cerebral manifestations have already been mentioned under uræmia. Headache, sometimes of the migraine type, may be an early and persistent feature of chronic Bright's disease. Cerebral apoplexy is closely related to interstitial nephritis. The hæmorrhage may take place into the meninges or the cerebrum. It is usually associated with marked changes in the vessels. Neuralgias, in various regions, are not uncommon.

SPECIAL SENSES.—Troubles in vision may be the first symptom of the disease. It is remarkable in how many cases of interstitial nephritis the condition is diagnosed first by the ophthalmic surgeon. The flame-shaped retinal hæmorrhages are the most common. Less frequent is diffuse retinitis or papillitis. Sudden blindness may supervene without retinal changes—uræmic amaurosis. Diplopia is a rare event. Recurring conjunctival and palpebral hæmorrhages are fairly common. Auditory troubles are by no means infrequent in chronic Bright's disease. Ringing in the ears, with dizziness, is not uncommon. Various forms of deafness may occur. Epistaxis is not infrequent, either alone, or of a severe type in association with purpura.

SKIN.—Œdema is not common in interstitial nephritis. Slight puffiness of the ankles may be present, but in a majority of the cases dropsy does not supervene. When extensive, it is almost always the result of gradual failure of the hypertrophied heart. The skin is often dry and pale, and sweats are not common. In some instances the sweat may deposit a white frost of urea on the surface of the skin. Eczema is a common accompaniment of chronic interstitial nephritis. Tingling of the fingers or numbness and pallor—the dead fingers—are not, as some suppose, in any way peculiar to Bright's disease. Intolerable itching of the skin may be present, and cramps in the muscles are by no means rare.

Hæmorrhages are not infrequent; epistaxis may prove serious and extensive; purpura may occur. Broncho-pulmonary hæmorrhages are said, by some French writers, to be common, but no instance of it has come under my observation. Ascites is rare except in association with cirrhosis of the liver.

259

Diagnosis.—The autopsy often discloses the true nature of the disease, one of the many intercurrent affections of which may have proved fatal. The early stages of interstitial nephritis are not recognizable. In a patient with increased pulse tension (particularly if the vessel wall is sclerotic), with the apex beat of the heart dislocated to the left, the second aortic sound ringing and accentuated, the urine abundant and of low specific gravity, with a trace of albumin and an occasional hyaline or granular cast, the diagnosis of interstitial nephritis may be safely made. Of all the indications, that offered by the pulse is the most important. Persistent high tension with thickening of the arterial wall in a man under fifty means that serious mischief has already taken place, that cardio-vascular changes are certainly, and renal most probably, present. It is important in the diagnosis of this condition not to rest content with a single examination of the urine. Both the evening and the morning secretion should be studied. The sediment should be collected in a conical glass, and in looking for tube-casts a large surface should be examined with a tolerably low power and little light. The arterio-sclerotic kidney may exist for a long time without the occurrence of albumin, or the albumin may be in very small quantities. Toward the end it is impossible to differentiate the primary interstitial nephritis from an arterio-sclerotic kidney, nor clinically is it of any special value so to do. In middle-aged men, with very high tension, great thickening of the superficial arteries, and marked hypertrophy of the heart, the renal are more likely to be secondary to the arterial changes.

Prognosis.—Chronic Bright's disease is an incurable affection, and the anatomical conditions on which it depends are quite as much beyond the reach of medicines as wrinkled skin or gray hair. Interstitial nephritis, however, is compatible with the enjoyment of life for many years, and it is now universally recognized that increased tension, thickening of the arterial walls, and polyuria with a small quantity of albumin, neither doom a man to death within a short time nor necessarily interfere with the pursuits of an active life so long as proper care be taken. I know patients who have had high tension and a little albumin in the urine with hyaline casts for ten, twelve, and, in one instance, fifteen years. Serious indications are the occurrence of uræmic symptoms, dilatation of the heart, the onset of serous effusions, the onset of Cheyne-Stokes breathing, persistent vomiting, and diarrhœa.

Treatment.—Patients without local indications or in whom the condition has been accidentally discovered should so regulate their lives as to throw the least possible strain upon heart, arteries, and kidneys. A quiet life without mental worry, with gentle but not excessive exercise, and residence in an equable climate, should be recommended. In addition they should be told to keep the bowels regular, the skin active by a daily tepid bath with friction, and the urinary secretion free by drinking daily a definite amount of either distilled water or some pleasant mineral water. Alcohol should be strictly prohibited. Tea and coffee are allowable.

The diet should be light and nourishing, and the patient should be warned not to eat excessively, and not to take meat more than once a day. Care in food and drink is probably the most important element in the treatment of these early cases.

A patient in good circumstances may be urged to go away during the winter months, or, if necessary, to move altogether to a warm equable climate, like that of Southern California. There is no doubt of the value in these cases of removal from the changeable, irregular weather which prevails in the temperate regions from November until April.

At this period medicines are not required unless for certain special symptoms. Patients derive much benefit from an annual visit to certain mineral springs, such as Poland, Bedford, Saratoga, in this country, and Vichy and others in Europe. Mineral waters have no curative influence upon chronic Bright's disease; they simply help the interstitial circulation and keep the drains flushed. In this early stage, when the patient's condition is good, the tension not high, and the quantity of albumin small, medicines are not indicated, since no remedies are known to have the slightest influence upon the progress of the disease. Sooner or later symptoms arise which demand treatment. Of these the following are the most important:

(a) *Greatly Increased Arterial Tension.*—It is to be remembered that a certain increase of tension is not only necessary but unavoidable in chronic Bright's disease, and probably the most serious danger is too great lowering of the blood tension. The happy medium must be sought between such heightened tension as throws a serious strain upon the heart and risks rupture of the vessels and the low tension which, under these circumstances, is specially liable to be associated with serous effusions. In cases with persistent high tension the diet should be light, an occasional saline purge should be given, and sweating promoted by means of hot air or the hot bath. If these measures do not suffice, nitroglycerin may be tried, beginning with 1 minim of the 1-per-cent solution three times a day, and gradually increasing the dose if necessary. Patients vary so much in susceptibilty to this drug that in each case it must be tested, the limit of dosage being that at which the patient experiences the physiological effect. As much as 10 minims of the 1-percent solution may be given three times a day. In many cases I have given it in much larger doses for weeks at a time. I have never seen any ill effects from it. If the dose is excessive the patients complain at once of flushing or headache. Its use may be kept up for six or seven weeks, then stopped for a week and resumed. Its value is seen not only in the reduction of the tension, but also in the striking manner in which it relieves the headache, dizziness, and dyspnœa. The sodium nitrite may be given in doses of grs. iii–v three times a day.

(b) More or less *anæmia* is present in advanced cases, and is best met by the use of iron. Weir Mitchell, who has had a unique experience in certain forms of chronic Bright's disease, gives the tincture of the perchloride of iron in large doses—from half a drachm to a drachm three times a day. He thinks that it not only benefits the anæmia, but that it also is an important means of reducing the arterial tension.

(c) Many patients with Bright's disease present themselves for treatment with signs of cardiac dilatation; there is a gallop rhythm or the heartsounds have a fœtal character, the breath is short, the urine scanty and highly albuminous, and there are signs of local dropsy. In these cases the treatment must be directed to the heart. A morning dose of salts or calomel may be given, and digitalis in 10-minim doses, three or four times a day. Strychnia may be used with benefit in this condition. In some instances other cardiac tonics may be necessary, but as a rule the digitalis acts promptly and well.

(*d*) *Urœmic Symptoms.*—Even before marked manifestations are present there may be extreme restlessness, mental wandering, a heavy, foul breath, and a coated tongue. Headache is not often complained of, though intense frontal headache may be an early symptom of uræmia. In this condition, too, the patient may complain of palpitation, feelings of numbness, and sometimes nocturnal cramps. For these symptoms the saline purgatives should be ordered, and hot baths, so as to induce copious sweating. Grandin states that irrigation of the bowel with water at a temperature from 120° to 150° is most useful. Nitroglycerin also may be freely used to reduce the tension. For the uræmic convulsions, if severe, inhalations of chloroform may be used. If the patient is robust and full-blooded, from 12 to 20 ounces of blood should be removed. The patient should be freely sweated, and if the convulsions tend to recur chloral may be given, either by the mouth or per rectum, or, better still, morphia. Uræmic coma must be treated by active purgation, and sweating should be promoted by the use of pilocarpine or the hot bath. For the restlessness and delirium morphia is indispensable. Since its recommendation in uræmic states some years ago, by Stephen MacKenzie, I have used this remedy extensively and can speak of its great value in these cases. I have never seen ill effects or any tendency to coma follow. It is of special value in the dyspnœa and Cheyne-Stokes breathing of advanced arterio-sclerosis with chronic uræmia.

SURGICAL TREATMENT.—Edebohls has introduced the operation of decapsulization of the kidneys in Bright's disease in order to establish new vascular connections, and so influence the nutrition and work of the organs. In his work (Surgical Treatment of Bright's Disease, 1904) records are given of 72 cases; 7 died within two weeks, 22 died at periods more or less remote, 3 disappeared from observation, and 40 were known to be living—one eleven years and eight months after the operation. As Edebohls says, the difficult thing to determine is the existence of chronic Bright's disease before operation. No case should be regarded as such on the urine examination alone. The cardiovascular condition should be studied and the retinæ. There is probably a small group of suitable cases—the subacute and chronic forms which follow the acute infections—in which the outlook is hopeless from medical treatment.

VIII. AMYLOID DISEASE.

Amyloid (lardaceous or waxy) degeneration of the kidneys is simply an event in the process of chronic Bright's disease, most commonly in the chronic parenchymatous nephritis following fevers, or of cachectic states. It has no claim to be regarded as one of the varieties of Bright's disease. The affection of the kidneys is generally a part of a wide-spread amyloid degeneration occurring in prolonged suppuration, as in disease of the bone, in syphilis, tuberculosis, and occasionally leukæmia, lead poisoning, and gout. It varies curiously in frequency in different localities.

Anatomically the amyloid kidney is large and pale, the surface smooth, and the venæ stellatæ well marked. On section the cortex is large and may show a peculiar glistening, infiltrated appearance, and the glomeruli are very distinct. The pyramids, in striking contrast to the cortex, are of a deep red color. A section soaked in dilute tincture of iodine shows spots of a walnut or mahogany brown color. The Malpighian tufts and the straight vessels may be most affected. In lardaceous disease of the kidneys the organs are not always enlarged. They may be normal in size or small, pale, and granular. The amyloid change is first seen in the Malpighian tufts, and then involves the afferent and efferent vessels and the straight vessels. It may be confined entirely to them. In later stages of the disease the tubules are affected, chiefly the membrane, rarely, if ever, the cells themselves. In addition, the kidneys always show signs of diffuse nephritis. The Bowman's capsules are·thickened, there may be glomerulitis, and the tubal epithelium is swollen, granular, and fatty.

Symptoms.—The renal features alone may not indicate the presence of this degeneration. Usually the associated condition gives a hint of the nature of the process. The urine, as a rule, shows important changes; the quantity is increased, and it is pale, clear, and of low specific gravity. The albumin is usually abundant, but it may be scanty, and in rare instances absent. Possibly the variations in the situation of the amyloid changes may account for this, since albumin is less likely to be present when the change is confined to the vasa recta. In addition to ordinary albumin globulin may be present. The tube-casts are variable, usually hyaline, often fatty or finely granular. Occasionally the amyloid reaction can be detected in the hyaline casts. Dropsy is present in many instances, particularly when there is much anæmia or profound cachexia. It is not, however, an invariable symptom, and there are cases in which it does not develop. Diarrhœa is a common accompaniment.

Increased arterial tension and cardiac hypertrophy are not usually present, except in those cases in which amyloid degeneration occurs in the secondary contracted kidney; under which circumstances there may be uræmia and retinal changes, which, as a rule, are not met with in other forms.

Diagnosis.—By the condition of the urine alone it is not possible to recognize amyloid changes in the kidney. Usually, however, there is no difficulty, since the Bright's disease comes on in association with syphilis, prolonged suppuration, disease of the bone, or tuberculosis, and there is evidence of enlargement of the liver and spleen. A suspicious circumstance is the existence of polyuria with a large amount of albumin in the urine and few casts, or when, in these constitutional affections, a large quantity of clear, pale urine is passed, even without the presence of albumin.

The prognosis depends rather on the condition with which the nephritis is associated.. As a rule it is grave.

IX. PYELITIS.

(Consecutive Nephritis; Pyelonephritis; Pyonephrosis.)

Definition.—Inflammation of the pelvis of the kidney and the conditions which result from it.

Etiology.—Pyelitis in almost all cases is induced by bacterial invasion and multiplication, rarely by the irritation of various substances such as turpentine, cubebs, or sugar (diabetes). Normally the kidney can eliminate without harm to itself, apparently, various bacteria carried to it by the blood-current from the intestinal tract or some focus of infection; and it probably becomes infected only where its resistance is lowered, as a result of some general cause, as anæmia, malnutrition, or intercurrent disease, or of some local cause, as nephritis, displacement, congestion due to pressure of neoplasms upon the ureter, twisted ureter (Dietl's crisis), or of operation, or where the number or virulence of the micro-organisms is increased. These same factors probably play an important *rôle* also in the other common causes of pyelitis, ascending infection from an infected bladder (cystitis), and tuberculous infection. Other causes described are various fevers, cancer, hydatids, the ova of certain parasites, cold, and overexertion. Calculus seems not to be a common cause. It is a not uncommon complication of pregnancy (French, Goulstonian Lectures, 1908). In T. R. Brown's series of 20 cases, the colon bacillus was obtained 7 times, the tubercle bacillus 6, the proteus bacillus 4, a white staphylococcus twice, while in 1 case cultures were negative.

Morbid Anatomy.—In the early stages of pyelitis the mucous membrane is turbid, somewhat swollen, and may show ecchymoses or a grayish pseudomembrane. The urine in the pelvis is cloudy, and, on examination, numbers of epithelial cells are seen.

In the calculous pyelitis there may be only slight turbidity of the membrane, which has been called by some catarrhal pyelitis. More commonly the mucosa is roughened, grayish in color, and thick. Under these circumstances there is almost always more or less dilatation of the calyces and flattening of the papillæ. Following this condition there may be (*a*) extension of the suppurative process to the kidney itself, forming a pyelonephritis; (*b*) a gradual dilatation of the calyces with atrophy of the kidney substance, and finally the production of the condition of pyonephrosis, in which the entire organ is represented by a sac of pus with or without a thin shell of renal tissue. (*c*) After the kidney structure has been destroyed by suppuration, if the obstruction at the orifice of the pelvis persists, the fluid portions may be absorbed and the pus become inspissated, so that the organ is represented by a series of sacculi containing grayish, putty-like masses, which may become impregnated with lime salts.

Tuberculous pyelitis, as already described, usually starts upon the apices of the pyramids, and may at first be limited in extent. Ultimately the condition produced may be similar to that of calculous pyelitis. Pyonephrosis is quite as frequent a sequence, while the final transformation of the pus into a putty-like material impregnated with salts, forming the so-called scrofulous kidney, is even commoner.

The pyelitis consecutive to cystitis is generally bilateral, and the kidneys are sometimes involved, forming the so-called *surgical kidneys*—acute suppurative nephritis. There are lines of suppuration extending along the pyramids, or small abscesses in the cortex, often just beneath the capsule; or there may be wedge-shaped abscesses. The pus organisms either pass up the tubules or, as Steven has shown, through the lymphatics.

Symptoms.—The forms associated with the fevers rarely cause any symptoms, even when the process is extensive. In mild grades there is pain in the back or there may be tenderness on deep pressure on the affected side. The urine, turbid and containing pus cells, some mucus, and occasional red blood-cells, is acid or alkaline, depending on the infecting microbe; usually the albuminuria is of higher grade comparatively than the pyuria.

Before the condition of pyuria is established there may be attacks of pain on the affected side (not reaching the severe agony of renal colic), rigors, high fever, and sweats. Under these circumstances the urine, which may have been clear, becomes turbid or smoky from the presence of blood, and may contain large numbers of mucus cells and transitional epithelium. These cases are not common, but I have twice had opportunity of studying such attacks for a prolonged period. In one patient the occurrence of the rigor and fever could sometimes be predicted from the change in the condition of the urine. Such cases occur, I believe, in association with calculi in the pelvis.

The statement is not infrequently made that the epithelium in the urine in pyelitis is distinctive and characteristic. This is erroneous, as may be readily demonstrated by comparing scrapings of the mucosa of the renal pelvis and of the bladder. In both the epithelium belongs to what is called the transitional variety, and in both regions the same conical, fusiform, and irregular cells with long tails are found, and yet in pyelitis more of these tailed cells occur, for in cystitis one must often search long for them.

When the pyelitis, whether calculous or tuberculous, has become chronic and discharges, the symptoms are:

(1) *Pyuria.*—The pus is in variable amount, and may be intermittent. Thus, as is often the case when only one kidney is involved, the ureter may be temporarily blocked, and normal urine is passed for a time; then there is a sudden outflow of the pent-up pus and the urine becomes purulent. Coincident with this retention, a tumor mass may be felt on the side affected. The pus has the ordinary characters, but the transitional epithelium is not so abundant at this stage and comes from the bladder or from the pelvis of the healthy side. Occasionally in rapidly advancing pyelonephritis, portions of the kidney tissue, particularly of the apices of the pyramids, may slough away and appear in the urine; or, as in a remarkable specimen shown to me by Tyson, solid cheesy moulds of the calyces are passed. Casts from the kidney tubules are sometimes present. The reaction of the urine depends entirely upon the infecting microbe, whether the condition is unilateral or bilateral, and whether the bladder is also infected, when vesical irritability and frequent micturition may be present. Polyuria is usually present in the chronic cases.

(2) Intermittent fever associated with rigors is usually present in cases of suppurative pyelitis. The chills may recur at regular intervals, and the cases are often mistaken for malaria. Owen-Rees called attention to the frequent occurrence of these rigors, which form a characteristic feature of both calculous and tuberculous pyelitis. Ultimately the fever assumes a hectic type and the rigors may cease.

(3) The general condition of the patient often indicates prolonged suppuration. There is more or less wasting with anæmia and a progressive failure of health. Secondary abscesses may develop and the clinical picture becomes that of pyæmia. In some instances, particularly of tuberculous pyelitis, the clinical course may resemble that of typhoid fever. There are instances of pyuria recurring, at intervals, for many years without impairment of the bodily vigor. Some of the chronic cases have practically no discomfort.

(4) Physical examination in chronic pyelitis usually reveals tenderness on the affected side or a definite swelling, which may vary much in size and

46

ultimately attain large dimensions if the kidney becomes enormously distended, as in pyonephrosis.

(5) Occasionally nervous symptoms, which may be associated with dyspnœa, supervene, or the termination may be by coma, not unlike that of diabetes. These have been attributed to the absorption of the decomposing materials in the urine, whence the so-called ammoniæmia. A form of paraplegia has been described in connection with some cases of abscess of the kidney, but whether due to a myelitis or to a peripheral neuritis has not yet been determined.

In suppurative nephritis or surgical kidney following cystitis, the patient complains of pain in the back, the fever becomes high, irregular, and associated with chills, and in acute cases a typhoid state may precede the fatal event.

Diagnosis.—Between the tuberculous and the calculous forms of pyelitis it may be difficult or impossible to distinguish, except by the detection of tubercle bacilli in the pus. The examination for bacilli should be made systematically, and in suspicious cases intraperitoneal injections of guinea-pigs should also be made. From perinephric abscess pyonephrosis is distinguished by the more definite character of the tumor, the absence of œdematous swelling in the lumbar region, and, most important of all, the history of the case. The urine, too, in perinephric abscess may be free from pus. There are cases, however, in which it is difficult indeed to make a satisfactory diagnosis. A patient, whom I saw with Fussell, had had cystitis through her pregnancy, subsequently pus in the urine for several months, and then a large fluctuating abscess developed in the right lumbar region. It did not seem possible, either before or during the operation, to determine whether the case was a simple pyonephrosis or whether there had been a perinephric abscess caused by the pyelitis.

Suppurative pyelitis and cystitis are apt to be confounded, and perineal section is not infrequently performed on the supposition of the existence of the latter. The two conditions may, of course, coexist and prove puzzling, but the history, the higher relative grade of albuminuria in pyelitis (Rosenfeld, Goldberg, T. R. Brown), the polyuria, the mode of development, the local signs in one lumbar region, and the absence of pain in the bladder, should be sufficient to differentiate the affections. In women, by catheterization of the ureters, it may be definitely determined whether the pus comes from the kidneys or from the bladder. The cystoscope may be used for this purpose.

Prognosis.—Cases coming on during the fevers usually recover. Tuberculous pyelitis may terminate favorably by inspissation of the pus and conversion into a putty-like substance with deposition of lime salts. With pyonephrosis the dangers are increased. Perforation may occur into the peritonæum, the patient may be worn out by the hectic fever, or amyloid disease may develop.

Treatment.—In mild cases fluids should be taken freely, particularly the alkaline mineral waters, to which potassium citrate may be added.

The treatment of the calculous form will be considered later. Practically there are no remedies which have much influence upon the pyuria. Some of the recently described urinary antiseptics, as urotropin, etc., seem to be of value, especially in the acute cases. Tonics should be given, a nourishing diet, and milk and butter-milk may be taken freely. When the tumor has formed or even before it is perceptible, if the symptoms are serious and severe, the kidney should be explored, and, if necessary, nephrotomy or nephrectomy should be performed.

X. HYDRONEPHROSIS.

Definition.—Dilatation of the pelvis and calyx of the kidney with atrophy of its substance, caused by the accumulation of non-purulent fluids, the result of obstruction.

Etiology.—The condition may be congenital, owing to some abnormality in the ureter or urethra. The tumor produced may be large enough to retard labor. Sometimes it is associated with other malformations. There is a condition of moderate dilatation, apparently congenital, which is not connected with any obstruction in the ducts.

In some instances there has been contraction or twisting of the ureter, or it has been inserted into the kidney at an acute angle or at a high level. In adult life the condition may be due to lodgment of a calculus, or to a cicatricial stricture following ulcer.

There is a remarkable condition of hypertrophy and dilatation of the bladder and ureters associated with congenital defect of the abdominal muscles. The bladder may form a large abdominal tumor and the ureters may be as large and visible as coils of the small intestine.

New growths, such as tubercle or cancer, occasionally induce hydronephrosis; more commonly, pressure upon the ureter from without, particularly tumors of the ovaries and uterus. Occasionally cicatricial bands compress the ureter. Obstruction within the bladder may result from cancer, from hypertrophy of the prostate with cystitis, and in the urethra from stricture. It is stated that slight grades of hydronephrosis have been found in patients with excessive polyuria.

In whatever way produced, when the ureter is blocked the secretion accumulates in the pelvis and infundibula. Sometimes acute inflammation follows, but more commonly the slow, gradual pressure causes atrophy of the papillæ with gradual distention and wasting of the organ. In acquired cases from pressure, even when dilatation is extreme, there may usually be seen a thin layer of renal structure. In the most extreme stages the kidney is represented by a large cyst, which may perhaps show on its inner surface imperfect septa. The fluid is thin and yellowish in color, and contains traces of urinary salts, urea, uric acid, and sometimes albumin. The secretion may be turbid from admixture with small quantities of pus.

Total occlusion does not always lead to a hydronephrosis, but may be followed by atrophy of the kidney. It appears that when the obstruction is intermittent or not complete the greatest dilatation is apt to follow. The sac may be enormous, and cause an abdominal tumor of the largest size. The condition has even been mistaken for ascites. Enlargement of the other kidney may compensate for the defect. Hypertrophy of the left side of the heart usually follows.

Symptoms.—When small, it may not be noticed. The congenital cases when bilateral usually prove fatal within a few days; when unilateral, the

diseases of the kidneys

When the seventh edition of *The Principles and Practice of Medicine* was published in 1909, controversy as to the mechanism of urine formation divided renal physiologists into two camps: those who adhered to Ludwig's theory of mechanical (hydrostatic) filtration through the glomerulus with "chemical" (endosmotic) reabsorption of water and salts back into the peritubular capillaries; and those who favored Heidenhain and believed that the glomerulus secreted water and the tubule cells secreted the other urinary constituents. Not until the midtwenties were A. N. Richards and his associates to demonstrate that the fluid in Bowman's capsule had the characteristics of an ultrafiltrate of plasma and Marshall and Vickers to provide experimental evidence that tubular secretion (as well as reabsorption) took place. Shortly thereafter Rehberg devised a method for estimating glomerular filtration rate in intact man, and subsequently Homer Smith introduced methods for estimating renal blood flow and quantitating tubular secretion and reabsorption. In midcentury Wirz, Hargitay, and Kuhn elucidated the mechanism of urinary concentration, and Gottschalk, reintroducing tubular micropuncture, clearly showed the site of urinary dilution.

These enormous changes in our understanding of the physiology of the kidney stand distinct from those concerning renal disease.

The section on "Acute Bright's Disease" includes numerous types: post-streptococcal, acute tubular necrosis secondary to chemical poisons or to trauma, and the group associated with "exudative erythema and the allied purpuric affections." Today the last would no doubt be subdivided according to our present nosological classification as associated with various vascular disorders, such as systemic lupus erythematosus, Schönlein-Henoch syndrome, thrombotic thrombocytopenic purpura, polyarteritis nodosa, and allergic vasculitis. However, as he pointed out in his 1904 paper, Osler was seeking similarities, not diversities.

It is of particular interest to note Osler's recognition of trauma as a cause of acute "Bright's disease," since this had to be rediscovered by Minami during the first world war, was promptly forgotten, and then resurrected during the second world war as the "crush syndrome," now designated acute tubular necrosis.

Osler's description of the course of scarlatinal (post-streptococcal) glomerulonephritis is detailed and can hardly be improved. We might add to his concept of its being caused by the "poison" of scarlet fever by suggesting that the poison is an antigen and that the glomerular damage is due to an antigen-antibody reaction, but we can hardly fill in the details.

"As there is marked retention of the chlorides, which seem to bear a relation to the dropsy, salt should be withheld." No clearer statement of this most important aspect of the treatment of acute glomerulonephritis could be made, yet it seems to have been overlooked in the succeeding decades until rediscovery in the 1930s.

"No remedies, so far as known, control directly the changes which are going on in the kidneys. The indications are: (1) to give the excretory function of the kidney rest by utilizing the skin and the bowels, in the hope that the natural processes may be sufficient to effect a cure; (2) to meet the symptoms as they arise."

Here, indeed, we can amplify as a result of newer knowledge and technics developed during the 1940s, but the principles remain unchanged. Since the excretory function of the kidney is largely limited to the disposal of end products of protein catabolism (nitrogen, hydrogen ion, sulfate, phosphate, and particularly potassium) we avoid all protein intake in the severely oliguric patient and reduce endogenous protein (cellular) catabolism to a minimum by furnishing an adequate supply of carbohydrate around the clock. The second major excretory function is the removal of water and salts which, surplus to the needs of the body, the mouth takes in, or the physician infuses. By eliminating the intake of such surpluses we can, in a sense, obviate the need for this second renal excretory function.

Measures outlined above usually suffice for the management of most patients with acute Bright's disease unless there should be severe and prolonged oliguria. In such cases, hyperkalemia may not be controlled unless "the bowels are utilized." For this, the nonmetabolizable osmotic purgative, sorbitol, is today preferred to Osler's "morning saline purge."

Peritoneal dialysis and hemodialysis, the latter proposed by Osler's colleagues at Hopkins in 1913, are now easily accomplished and can be employed with minimal risk whenever the comfort or life of the patient with acute renal failure is threatened.

The section on chronic parenchymatous nephritis (nephrotic syndrome), including the transition of some cases to the picture of chronic renal insufficiency, is a marvel of precision and concision. The varied etiologies and histopathological changes, the ominous prognosis in adults, and the treatment with "a salt-free diet" and diuretics hold today. To be sure

Diseases of the kidneys

Osler did not have the advantage of being able to examine tissue obtained by renal biopsy, a technique introduced at the midcentury mark, nor were the diuretic agents of his day as potent as the parenteral mercurials introduced in 1920. (Richard Bright's monograph of 1827 had described the use of mercury compounded with other ingredients as an oral diuretic pill.) Less than a decade ago the benzothiadiazides and more recently ethacrynic acid have added to our ability to control edema but also to initiate iatrogenic morbidity.

The section on chronic interstitial nephritis is concerned largely with two disorders: arteriolar nephrosclerosis and chronic glomerulonephritis. Of these Osler considered the former the more common. The polyuria of low specific gravity, the nyctyria, and the thirst come in for mention as characteristic of nonarteriosclerotic kidney, and in treatment the necessity of "drinking daily a definite amount of either distilled water or some pleasant mineral water" is emphasized. Although one cannot be certain, it may well be that Osler recognized the tendency of these individuals to become dehydrated because of their polyuria. Since it is now apparent that many nonedematous patients with chronic renal disease are obligatory salt-wasters if their sodium chloride intake is sharply curtailed, the suggested use of mineral water may be equivalent to the prescription of chilled isotonic saline employed in such patients today.

Pyelitis is differentiated from pyelonephritis inasmuch as in the former invasion of the kidney parenchyma has not occurred. As one reads the section reprinted here one gains the impression that in the absence of renal calculus or of tuberculous infection the prognosis was good and recovery with no treatment other than a large fluid intake was the rule. Whether or not the widespread use of antibiotics has changed this remains to be seen.

In this brief survey of progress over the past 58 years, much must be omitted, particularly since complete evaluation has yet to be accomplished in such areas as renovascular hypertension and the treatment of chronic irreversible renal disease by hemodialysis or by renal transplantation. An important and unexpected finding in connection with isogeneic kidney grafts (between identical twins) in glomerulonephritis, has been the tendency of the graft, after a variable time interval, to develop the *same* type of glomerulonephritis that had originally destroyed the recipient's kidneys, and this despite the removal of the latter at or shortly after the grafting procedure.

270

Diseases of the kidneys

For uremic symptoms in chronic Bright's disease, if the patient was robust and full-blooded, Osler recommended the removal of 12 to 20 ounces of blood, as had Richard Bright a century earlier. No doubt both would be perplexed were they to observe the custom of today when even frail and pale patients are bled daily of an ounce or so by white-coated technicians! On the other hand Huang Ti (twenty-seventh century BC) would presumably consider our plunging of needles of varying lengths and designs into arms, legs, kidneys, livers, and lungs as but a slight modification of the acupuncture of his day!

Maurice B. Strauss

REFERENCES

Abel, J.J., Rowntree, L.G., and Turner, B.B. The removal of diffusible substances from the circulating blood by means of dialysis. Trans. Ass. Am. Physicians, 28:51, 1913.

Dammin, G.J. Immunological injury of the kidney. In Renal Transplants: Correlation of Histological Pattern with Function (in press).

Gottschalk, C., and Mylle, M. Micropuncture of tubular function in the mammolian kidney. Physiologist, 4:35, 1961.

Iverson, P., and Brun, C. Aspiration biopsy of the kidney. Amer. J. Med., 11:324, 1951.

Marshall, E.K., Jr., and Vickers, J.L. The mechanism of the elimination of phenolsulphonephthalein by the kidney; a proof of secretion by the convoluted tubules. Bull. Hopkins Hosp., 34:1, 1923.

Rehberg, P.B. Studies on kidney function. I. The rate of filtration and reabsorption in the human kidney. Biochem. J., 20:447, 1926.

Smith, H.W., Goldring, W., and Chasis, H. The measurement of the tubular excretory mass, effective blood flow, and filtration rate in the normal human kidney. J. Clin. Invest., 17:263, 1938.

Wearn, J.T., and Richards, A.N. Observations on the composition of glomerular urine, with particular reference to the problem of reabsorption in the renal tubules. Amer. J. Physiol., 71:209, 1924.

Wirz, H., Hargitay, B., and Kuhn, W. Lokalisation des Konzentrierungsprozesses in der Niere durch direkte Kryoskopie. Helv. Physiol. Pharmacol. Acta, 9:196, 1951.

of the very large corpuscles, such as one sees in pernicious anæmia, is not noted, the average size appearing to be rather smaller than normal.

Nucleated red corpuscles are usually scanty. In long-continued chronic secondary anæmias occasional larger nucleated red corpuscles may be seen, bodies with larger palely staining nuclei; in some of these cells karyokinetic figures occur. Nucleated red corpuscles with fragmentary nuclei may also be seen.

The leucocytes may be increased in number, though in some severe chronic cases there may be a diminution.

(3) **Anæmia from Inanition.**—This may be brought about by defective food supply, or by conditions which interfere with the proper reception and preparation of the food, as in cancer of the œsophagus and chronic dyspepsia. The reduction of the blood mass may be extreme, but the plasma suffers proportionately more than the corpuscles, which, even in the wasting of cancer of the œsophagus, may not be reduced more than one-half or three-fourths. The reduction in the plasma may be·so great that the corpuscles show a relative increase.

(4) **Toxic anæmia** is induced by the action of certain poisons on the blood, such as lead, mercury, and arsenic, among inorganic substances, and the virus of syphilis and malaria among organic poisons. They act either by directly destroying the red blood-corpuscles, as in malaria, or by increasing the rate of ordinary consumption. The anæmia of pyrexia may in part be due to a toxic action, but is also caused in part by the disturbance of digestion and interference with the function of the blood-making organs.

PRIMARY OR ESSENTIAL ANÆMIA.

1. *Chlorosis.*

Definition.—An anæmia of unknown cause, occurring in young girls, characterized by a marked relative diminution of the hæmoglobin.

Etiology.—It is a disease of girls, more often of blondes than of brunettes. It is doubtful if males are ever affected. I have never seen true chlorosis in a boy. The age of onset is between the fourteenth and seventeenth years; under the age of twelve cases are rare. Recurrences, which are common, may extend into the third decade. Of the essential cause of the disease we know nothing. There exists a lowered energy in the blood-making organs, associated in some obscure way with the evolution of the sexual apparatus in women. Hereditary influences, particularly chlorosis and tuberculosis, play a part in some cases. Sometimes, as Virchow pointed out, the condition exists with a defective development (hypoplasia) of the circulatory and generative organs.

The disease is most common among the ill-fed, overworked girls of large towns, who are confined all day in close, badly lighted rooms, or have to do much stair-climbing. Cases occur, however, under the most favorable conditions of life, but not often in country-bred girls, as Maudlin sings in the *Compleat Angler*. Lack of proper exercise and of fresh air, and the use of improper food are important factors. Emotional and nervous disturbances may be prominent—so prominent that certain writers have regarded the disease as a neurosis. De Sauvages speaks of a *chlorose par amour*. Newly

47

arrived Irish girls were very prone to the disease in Montreal. The "corset and chlorosis" expresses O. Rosenbach's opinion. Menstrual disturbances are not uncommon, but are probably a sequence, not a cause, of chlorosis. Sir Andrew Clark believed that constipation plays an important *rôle,* and that the condition is in reality a *copræmia* due to the absorption of poisons—leucomaines and ptomaines—from the large bowel, a view which does not seem very reasonable, considering the great frequency of constipation both in women and in men.

Symptoms.—(*a*) GENERAL.—The symptoms of chlorosis are those of anæmia. The subcutaneous fat is well retained or even increased in amount. The complexion is peculiar; neither the blanched aspect of hæmorrhage nor the muddy pallor of grave anæmia, but a curious yellow-green tinge, which has given to the disease its name, and its popular designation, the green sickness. Occasionally the skin shows areas of pigmentation, particularly about the joints. In cases of moderate grade the color may be deceptive, as the cheeks have a reddish tint, particularly on exertion (chlorosis rubra). The subjects complain of breathlessness and palpitation, and there may be a tendency to fainting—symptoms which often lead to the suspicion of heart or lung disease. Puffiness of the face and swelling of the ankles may suggest nephritis. The disposition often changes, and the girl becomes low-spirited and irritable. The eyes have a peculiar brilliancy and the sclerotics are of a bluish color.

(*b*) SPECIAL FEATURES.—*Blood.*—The drop as expressed looks pale. Johann Duncan, in 1867, first called attention to the fact that the essential feature was not a great reduction in the number of the corpuscles, but a quantitative change in the hæmoglobin. The corpuscles themselves look pale. In 63 consecutive cases examined at my clinic by Thayer, the average number per cubic millimetre of the red blood-corpuscles was 4,096,544, or over 80 per cent, whereas the percentage of hæmoglobin for the total number was 42.3 per cent. The accompanying chart illustrates well these striking differences. There may, however, be well-marked actual anæmia. The lowest blood-count in the series of cases referred to above was 1,932,000. There may be all the physical characteristics and symptoms of a profound anæmia with the number of the blood-corpuscles nearly at the normal standard. Thus in one instance the globular richness was over 85 per cent, with the hæmoglobin about 35. No other form of anæmia presents this feature, at least with the same constancy and in the same degree. The importance of the reduction in the hæmoglobin depends upon the fact that it is the iron-containing elements of the blood with which in respiration the oxygen enters into combination. This marked diminution in the iron has also been determined by chemical analysis of the blood. The microscopical characteristics of the blood are as follows: In severe cases the corpuscles may be extremely irregular in size and shape—poikilocytosis, which may occasionally be as marked as in some cases of pernicious anæmia. The large forms of red blood-cells are not as common, and the average size is stated to be below normal. The color of the corpuscles is noticeably pale and the deficiency may be seen either in individual corpuscles or in the blood mixture prepared for counting. Nucleated red corpuscles (normoblasts) are not very uncommon, and may vary greatly in numbers in the same case at different periods. The leucocytes may show a slight increase; the average in the 63 cases above referred to was 8,467 per cubic millimetre.

(*c*) GASTRO-INTESTINAL SYMPTOMS.—The appetite is capricious, and patients often have a longing for unusual articles, particularly acids. In some instances they eat all sorts of indigestible things, such as chalk or even earth. Superacidity of the gastric juice is commonly associated with chlorosis. In 19 out of 21 cases in Riegel's clinic this condition was found to exist. In the other two instances the acidity was normal or a trifle increased. Distress

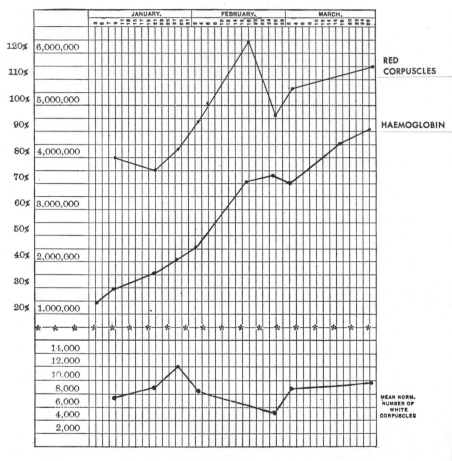

CHART XVII.—CHLOROSIS.

after eating and even cardialgic attacks may be associated with it. Constipation is a common symptom, and, as already mentioned, has been regarded as an important element in causing the disease. A majority of chlorotic girls who wear corsets have gastroptosis, and on inflation the stomach will be found vertically placed; sometimes the organ is very much dilated. The motor power is usually well retained. Enteroptosis with palpable right kidney is not uncommon.

(*d*) Circulatory Symptoms.—Palpitation of the heart occurs on **exertion**, and may be the most distressing symptom of which the patient complains. Percussion may show slight increase in the transverse dulness. A systolic murmur is heard at the apex or at the base; more commonly at the latter, but in extreme cases at both. A diastolic murmur is rarely heard. The systolic murmur is usually loudest in the second left intercostal space, where there is sometimes a distinct pulsation. The exact mode of production is still in dispute. Balfour holds that it is produced at the mitral orifice by relative insufficiency of the valves in the dilated condition of the ventricle. On the right side of the neck over the jugular vein a continuous murmur may be heard, the *bruit de diable*, or humming-top murmur.

Tho pulso is usually full and soft. Visible impulse is present in the veins of the neck, as noted by Lancisi. Pulsation in the peripheral veins is sometimes seen. Thrombosis in the veins may occur, most commonly in the femoral, but in other instances in the cerebral sinuses there may be multiple thrombi. In 86 cases the veins of the legs were affected in 48, the cerebral sinuses in 29 (Lichtenstern). The chief danger in thrombosis of the extremities is pulmonary embolism, which occurred in 13 of 52 cases collected by Welch.

As in all forms of essential anæmia, fever is not uncommon. Chlorotic patients suffer frequently from headache and neuralgia, which may be paroxysmal. The hands and feet are often cold. Dermatographia is common. Hysterical manifestations are not infrequent. Menstrual disturbances are very common—amenorrhœa or dysmenorrhœa. With the improvement in the blood condition this function is usually restored.

Diagnosis.—The green sickness, as it is sometimes called, is in many instances recognized at a glance. The well-nourished condition of the girl, the peculiar complexion, which is most marked in brunettes, and the white or bluish sclerotics are very characteristic. A special danger exists in mistaking the apparent anæmia of the early stage of pulmonary tuberculosis for chlorosis. Mistakes of this sort may often be avoided by the very simple test furnished by allowing a drop of blood to fall on a white towel or a piece of blotting paper—a deficiency in hæmoglobin is readily appreciated. The palpitation of the heart and shortness of breath frequently suggest heart-disease, and the œdema of the feet and general pallor cause the cases to be mistaken for Bright's disease. In the great majority of cases the characters of the blood readily separate chlorosis from other forms of anæmia.

2. *Idiopathic or Progressive Pernicious Anæmia.*

The disease was first clearly described by Addison, who called it idiopathic anæmia. Channing and Gusserow described the cases occurring post partum, but to Biermer we owe a revival of interest in the subject.

Etiology.—The existence of a separate disease worthy of the term progressive pernicious anæmia has been doubted, but there are very many cases in which, as Addison says, there exist none of the usual causes or concomitants of anæmia. Clinically there are several different groups which present the characters of a progressive and pernicious anæmia and are etiologically different. Thus, a fatal anæmia may be due to the presence of parasites, or may follow hæmorrhage, or be associated with chronic atrophy of the stomach; but when we have excluded all these causes there remains a group which, in the words of Addison, is characterized by a "general anæmia occurring without any discoverable cause whatever, cases in which there had been no previous loss of blood, no exhausting diarrhœa, no chlorosis, no purpura, no renal, splenic, miasmatic, glandular, strumous, or malignant disease."

William Hunter considers that the idiopathic anæmia described by Addison and the progressive pernicious anæmia of Biermer are different affections. That described by Addison is a distinct disease, while that described by Biermer is "a frequently recurring group of symptoms met with in very different conditions of disease." Hunter holds that there are two important factors in the disease, (*a*) hæmolysis and (*b*) a chronic septic infection often associated with a specific glossitis, and oral, gastric, and intestinal sepsis.

Idiopathic anæmia is widely distributed. It is of frequent occurrence in the Swiss cantons, and it is common in the United States. It affects middle-aged persons, but instances in children have been described. Of the 81 cases in my hospital series 36 were above fifty years of age; only 1 was under twenty. Griffith mentions about 10 cases occurring under twelve years of age. The youngest patient I have seen was a boy of ten. Males are more frequently affected than females. Of 550 cases collected by Colman, 323 were in men and 227 in women. Sinkler and Eshner record 3 cases in one family, the father and two girls.

With the following conditions may be associated a profound anæmia not always to be distinguished clinically from Addison's idiopathic form:

(*a*) *Pregnancy and Parturition.*—The symptoms may occur during pregnancy, as in 19 of 29 cases of this group in Eichhorst's table. More commonly, in my experience, the condition has been post partum.

(*b*) *Atrophy of the Stomach.*—This condition, early recognized by Flint and Fenwick, may certainly cause a progressive pernicious anæmia. By modern methods it may now be possible to exclude this extreme gastric atrophy.

(*c*) *Parasites.*—The most severe form may be due to the presence of parasites, and the accounts of cases depending upon the anchylostoma and the bothriocephalus describe a progressive and often pernicious anæmia.

After the exclusion of these forms there remain a large proportion, which correspond to Addison's description. The researches of Quincke and his student Peters showed that there was an enormous increase in the iron in the liver, and they suggested that the affection was probably due to increased hæmolysis. This has been strongly supported by the extensive observations of Hunter, who has also shown that the urine excreted is darker in color and contains pathological urobilin. The lemon tint of the skin or the actual jaundice is attributed, on this view, to an overproduction. To explain the hæmolysis, it has been thought that in the condition of faulty gastro-intestinal digestion, which is so commonly associated with these cases, poisonous materials are developed, which when absorbed cause destruction of the corpuscles. Certainly the case for hæmolysis is very strong, and is supported by the experimental work of Bunting, who has been able to produce in animals a condition the counterpart of pernicious anæmia in man.

Stockman suggests that repeated small capillary hæmorrhages—chiefly internal—play an important *rôle* in the causation of the disease, which also explains, he holds, the existence of a great excess of iron in the liver.

On the other hand, F. P. Henry, Stephen Mackenzie, Rindfleisch, and other authorities incline to the belief that the essence of the disease is in defective hæmogenesis, in consequence of which the red blood-corpuscles are abnormally vulnerable.

Morbid Anatomy.—The body is rarely emaciated. A lemon tint of the skin is present in a majority of the cases. The muscles often are intensely red in color, like horse-flesh, while the fat is light yellow. Hæmorrhages are common on the skin and serous surfaces. The heart is usually large, flabby, and empty. In one instance I obtained only 2 drachms of blood from the right heart, and between 3 and 4 from the left. The muscle substance of the heart is intensely fatty, and of a pale, light-yellow color. In no affection do we see more extreme fatty degeneration. The lungs show no special changes. The stomach in many instances is normal, but in some cases of fatal anæmia the mucosa has been extensively atrophied. In the case described by Henry and myself the mucous membrane had a smooth, cuticular appearance, and there was complete atrophy of the secreting tubules. The liver may be enlarged and fatty. In most of my autopsies it was normal in size, but usually fatty. The iron is in excess, a striking contrast to the condition in cases of secondary anæmia. It is deposited in the outer and middle zones of the lobules, and in two specimens, which I examined, seemed to have such a distribution that the bile capillaries were distinctly outlined. This, Hunter states, is a special and characteristic lesion, possibly peculiar to pernicious anæmia.

The spleen shows no important changes. In one of Palmer Howard's cases the organ weighed only 1 ounce and 5 drachms. The iron pigment is usually in excess. The lymph-glands may be of a deep red color. The amount of iron pigment is increased in the kidneys, chiefly in the convoluted tubules. The bone-marrow is usually red, lymphoid in character, showing great numbers of nucleated red corpuscles, especially the larger forms called by Ehrlich gigantoblasts. Cases in which the bone-marrow shows no signs of activity have been described as *aplastic anæmia.* Lichtheim and others have found sclerosis in the posterior columns of the cord.

Symptoms.—The patient may have been in previous good health, but in many cases there is a history of gastro-intestinal disturbance, mental shock, or worry. The description given by Addison presents the chief features of the disease in a masterly way. "It makes its approach in so slow and insidious a manner that the patient can hardly fix a date to the earliest feeling of that languor which is shortly to become so extreme. The countenance gets pale, the whites of the eyes become pearly, the general frame flabby rather than wasted, the pulse perhaps large, but remarkably soft and compressible, and occasionally with a slight jerk, especially under the slightest excitement. There is an increasing indisposition to exertion, with an uncomfortable feeling of faintness or breathlessness in attempting it; the heart is readily made to palpitate; the whole surface of the body presents a blanched, smooth, and waxy appearance; the lips, gums, and tongue seem bloodless, the flabbiness of the solids increases, the appetite fails, extreme languor and faintness supervene, breathlessness and palpitations are produced by the most trifling exertion or emotion; some slight œdema is probably perceived about the ankles; the debility becomes extreme—the patient can no longer rise from bed; the mind occasionally wanders; he falls into a prostrate and half-torpid state, and at length expires; nevertheless, to the very last, and after a sickness of several months' duration, the bulkiness of the general frame and the amount of obesity often present a most striking contrast to the failure and exhaustion observable in every other respect."

THE BLOOD.—The red corpuscles may fall to one-fifth or less of the normal number. The average count in my 81 (in 102 admissions) hospital cases was 1,575,000 per cubic millimetre—that is, in 81 per cent of the cases under

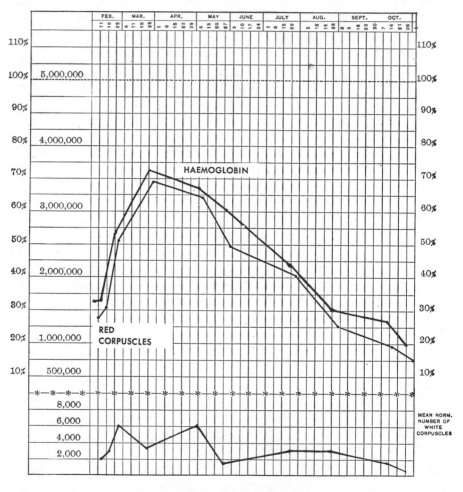

CHART XVIII.—PERNICIOUS ANÆMIA.

2,000,000 and in 12 per cent under 1,000,000 cells—and the hæmoglobin was about 30 per cent. The hæmoglobin is relatively increased, so that the individual globular richness is plus, a condition exactly the opposite to that which occurs in chlorosis and the secondary anæmia, in which the corpuscular rich-

278

ness in coloring matter is minus. The relative increase in the hæmoglobin is probably associated with the average increase in the size of the red blood-corpuscles. Chart XVIII, page 727, illustrates these points. Microscopically the red blood-corpuscles present a great variation in size, and there can be seen large giant forms, megalocytes, which are often ovoid in form, measuring 8, 11, or even 15 μ in diameter—a circumstance which Henry regards as indicating a reversion to a lower type. Laache thinks these pathognomonic, and they certainly form a constant feature. There are also small round cells, microcytes, from 2 to 6 μ in diameter, and of a deep red color. The corpusces show a remarkable irregularity in form; they are elongated and rodlike or pyriform; one end of a corpuscle may retain its shape while the other is narrow and extended. To this condition of irregularity Quincke gave the name poikilocytosis.

Nucleated red blood-corpuscles are almost always present, as pointed out by Ehrlich. It may require a long search to find them. There are two types, normoblasts and megaloblasts, which Ehrlich regards as almost distinctive of this anæmia. There are frequently forms intermediate between these two groups which often have irregular nuclei. A relatively large number of megaloblasts usually indicates a grave outlook. Though these large forms are most characteristic, occasionally forms closely similar to them may be found in the graver secondary anæmias—e. g., bothriocephalus anæmia, anchylostomiasis—and in leukæmia. Karyokinetic figures may be seen in these bodies. Red corpuscles with fragmenting nuclei are common in pernicious anæmia. *Blood crises* were first described under this name by v. Noorden. He considered the phenomenon one of active blood regeneration, causing the appearance in the peripheral blood of large numbers of nucleated reds, which remain for a few days, and are followed by a decided gain in the blood-count. This may be true in secondary anæmias, but in pernicious anæmia they are often part of the terminal picture with declining count of red corpuscles and leucocytes, and the presence of large numbers of nucleated reds which may continue even for nineteen weeks, as if the marrow were making convulsive but fruitless efforts to restore the blood. There were 20 crises in 13 of my 81 cases, and in 5 they were terminal events. Three-fourths of these crises were megaloblastic in character, in the others the cells were chiefly normoblasts. In the highest crisis there were 14,388 normoblasts, 460 intermediates, and 138 megaloblasts per cubic millimetre. Bensançon and Labbé mention a crisis with 10,000 normoblasts and 960 megaloblasts per cubic millimetre (the intermediates were probably counted with the latter). Only 5 of the 20 crises were followed by a real gain in the count of red cells, and these were of normoblastic type. The leucocytes are generally normal or diminished in number, even to 500 per cubic millimetre; and a marked relative increase in the small mononuclear forms—in one of my cases even 79 per cent, yet with absolute number normal—with a diminution in the polynuclear leucocytes, is often noted. Myelocytes are usually found, and in one of my cases were 8 per cent. The blood-plates are either absent or very scanty.

The *cardio-vascular* symptoms are important and are noted in the description given above. Hæmic murmurs are usually present. The larger arteries pulsate visibly and the throbbing in them may be distressing to the patient. The pulse is full and frequently suggests the water-hammer beat of aortic insufficiency. The capillary pulse is frequently to be seen. The superficial veins are often prominent, and I have seen well-marked pulsation in them. Hæmorrhages occurred, either in the skin or from the mucous surfaces, in 12 cases of my series. Retinal hæmorrhages are common. There are rarely symptoms in the respiratory organs.

Gastro-intestinal symptoms, such as dyspepsia, nausea, and vomiting, may be present throughout the disease. Diarrhœa is not infrequent. The urine is usually of a low specific gravity and sometimes pale, but in other instances it is of a deep sherry color, shown by Hunter and Mott to be due to great excess of urobilin. Fever was present in three-fourths of my cases.

The *skin* has most frequently a lemon-tint, sometimes positively icteroid; in a few cases there is pallor without any change in color, while in a third group the skin is pigmented, so that Addison's disease is suspected. This occurs in a few instances in which arsenic has not been given; as a rule it follows the administration of this drug. The pigmentation may be patchy and associated with areas of leucoderma. The *nervous* symptoms are of great interest. Extensive changes may be present in the cord without any symptoms during life. In a majority of the cases the numbness comes on in the legs and feet, less often in the hands, and in a few instances there is pain of great severity. Gradually the signs of postero-lateral sclerosis become well marked. In a third group, described by Risien Russell, Batten, and Collier, the nervous symptoms—indicating a postero-lateral sclerosis—come first and the anæmia follows; but the cases have not always the features of the progressive pernicious disease.

Diagnosis.—The disease is not often recognized by the general practitioner. The lemon-yellow tint of the skin leads to the diagnosis of *jaundice*; the pigmentation suggests *Addison's disease*; the anæmia, puffy face, swollen ankles, and albumin in the urine, *Bright's disease*; the shortness of breath and palpitation, *heart-disease*; the pallor and gastric symptoms, *cancer of the stomach*. The retention of fat, the insidious onset, the absence of signs of local disease, and the blood features already discussed are the most important diagnostic points. From cancer of the stomach it is distinguished by (1) the absence of wasting; (2) the high-color index of the blood and the lower corpuscular count, reaching frequently below one million per cubic millimetre; (3) the absence of the fairly characteristic reactions of the stomach contents; and (4) the marked improvement in the first attacks with rest, fresh air, diet, and arsenic.

Prognosis.—In the true Addisonian cases the ultimate outlook is bad; of late years the proportion of cases of temporary recovery has increased. Of the 81 cases from my wards, death occurred in 27 while under observation. Counts taken in 18 of the fatal cases on the day of death were all below 700,000 red cells per cmm. The average duration of these was one year. One patient recovered completely. He was admitted in 1890 with a history of one year, was discharged well, and returned in 1896 with cancer of the stomach. One patient is in good health six years and another four years after the onset. In Pye-Smith's article in the Guy's Hospital Reports he mentions 20 cases of recovery. Colman, in a recent article, states that one of these cases treated with arsenic in 1880 was alive and well in March, 1900. The history is usually not one of progressive advance but of alternate periods of gain and loss. In my series

280

a red count below one million has been a bad omen. The presence of many megaloblasts is unfavorable. They were relatively eleven times more numerous in the fatal cases of my series than in those that recovered. That a large relative percentage of small mononuclears was of bad import is not supported by my cases. Those that recovered had a slightly higher average percentage than the fatal cases. The blood crises are usually of ill omen. Patients who do not take arsenic well usually do badly. Gastro-intestinal disturbances are serious. There are remarkable acute cases which may prove fatal within ten days, as in a patient I saw with Finley, of Montreal.

Treatment of Anæmia.—SECONDARY ANÆMIA.—The traumatic cases do best, and with plenty of good food and fresh air the blood is readily restored. The extraordinary rapidity with which the normal percentage of red blood-corpuscles is reached without any medication whatever is an important lesson. The cause of the hæmorrhage should be sought and the necessary indications met. The large group depending on the drain on the albuminous materials of the blood, as in Bright's disease, suppuration, and fever, is difficult to treat successfully, and so long as the cause keeps up it is impossible to restore the normal blood condition. The anæmia of inanition requires plenty of nourishing food. When dependent on organic changes in the gastro-intestinal mucosa not much can be expected from either food or medicine. In the toxic cases due to mercury and lead, the poison must be eliminated and a nutritious diet given with full doses of iron. In a great majority of these cases there is deficient blood formation, and the indications are briefly three: plenty of food, an open-air life, and iron. As a rule it makes but little difference what form of the drug is administered.

CHLOROSIS.—The treatment of chlorosis affords one of the most brilliant instances—of which we have but three or four—of the specific action of a remedy. Apart from the action of quinine in malarial fever, and of mercury and iodide of potassium in syphilis, there is no other drug the beneficial effects of which we can trace with the accuracy of a scientific experiment. It is a minor matter *how* the iron cures chlorosis. In a week we give to a case as much iron as is contained in the entire blood, as even in the worst case of chlorosis there is rarely a deficit of more than 2 grammes of this metal. Iron is present in the fæces of chlorotic patients before they are placed upon any treatment, so that the disease does not result from any deficiency of available iron in the food. Bunge believes that it is the sulphur which interferes with the digestion and assimilation of this natural iron. The sulphides are produced in the process of fermentation and decomposition in the fæces, and interfere with the assimilation of the normal iron contained in the food. By the administration of an inorganic preparation of iron, with which these sulphides unite, the natural organic combinations in the food are spared.

In studying charts of chlorosis, it is seen that there is an increase in the red blood-corpuscles under the influence of the iron, and in some instances the globular richness rises above normal. The increase in the hæmoglobin is slower and the maximum percentage may not be reached for a long time. I have for years in the treatment of chlorosis used with the greatest success Blaud's pills, made and given according to the formula in Niemeyr's text-book, in which each pill contains 2 grains of the sulphate of iron. During the first week one pill is given three times a day; in the second week, two pills; in the third week, three pills, three times a day. This dose should be continued for four or five weeks at least before reduction. An important feature in the treatment is to persist in the use of the iron for at least three months, and, if necessary, subsequently to resume it in smaller doses, as recurrences are so common. The diet should consist of good, easily digested food. Special care should be directed to the bowels, and if constipation is present a saline purge should be given each morning. Such stress did Sir Andrew Clark lay on the importance of constipation in chlorosis, that he stated that if limited to the choice of one drug in the treatment of the disease he would choose a purgative. In many instances the dyspeptic symptoms may be relieved by alkalies. Dilute hydrochloric acid, manganese, phosphorus, and oxygen have been recommended. Rest in bed is important in severe cases.

TREATMENT OF PERNICIOUS ANÆMIA.—There are five essentials: first, a diagnosis; secondly, rest in bed for weeks or even months, if possible (thirdly) in the open air; fourthly, all the good food the patient can take; the outlook depends on the stomach; fifthly, arsenic; Fowler's solution in increasing doses, beginning with ♏ iii or v three times a day, and increasing ♏ i each week until the patient takes ♏ xv or xx three times a day. Other forms of arsenic may be tried, as the sodium cacodylate or the atoxyl hypodermically. Accessories are oil inunctions; bone-marrow, which has the merit of a recommendation by Galen; in some cases iron seems to do good. Care should be taken of the mouth and teeth. After recovery the patient should be told to watch the earliest indications of return of the trouble and at once resume the arsenic.

II. LEUKÆMIA.

Definition.—An affection characterized by persistent increase in the white blood-corpuscles, associated with changes, either alone or together, in the spleen, lymphatic glands, or bone-marrow.

The disease was described almost simultaneously by Virchow and by Bennett, who gave to it the name leucocythæmia. It is ordinarily seen in two main types, though combinations and variations may occur:

(1) Spleno-medullary leukæmia, in which the changes are especially localized in the spleen and the bone-marrow, while the blood shows a great increase in elements which are derived especially from the latter tissue, a condition which Müller has termed "myelæmia." Ehrlich prefers to call this type of the disease "myelogenous leukæmia," believing the part played by the spleen in the process to be purely passive.

(2) Lymphatic leukæmia, in which the changes are chiefly localized in the lymphatic apparatus, the blood showing an especial increase in those elements derived from the lymph-glands.

Etiology.—We know nothing of the conditions under which the disease arises. It is not uncommon in America. There have been 37 cases in my wards in fifteen years, of which 24 were of the spleno-myelogenous and 13 of the lymphatic type. There were 21 males and 16 females. Four were colored. There were 24 below the age of forty years. The disease is most common in the middle period of life. The youngest of my patients was a child of eight months, and cases are on record of the disease as early as the eighth or tenth week. It may occur as late as the seventieth year. Males

pernicious anemia

Osler first wrote about the disease in 1877, and by 1909, when the seventh edition of his textbook appeared, he had seen 81 cases of "idiopathic" or "progressive pernicious anaemia." The latter term, a catchy one, had been coined by Biermer in 1872 to include several kinds of anemia that we readily distinguish today. The anemia described by Addison of Guy's in 1855 was attributed by an American contemporary, Austin Flint, Sr., in 1860 to atrophy of the stomach. In 1870 Fenwick confirmed with the microscope Flint's surmise as to "degenerative disease of the glandular tubuli of the stomach" and also demonstrated a lack of peptic activity in mucosal scrapings of a postmortem specimen from such a patient.

Although in 1886 Osler had reported a case of atrophy of the stomach with the clinical features of pernicious anemia, he still followed Addison in insisting upon the inscrutable nature of the true disease. Thus, he cites as "not always to be distinguished clinically from Addison's idiopathic form" such anemias as those related to pregnancy and parturition, atrophy of the stomach, and parasites (*Ancylostoma* and *Bothriocephalus*). He quotes with conventional admiration Addison's classic description, which except for its depiction of the insidious onset and of obesity strikingly retained until the fatal termination of a long illness, is merely that of any chronic anemia. With all the respect due a great clinical observer (who had his eye on the suprarenal capsules) it must be pointed out that Addison did not mention the clinical features of the disease that best define it: glossitis, icterus, and neural changes. These were, however, cardinal points in Osler's textbook description. Glossitis and digestive disturbances had been emphasized in the decade before 1900 by William Hunter, who ascribed them to a chronic streptococcal infection of the tongue with a potential for direct extension to the esophagus, stomach, and intestine. The characteristic icterus and urobilinuria were also enlisted by Hunter in support of his theory of the infective origin of pernicious anemia as a hemolytic process. He pointed to the earlier work of Quincke in 1876 who had shown, well before the days of transfusion, an enormous accumulation of iron in the liver, which he attributed to hemolysis. Recognition of the significant association of posterolateral sclerosis of the spinal cord followed its clear description by Russell and his colleagues in 1900, who noted its appearance before the anemia in some patients. It was not until the early 1920s however, that the cumulative work of Faber, Hurst, Levine and others established during life the constancy and primacy of achylia gastrica as the hallmark of pernicious anemia.

Osler described admirably the hematological features

Pernicious anemia

of the disease. He emphasized the severe reduction of the red cell count and the contrast between the hyperchromia and oval macrocytes of pernicious anemia and those of chlorosis and secondary anemia, and he found it difficult to detect Ehrlich's nucleated megaloblasts in the blood without prolonged search. He appreciated that the "blast crises," of which no one speaks today, were an agonal event. He correctly noted leukopenia with "relative increase in the small mononuclear forms" and the scanty number of platelets. No mention was made of reticulocytes, although the predictive significance of these young cells had been experimentally defined by Theobald Smith as early as 1891. Recognition of the diagnostic significance of an increase in the number of nuclear lobes of the granulocytes is a more recent event.

Osler mentioned fever and cardiovascular, gastrointestinal, and urinary symptoms and signs as well as retinal hemorrhages and skin pigmentation. This last was then usually, but not always, due to therapy with Fowler's solution. He pointed out that, even as today (if the general practitioner does not determine the hemoglobin level or look at a blood smear), the patient is often wrongly thought to have heart, liver, or kidney disease. Even with the correct diagnosis, Osler knew that the outlook was bad, despite his other four essentials of treatment: prolonged bed rest, open air, good food in plenty ("the outlook depends on the stomach"), and Fowler's solution in increasing doses.

Significant progress in the understanding of pernicious anemia came about only after the brilliant success of its empirical treatment with liver at the end of the first quarter of the present century. For that great event in the era of the "newer knowledge of nutrition," the experimental work of G. H. Whipple and his associates in the years after 1918 provided an essential stimulus. They analyzed quantitatively the effect of various supplements to a basal diet in augmenting hemoglobin regeneration in chronically bled dogs. Of these, liver was the most potent, for reasons then not at all clear. Fortunately, this uncertainty led several clinicians to try liver feeding in a quite different condition — pernicious anemia — sometimes with improvement that they found difficult to distinguish from "spontaneous remission." However, it was G. R. Minot's prior and persistent conviction "that something in food might be of advantage" and especially the understanding use of the so-called reticulocyte response that enabled him and W. P. Murphy in Boston in 1926 firmly to relate liver feeding (in amounts up to half a pound daily) to prompt remission and progressive red cell rises in 45 patients with pernicious anemia.

Collaboration with Harvard's physical chemist E. J. Cohn and the help of the reticulocyte response soon led to the production of an experimental "Fraction G" as a pharmaceutical powdered liver extract. It was hematopoietically effective in only 12.75 grams daily. In 1930 Gänsslen in Germany developed the first practical parenteral liver extract of which about 0.35 grams daily in solution were surprisingly active. In 1937, after Dakin and West had developed a more purified injectable preparation, it was found by Lucy Wills to be ineffective in the nutritional macrocytic anemias in Bombay that responded well to less refined preparations and to autolyzed yeast. Her work eventually led to the recognition of two types of megaloblastic anemia specifically responsive to two different substances in liver. Thus, in 1945 pteroylglutamic (folic) acid was isolated from yeast; and in 1948 vitamin B_{12} was isolated from liver in the form of cyanocobalamin as a result of research by the pharmaceutical industry in the United States and in England almost simultaneously. Spies first demonstrated the clinical effectiveness of folic acid; West, that of vitamin B_{12}. Folic acid is active in Osler's macrocytic anemia of "pregnancy and the puerperium" in 200 microgram amounts daily; vitamin B_{12} in that of "atrophy of the stomach" when injected in 1 microgram amounts daily. Normally each vitamin functions as a specific coenzyme, with mutual dependence in some reactions. Today microbiological assays of the decreased serum levels of each vitamin permit exact diagnosis of the nature of the anemia, prior to a therapeutic trial. Deficiency of either vitamin leads to delay in the synthesis of the deoxyribonucleic acid of the cells of the bone marrow, with consequent lethargic nuclear maturation and division reflected in the megaloblastic series of red cells. Granulocyte and platelet production are similarly jeopardized, as are the epithelial cells of the tongue, intestine, and other proliferating tissues. The biochemical mechanism of the spinal cord lesions, which occur only with lack of vitamin B_{12}, is still unknown. However, their development may be accelerated in pernicious anemia by folic acid administration in milligram daily doses, probably as a result of forcing the metabolic utilization of remaining traces of vitamin B_{12}.

As early as 1922 Whipple pointed to the excessive production of bile pigment in pernicious anemia as indicating a source other than the breakdown of circulating red cell hemoglobin; and this was confirmed by London and West in 1950 with N^{15}-labeled glycine. In 1930 Jedlicka had expressed the view that the site of hemoglobin destruction involved reticulocytes and their nucleated precursors in the bone marrow, and this was demonstrated in 1956 by the ferrokinetic studies of Finch, showing rapid clearance of radioactive iron from the plasma by the bone marrow, but its slow reappearance as labeled hemoglobin. This discrepancy was termed by him "ineffective erythropoiesis." Together these histological and biochemical studies, by demonstrating a modicum of truth for each point of view, settled

Pernicious anemia

the 60 years war between those seeking to explain the immaturity and hyper-cellularity of the bone marrow, on the one hand as a primary "maturation arrest" or on the other as a secondary response to a hemolytic anemia. Today, it is evident that the first process determines the quality of the peripheral blood, the second largely its quantity.

Minot and Murphy's work at once made it clear that pernicious anemia was a disease involving some type of nutritional or metabolic defect. In 1928 Castle and his collaborators, impressed with the universality of achylia gastrica and noting Elders' partial success with meat feeding in pernicious anemia, inferred that the normal stomach could produce from meat something different that was present in liver. Seemingly consistent with this was their demonstration of the hematopoietic effects of feeding mixtures of normal human gastric juice ("intrinsic factor") and of beef muscle ("extrinsic factor") to patients with pernicious anemia in whom either factor alone was inert. However, 20 years later, in 1948, the active principle of liver, isolated in the form of cyanocobalamin, was shown also to be the extrinsic factor of beef muscle.

In 1952 Heinle and Welch demonstrated with radio-active cyanocobalamin that intrinsic factor enhanced the absorption of the radioactivity, which was shown the following year by Schilling to be excreted thereafter in the urine as intact labeled cyanocobalamin. After 1955 with the help of studies of gastrectomized rats by Watson and Florey and of everted segments of intestine by Wilson, Herbert, and others it was shown that the essential property of intrinsic factor is to bind the minute amounts of vitamin B_{12} present in dietary animal protein. This complex is then absorbed in the distal ileum into the bloodstream through an energy-requiring process, possibly "pinocytosis." Intrinsic factor is secreted exclusively by the parietal cells of the human stomach and is thought to be a mucopolypeptide or muco-polysaccharide with a molecular weight in the vicinity of 50,000. Patients may develop vitamin B_{12} deficiency because of dietary defect (vegans), achylia gastrica, gastrectomy, competition for vitamin B_{12} by intestinal parasites (broad tapeworm or bacteria in intestinal diverticuli or blind loop), or because the distal ileum has been resected or is the site of destructive disease.

Although dried sheep thyroid had been used for thyroid atrophy since 1891, as has been pointed out by Dock, no one thought to try feeding desiccated stomach for gastric atrophy until its successful use by Sturgis and Isaacs in 1929. In 1950 its effectiveness was shown to be due to the presence of both native vitamin B_{12} and intrinsic factor, and soon cyanocobalamin was being added to semipurified commercial preparations of hog intrinsic factor for oral use. In 1957 Schwartz of Copenhagen discovered that some patients with pernicious anemia were becoming refractory to these preparations, and that their serums were inhibitory to hog intrinsic factor when given with it by mouth in the second stage of a so-called Schilling test. Almost at once Keith Taylor in Oxford showed that this antagonistic property of the serum was not due to prior administration of hog stomach. This opened the latest chapter in the story of pernicious anemia, which must here be summarized in a few words. Doniach, Taylor, Irvine, Jeffries, and others have now shown that the serum of about half of patients with pernicious anemia contains an anti-intrinsic factor antibody in the form of a gamma globulin and that all but a tenth display a serum autoantibody directed against gastric parietal cells. Moreover, the parietal cell antibody is accompanied in about half the patients and their relatives by a thyroid acinar cell antibody. In patients with Hashimoto's disease or primary myxedema, as well as among their relatives, these two antibodies occur in about a third and in over three quarters of the subjects, respectively. The tentative explanation offered is that a hereditary tendency to develop an autoimmune process is characteristic of both pernicious anemia and myxedema patients and their relatives. It is possible, but not proved, that the antibodies are the cause of the atrophy of the stomach and of the thyroid cells, respectively. The resulting vitamin and endocrine deficiencies sometimes occur together in the same patient. The intrinsic factor antibody is found almost exclusively in the serum of patients with developed pernicious anemia. It has nothing to do with their inability to assimilate vitamin B_{12} unless leakage of serum into the gastrointestinal tract should occur. Refractoriness to hog intrinsic factor preparations is probably the result of the development of local resistance in the intestine.

Today pernicious anemia, requiring only monthly injections of 30 to 100 micrograms of vitamin B_{12}, is the simplest chronic disease to treat with the least disability, unless neural lesions have become well established.

William B. Castle

Pernicious anemia

REFERENCES

Beck, W.S. The metabolic basis of megaloblastic erythropoiesis. Medicine, 43:715, 1964.

Berk, L., Castle, W.B., Welch, A.D., Heinle, R.W., Anker, R., and Epstein, M. Observations on the etiologic relationships of achylia gastrica to pernicious anemia. X. Activity of vitamin B_{12} as food (extrinsic) factor. New Eng. J. Med., 239:911, 1948.

Castle, W.B. A century of curiosity about pernicious anemia. Trans. Amer. Clin. Climat. Ass., 73:54, 1961. (All references not listed are included here.)

Doniach, D., and Roitt, I.M. An evaluation of gastric and thyroid auto-immunity in relation to hematologic disorders. Seminars in Hematology, 1:313, 1964.

Elders, C. Tropical sprue and pernicious anaemia. Aetiology and treatment. Lancet, 1:75, 1925.

Glass, G.B.J. Gastric intrinsic factor and its function in the metabolism of vitamin B_{12}. Physiol. Rev., 43:529, 1963.

Henry, F.P., and Osler, W. Atrophy of the stomach, with the clinical features of progressive pernicious anaemia. Amer. J. Med. Sci., 91:498, 1886.

Hoedemaker, P.J., Abels, J., Wachters, J.J., et al. Investigations about the site of production of Castle's intrinsic factor. Lab. Invest., 13:1394, 1964.

Hunter, W. Pernicious Anaemia. London, Charles Griffin, 1900.

Irvine, W.J. Immunologic aspects of pernicious anemia. New Eng. J. Med., 273:432, 1965.

Jeffries, G.H., and Sleisinger, M.H. Studies of parietal cell antibody in pernicious anemia. J. Clin. Invest., 44:2021, 1965.

Jones, O.P. Origin of neutrophils in pernicious anemia (Cooke's macropolycytes). Biopsies of bone marrow. Ann. Intern. Med., 60:1002, 1937.

Kaplan, M.E., Zalusky, R., Rimington, J., and Herbert, V. Immunologic studies with intrinsic factor in man. J. Clin. Invest., 42:368, 1963.

Quincke, H. Sammlung Klinischer Vortrage, No. 100. Leipzig, Breitkopf und Hartel, 1876, p. 797.

Schwartz, M., Lous, P., and Meulengracht, E. Reduced effect of heterologous intrinsic factor after prolonged oral treatment in pernicious anaemia. Lancet, 1:751, 1957.

Smith, T. On changes in the red blood-corpuscles in the pernicious anaemia of Texas cattle fever. Trans. Ass. Amer. Physicians, 6:263, 1891.

Strauss, E.W., and Wilson, T.H. Effect of intrinsic factor on vitamin B_{12} uptake by rat intestine in vitro. Proc. Exp. Biol. Med., 99:224, 1928.

Vilter, R.W. Interrelationships between folic acid, vitamin B_{12} and ascorbic acid in the megaloblastic anemias. Medicine, 43:727, 1964.

Watson, G.M., and Florey, H.W. The absorption of vitamin B_{12} in gastrectomised rats. Brit. J. Exp. Path., 36:479, 1955.

the third week, three pills, three times a day. This dose should be continued for four or five weeks at least before reduction. An important feature in the treatment is to persist in the use of the iron for at least three months, and, if necessary, subsequently to resume it in smaller doses, as recurrences are so common. The diet should consist of good, easily digested food. Special care should be directed to the bowels, and if constipation is present a saline purge should be given each morning. Such stress did Sir Andrew Clark lay on the importance of constipation in chlorosis, that he stated that if limited to the choice of one drug in the treatment of the disease he would choose a purgative. In many instances the dyspeptic symptoms may be relieved by alkalies. Dilute hydrochloric acid, manganese, phosphorus, and oxygen have been recommended. Rest in bed is important in severe cases.

TREATMENT OF PERNICIOUS ANÆMIA.—There are five essentials: first, a diagnosis; secondly, rest in bed for weeks or even months, if possible (thirdly) in the open air; fourthly, all the good food the patient can take; the outlook depends on the stomach; fifthly, arsenic; Fowler's solution in increasing doses, beginning with ℥ iii or v three times a day, and increasing ℥ i each week until the patient takes ℥ xv or xx three times a day. Other forms of arsenic may be tried, as the sodium cacodylate or the atoxyl hypodermically. Accessories are oil inunctions; bone-marrow, which has the merit of a recommendation by Galen; in some cases iron seems to do good. Care should be taken of the mouth and teeth. After recovery the patient should be told to watch the earliest indications of return of the trouble and at once resume the arsenic.

II. LEUKÆMIA.

Definition.—An affection characterized by persistent increase in the white blood-corpuscles, associated with changes, either alone or together, in the spleen, lymphatic glands, or bone-marrow.

The disease was described almost simultaneously by Virchow and by Bennett, who gave to it the name leucocythæmia. It is ordinarily seen in two main types, though combinations and variations may occur:

(1) Spleno-medullary leukæmia, in which the changes are especially localized in the spleen and the bone-marrow, while the blood shows a great increase in elements which are derived especially from the latter tissue, a condition which Müller has termed "myelæmia." Ehrlich prefers to call this type of the disease "myelogenous leukæmia," believing the part played by the spleen in the process to be purely passive.

(2) Lymphatic leukæmia, in which the changes are chiefly localized in the lymphatic apparatus, the blood showing an especial increase in those elements derived from the lymph-glands.

Etiology.—We know nothing of the conditions under which the disease arises. It is not uncommon in America. There have been 37 cases in my wards in fifteen years, of which 24 were of the spleno-myelogenous and 13 of the lymphatic type. There were 21 males and 16 females. Four were colored. There were 24 below the age of forty years. The disease is most common in the middle period of life. The youngest of my patients was a child of eight months, and cases are on record of the disease as early as the eighth or tenth week. It may occur as late as the seventieth year. Males are more prone to the affection than females. Birch-Hirschfeld states that of 200 cases collected from the literature, 135 were males and 65 females.

A tendency to hæmorrhage has been noted in many cases, and some of the patients have suffered repeatedly from nose-bleeding. In women the disease is most common at the climacteric. There are instances in which it has occurred during pregnancy. The case described by J. Chalmers Cameron, of Montreal, is in this respect remarkable, as the patient passed through three pregnancies, bearing on each occasion non-leukæmic children. The case is interesting, too, as showing the hereditary character of the affection, as the grandmother and mother, as well as a brother, suffered from symptoms strongly suggestive of leukæmia. One of the patient's children had leukæmia before the mother showed any signs, and a second died of the disease. This patient gradually recovered from the third confinement, and the red blood-corpuscles had risen to 4,000,000 per cubic millimetre, and the ratio of white to red was 1 to 200. Sänger has reported a case in which a healthy mother bore a leukæmic child.

Malaria is believed by some to be an etiological factor. Of 150 cases analyzed by Gowers, there was a history of malaria in 30; of my hospital cases comparatively few gave a history of it. The disease has followed injury or a blow. The lower animals are subject to the affection, and cases have been described in horses, dogs, oxen, cats, swine, and mice.

Morbid Anatomy.—The wasting may be extreme, and dropsy is sometimes present. There is in many cases a remarkable condition of polyæmia; the heart and veins are distended with large blood-clots. In Case XI of my series the weight of blood in the heart chambers alone was 620 grammes. There may be remarkable distention of the portal, cerebral, pulmonary, and subcutaneous veins. The blood is usually clotted, and the enormous increase in the leucocytes gives a pus-like appearance to the coagula, so that it has happened more than once, as in Virchow's memorable case, that on opening the right auricle the observer at first thought he had cut into an abscess. The coagula have a peculiar greenish color, somewhat like the fat of a turtle. Sometimes this is so intense as to suggest the color of chloroma, described later. The alkalinity of the blood is diminished. The fibrin is increased. The character of the corpuscles will be described under the symptoms. Charcot's octahedral crystals may separate from the blood after death. The specific gravity of the blood is somewhat lowered. There may be pericardial ecchymoses.

In the spleno-medullary form the spleen is greatly enlarged. Strong adhesions may unite it to the abdominal wall, the diaphragm, or the stomach. The capsule may be thickened; the vessels at the hilus are enlarged. The weight may range from 2 to 18 pounds. The organ is in a condition of chronic hyperplasia. It cuts with resistance, has a uniformly reddish-brown color, and the Malpighian bodies are invisible. Grayish-white, circumscribed, lymphoid tumors may occur throughout the organ, contrasting strongly with the reddish-brown matrix. In the early stage the swollen spleen pulp is softer, and it is stated that rupture has occurred from the intense hyperæmia.

There is an extraordinary hyperplasia of the red marrow. Instead of a fatty tissue, the medulla of the long bones may resemble the consistent matter which forms the core of an abscess, or it may be dark brown in color. There may be hæmorrhagic infarctions. There may be much expansion of the shell of bone, and localized swellings which are tender and may even yield to firm pressure. Histologically, there are found in the medulla large numbers of nucleated red corpuscles in all stages of development, numerous cells with eosinophilic granules, both small polynuclear forms and large almost giant mononuclear elements. There are also many large cells with single large nuclei and neutrophilic granules—the *cellules médullaires* of Cornil—the *myelocytes* which are found in the blood. Great numbers of polynuclear leucocytes are also present, as well as a certain number of small mononuclear elements.

In the lymphatic forms of the disease there is a general lymphatic enlargement, which is usually associated with a certain amount of enlargement of the spleen. In the cases of lymphatic leukæmia the cervical, axillary, mesenteric, and inguinal groups may be much enlarged, but the glands are usually soft, isolated, and movable. They may vary considerably in size during the course of the disease. In acute cases the tonsils and the lymph follicles of the tongue, pharynx, and mouth may be enlarged.

In some instances there are leukæmic enlargements in the solitary and agminated glands of Peyer. In a case of Willcocks' there were growths on the surface of the stomach and gastro-splenic omentum. The thymus is rarely involved, though it has been enlarged in some of the acute cases. The bone-marrow in these cases may be replaced by a lymphoid tissue. Nucleated red corpuscles and the normal granular marrow elements may be greatly reduced in number.

The liver may be enlarged, and in a case described by Welch it weighed over 13 pounds. The enlargement is usually due to a diffuse leukæmic infiltration. The columns of liver cells are widely separated by leucocytes, which are partly within and partly outside the lobular capillaries. There may be definite leukæmic growths.

There are rarely changes of importance in the lungs. The kidneys are often enlarged and pale, the capillaries may be distended with leucocytes, and leukæmic tumors may occur. The skin may be involved, as in a case described by Kaposi.

Leukæmic tumors in the organs are not common. In 159 cases collected by Gowers there were only 13 instances of leukæmic nodules in the liver and 10 in the kidneys. These new growths probably develop from leucocytes which leave the capillaries. Bizzozero has shown that the cells which compose them are in active fission.

Symptoms.—The onset is insidious, and, as a rule, the patient seeks advice for progressive enlargement of the abdomen and shortness of breath, or for the enlarged glands or the pallor, palpitation, and other symptoms of anæmia. Bleeding at the nose is common. Gastro-intestinal symptoms may precede the onset. Occasionally the first symptoms are of a very serious nature. In one of the cases of my series the boy played lacrosse two days before the onset of the final hæmatemesis; and in another case a girl, who had, it was supposed, only a slight chlorosis, died of fatal hæmorrhage from the stomach before any suspicion had been aroused as to the true condition.

Anæmia is not a necessary accompaniment of all stages of the disease; the subjects may look very healthy and well.

As has been stated, the disease is most commonly seen in two main types, though combinations may occur.

(1) SPLENO-MEDULLARY LEUKÆMIA.—This is much the commonest type of the disease. The gradual increase in the volume of the spleen is the most prominent symptom in a majority of the cases. Pain and tenderness are common, though the progressive enlargement may be painless. A creaking fremitus may be felt on palpation. The enlarged organ extends downward to the right, and may be felt just at the costal edge, or when large it may extend as far over as the navel. In many cases it occupies fully one-half of the abdomen, reaching to the pubes below and extending beyond the middle line. As a rule, the edge, in some the notch or notches, can be felt distinctly. Its size varies greatly from time to time. It may be perceptibly larger after meals. A hæmorrhage or free diarrhœa may reduce the size. The pressure of the enlarged organ may cause distress after eating; in one case it caused fatal obstruction of the bowels. A murmur may sometimes be heard over the spleen, and Gerhardt has described a pulsation in it.

The pulse is usually rapid, soft, compressible, but often full in volume. There are rarely any cardiac symptoms. The apex beat may be lifted an interspace by the enlarged spleen. Toward the close œdema may occur in the feet or general anasarca. Hæmorrhage is common. There may be most extensive purpura, or hæmorrhagic exudate into pleura or peritonæum. Epistaxis is the most frequent form. Hæmoptysis and hæmaturia are rare. Bleeding from the gums may be present. Hæmatemesis proved fatal in two of my cases, and in a third a large cerebral hæmorrhage rapidly killed. The leukæmic retinitis is a part of the hæmorrhagic manifestations. J. Hughes Bennett's first leukæmic patient died suddenly, without obvious cause.

Local gangrene may develop, with signs of intense infection and high fever. There are very few pulmonary symptoms. The shortness of breath is due, as a rule, to the anæmia. Toward the end there may be œdema of the lungs, or pneumonia may carry off the patient. The gastro-intestinal symptoms are rarely absent. Nausea and vomiting are early features in some cases. Diarrhœa may be very troublesome, even fatal. Intestinal hæmorrhage is not common. There may be a dysenteric process in the colon. Jaundice rarely occurs, though in one case of my series there were recurrent attacks. Ascites may be a prominent symptom, probably due to the presence of the splenic tumor. A leukæmic peritonitis also may be present, due to new growths in the membranes.

The nervous system is not often involved. Facial paralysis has been noted. Headache, dizziness, and fainting spells are due to anæmia. The patients are usually tranquil. Coma may follow cerebral hæmorrhage.

The special senses are often affected. There is a peculiar retinitis, due chiefly to the extravasation of blood, but there may be aggregations of leucocytes, forming small leukæmic growths. Optic neuritis is rare. Deafness has frequently been observed; it may appear early and possibly is due to hæmorrhage. Features suggestive of Ménière's disease may come on quite suddenly, due to leukæmic infiltration or hæmorrhage into the semi-circular canal.

The urine presents no constant changes. The uric acid excreted is always in excess.

Priapism is a curious symptom which has been present in a large num-

292

ber of cases. It may, as in one of our cases, be the first symptom. In one of my cases it persisted for seven weeks. The cause is not known.

Fever was present in two-thirds of my series. Periods of pyrexia may alternate with prolonged intervals of freedom. The temperature may range from 102° to 103°.

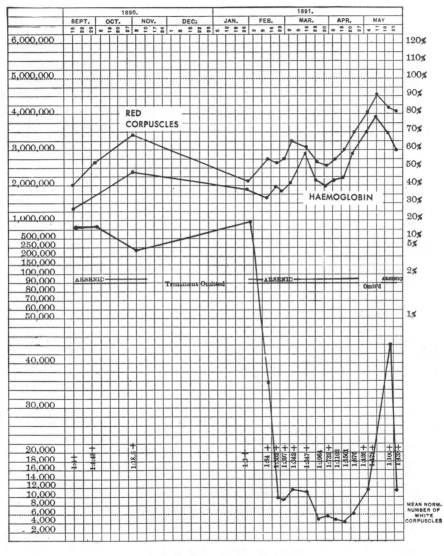

CHART XIX.—LEUKÆMIA.

Blood.—In all forms of the disease the diagnosis must be made by the examination of the blood, as it alone offers distinctive features.

The most striking change in the more common form, the spleno-myelogenous, is the increase in the colorless corpuscles. The average in one of my

293

series was 298,700 per cubic millimetre, and the average ratio to the red cells was 1 to 10. The proportion may be 1 to 5, or may even reach 1 to 1. There are instances on record in which the number of leucocytes has exceeded that of the red corpuscles. The leucocytes may vary greatly within short intervals.

The small mononuclear forms are little if at all increased; relatively they are greatly diminished. The eosinophiles are present in normal or increased relative proportion, so that there is a great total increase, and their presence is a striking feature in the stained blood-slide. The polynuclear neutrophiles may be in normal proportion; more frequently they are relatively diminished, and in the later stages they may form but a small proportion of the colorless elements. Marked differences in size between individual polynuclear leucocytes may be noted; the same is true of the eosinophiles. The most characteristic features of the blood in this form of leukæmia is the presence of cells which do not occur in normal blood. They appear to be derived from the marrow, and are called by Ehrlich *myelocytes.* They are large mononuclear neutrophilic cells, which may vary much in size. They comprise about 30 per cent of the colorless cells. Nicked nuclei are common. Müller has recently found many large mononuclear elements with karyokinetic figures in leukæmic blood and in the marrow. These probably correspond to the myelocytes of Ehrlich as well as to the "cellules médullaires" of Cornil. Polynuclear cells with coarse basophilic granules, "Mastzellen," are always present in this form of leukæmia in considerable numbers. The granules do not stain in Ehrlich's triacid mixture, and the cells may be recognized as polynuclear non-granular elements. These cells, which form only about 0.28 per cent of the leucocytes of normal blood, may be even more numerous than the eosinophiles.

Nucleated red blood-corpuscles are present in considerable numbers. These are usually "normoblasts," but cells with larger paler nuclei, some showing evidences of mitosis, may be seen. Red cells with fragmented nuclei are common, while true megaloblasts may be found. The average number of red cells in one of my series was 2,850,000 per cubic millimetre. In no case was the count below two million. The average hæmoglobin was 42 per cent. The blood chart on page 735 is from a case of leukæmia with an enormously enlarged spleen. Among other points about leukæmic blood may be mentioned the feebleness of the amœboid movement, as noted by Cavafy, which may be accounted for by the large number of mononuclear elements present, as the polynuclear alone are stated to possess this power. The blood-plates exist in variable numbers; they may be remarkably abundant. The fibrin network between the corpuscles is usually thick and dense. In blood slides which are kept for a short time, Charcot's octahedral crystals separate, and in the blood of leukæmia the hæmoglobin shows a remarkable tendency to crystallize.

2. LYMPHATIC LEUKÆMIA.—This form of leukæmia is rare. There were 13 out of 37 in my hospital series, of which 5 were acute. The superficial glands are usually most involved, but even when affected it is rare to see such large bunches as in Hodgkin's disease. External lymph tumors are rare. Lymphatic leukæmia is often more rapid and fatal in its course, though chronic cases may occur. It is more common in young subjects.

The histological characters of the *blood* in lymphatic leukæmia differ materially from those in the spleno-medullary form. The increase in the colorless elements is never so great as in the preceding form; a proportion of 1 to 10 would be extreme. The number of both white and red cells showed great variations in my series. This increase takes place solely in the lymphocytes, all other forms of leucocytes being present in greatly diminished relative proportion. In one of my cases over 99 per cent of all the leucocytes were lymphocytes. In some cases, as Cabot has pointed out, this increase takes place largely in the smaller forms, while in others the large lymphocytes—cells nearly as large as polynuclear leucocytes—predominate. Eosinophiles and nucleated red corpuscles are rare. Myelocytes are not present.

Combined forms of leukæmia are not common.

Leukanæmia.—This term was used by Leube to describe a condition which showed features both of leukæmia and severe anæmia. Some of the cases of acute leukæmia come under this head, but it must be regarded rather as a clinical term than a pathological condition. The symptoms are often suggestive of an acute infection. The onset may be sudden, and is frequently with severe tonsillitis, so that the throat condition is the most striking feature. The prominent symptoms are fever, weakness, hæmorrhages, extreme pallor, and a rapid downward course. General glandular enlargement is frequently, although not constantly present. The liver and spleen are usually enlarged. The duration varies from a few days to three months. The rapid fall in the hæmoglobin and in the number of red cells is striking. In half the reported cases the red count was below 1,500,000 per cmm. With this there is a high color index. The acute forms are usually of the lymphocytic type, although a few cases of acute myelogenous leukæmia have been reported. In the former the predominating lymphocyte is usually the large form, although in a few acute cases with hæmorrhages the small lymphocytes have been the more numerous.

Diagnosis.—The recognition of leukæmia can be determined only by microscopical examination of the blood. The clinical features may be identical with those of ordinary splenic anæmia, or of Hodgkin's disease. An interesting question arises whether real increase in the leucocytes is the only criterion of the existence of the disease. Thus, for instance, in the case whose chart is given on page 735, the patient came under observation in September, 1890, with 2,000,000 red blood-corpuscles per cubic millimetre, 30 per cent of hæmoglobin, and 500,000 white blood-corpuscles per cubic millimetre—a proportion of 1 to 4. As shown by the chart, throughout September, October, November, and December, this ratio was maintained. Early in January, under treatment with arsenic, the white corpuscles began to decrease, and gradually, as shown in the chart, the normal ratio was reached. At this time could it be said that the case was one of leukæmia without increase in the number of leucocytes? The blood examination showed that nucleated red corpuscles in large numbers as well as myelocytes, elements which are but rarely found in normal blood, were still present in numbers sufficient to suggest, if the patient had come under observation for the first time, that leukæmia might occur. In another of our cases the blood became normal and the spleen tumor disappeared twice in one year (McCrae). Altogether I have seen four cases in which the leucocyte count became normal, in three the splenic enlargement persisted.

Association with other Diseases.—Tuberculosis, of which Dock has collected 27 cases, occurs occasionally without any special influence on the course.

48

Intercurrent infections are not uncommon—influenza, typhoid fever, sepsis—often with remarkable influence, particularly on the leucocytes. In Dock's case within a couple of weeks after an attack of influenza they fell from 367,070 to 7,500 per cmm. Various other conditions influence the disease, and the excess of leucocytes has disappeared after the use of arsenic, quinine, tuberculin, nuclein, and the X-rays.

Prognosis.—Recovery occasionally occurs. A great majority of the cases prove fatal within two or three years. Unfavorable signs are a tendency to hæmorrhage, persistent diarrhœa, early dropsy, and high fever. Remarkable variations are displayed in the course, and a transient improvement may take place for weeks or even months. The pure lymphatic form seems to be of particular malignancy, some cases proving fatal in from three to eight weeks. In one of my cases the leukæmia lasted between eleven and twelve years. The diagnosis was made by the late W. H. Draper, and when I saw the patient, ten years after the onset, the cervical, axillary, and inguinal glands were greatly enlarged; the leucocytes were 242,000 per cubic millimetre, above 90 per cent of them being lymphocytes. The longest course of my hospital series of the lymphatic type was three years, and of the spleno-myelogenous about the same duration.

Treatment.—Fresh air, good diet, and abstention from mental worry and care, are the important general indications. The *indicatio morbi* can not be met. There are certain remedies which have an influence upon the disease. Of these, arsenic, given in large doses, is the best. I have repeatedly seen improvement under its use. On the other hand, there are curious remissions in the disease, as mentioned above, which render therapeutical deductions very fallacious.

Quinine may be given in cases with a malarial history. Iron may be of value in some cases, as may also inhalations of oxygen. Treatment with the X-rays should be tried. Some observers have reported very good results. Personally, I have not seen any very striking improvement.

Excision of the leukæmic spleen has been performed 43 times, with 5 recoveries (J. C. Warren).

Chloroma is a rare form of leukæmia in which there is a tumor-like hyperplasia of the bone-marrow with growths of a greenish color (" green cancer ") in the bones, particularly of the head and orbit, and in the organs. There is anæmia and marked leukæmia. Dock has collected 22 cases reported since 1893. The chief symptoms are progressive weakness, pallor, exophthalmos with the tumor formations. Sometimes there are skin eruptions, in Bramwell's case of a greenish color. The cause of the remarkable color is unknown.

III. HODGKIN'S DISEASE.

Definition.—An affection characterized by progressive enlargement of the lymphatic glands (beginning usually on one side of the neck) and spleen, with the formation in the liver, spleen, lungs, and other organs of nodular growths, associated with a secondary anæmia, without leukæmia.

Hodgkin, in 1832, recorded a series of cases of enlargement of the lymphatic glands and spleen. As with Addison's disease, to Wilks we owe a

leukemia
A half-century's progress does not alter Osler's sound concept of leukemia based on the bedside study of 37 patients. Probably 24 had chronic myelocytic ("spleno-medullary") leukemia and the remainder lymphatic, 5 of them acute. Leukemia has increased in the United States since Osler's day — from 1.5 cases per 100,000 population in 1910 to 6.1 in 1961.

Etiology

The cause of leukemia is still uncertain, but we now know some of the conditions under which it arises. Today it seems likely that leukemia results from uncontrolled multiplication of leukocytes due to genetic faults in hematopoiesis. Ionizing radiation, chemicals, and viruses cause leukemia in vertebrates, yet no one type of insult by itself can be proved to be the usual cause of clinical leukemia. The clearest relation of genetic damage and leukemia is seen in the observations by Nowell and Hungerford of the Philadelphia chromosome (partially deleted No. 21) in 90 percent of patients with chronic myelocytic leukemia. In another genetic defect of the same chromosome, Down's syndrome, the occurrence of leukemia is increased. Ionizing radiation caused a 30-fold increase in chronic myelocytic leukemia at Hiroshima. Court Brown and Abbatt have shown that patients receiving x-irradiation for ankylosing spondylitis have a (myelocytic) leukemia occurrence of 4 per 1,000. A number of chemicals induce leukemia in mice, but to date only benzol exposure is thought to be associated with human leukemia. In 1951 Gross transmitted leukemia in mice by a virus, and a number of murine leukemias are now known to be due to a group of RNA viruses. Similar particles have been found in lymph nodes (Dmochowski) and in blood of about 20 percent of leukemic patients (Dalton), but their significance is not known. Grace and others have been able to grow in tissue culture leukemic cells that produce herpes-like virus particles whose causative role cannot be stated. Earlier, Epstein had demonstrated herpes-like particles in the cultures of cells from patients with the African lymphoma described by Burkitt.

Pathophysiology

The morbid anatomy and symptoms of leukemia as it is known today do not differ from Osler's descriptions except where therapy has altered its course. For example, meningeal leukemia, rare in his day,

Leukemia

is now quite common because antileukemic drugs do not achieve leukemicidal concentrations in the cerebrospinal fluid and allow a selective proliferation in the meninges. The symptomatology of leukemia arises from interference with normal organ function by excess abnormal leukocytes. The major deficits are those of diminished function of the bone marrow and lymphocyte-producing tissues, leading to anemia, thrombocytopenia, granulocytopenia, and lymphocytopenia. Anemia, more common and severe than in Osler's patients, has been shown by Berlin, when not due to hemorrhage or drugs, to result from a variable combination of shortened red cell life span and diminished red cell production. Hemorrhage remains as a common cause of death in the acute leukemias, and Freireich's studies show a linear inverse relationship between platelet count and probability of bleeding. Osler, an early platelet scholar (1874), did not in this section comment on their relation to hemorrhage. Infection is now the major cause of death. Two mechanisms of host depletion leading to bacterial infection are granulocytopenia and diminished synthesis of immunoglobulins. The pattern of infections in leukemia has changed rapidly; malaria, typhoid fever, and tuberculosis yielded to pneumococcal, streptococcal, and staphylococcal infections, and these in turn have been replaced by septicemias due to gram-negative bacilli or fungi, and cytomegalic inclusion disease.

Diagnosis

Osler said it succinctly: "The recognition of leukemia can be determined only by microscopical examination of the blood." One need only add that if the physician suspects leukemia and the blood examination is not typical he can often settle the issue by study of bone marrow aspirates.

Treatment

Osler, cautious in therapeutic judgments, said that arsenic was the only useful therapy. X-irradiation might be tried, but he doubted its value. Since 1910 ionizing radiation, drugs, and physiological repair have brought symptomatic relief and longer survival. At the present time x-rays are used largely for the relief of symptoms due to localized disease, such as an enlarged spleen or a mass of lymph nodes. Lawrence in 1936 introduced the use of the radioisotope P^{32} for chronic myelocytic leukemia, and Osgood has shown that with it the disease can be suppressed for long periods. Drugs constitute the treatment of choice in the leukemias. The con-

298

trol of chronic leukemia by drugs began with nitrogen mustard. Although many alkylating agents affect chronic leukemia, at the present time chlorambucil is the treatment of choice for chronic lymphocytic leukemia and busulfan for chronic myelocytic leukemia. Eventually the chronic leukemias no longer respond to these or similar agents. Chronic myelocytic leukemia usually erupts into a blastic crisis, indistinguishable from acute leukemia. Chronic lymphocytic leukemia often ends in infection, due to inability to form immunoglobulins.

The ability to control the acute leukemias started in 1947 with Farber's discovery of the effectiveness of folic acid antagonists. Subsequently five other agents were found to induce complete remission: cortisone (and ACTH) in 1949 by Pearson and associates; 6-mercaptopurine in 1953 by Burchenal and colleagues; cyclophosphamide in 1960 by Fernbach and co-workers; vincristine in 1962 by Karon et al.; and methylglyoxal bis guanylhydrazone in 1962 by Freireich and colleagues. Methotrexate is now the preferred folic acid antagonist, and prednisone the usual corticosteroid. Each of these agents, except methylglyoxal bis guanylhydrazone, is effective in acute lymphocytic leukemia. Acute myelocytic leukemia is sensitive to 6-mercaptopurine, methotrexate, and methylglyoxal bis guanylhydrazone. There is extraordinary activity in the investigation of the best way to use these agents. Freireich and associates in 1964 reported long remissions with a combination of four drugs. As of January 1966 the best reported results in acute lymphocytic leukemia are those of Selawry and colleagues (1965), with 81 percent of the patients treated surviving two years. They induced remissions with a combination of vincristine and prednisone and maintained remission by intermittent parenteral methotrexate. The best results in acute myelocytic leukemia are those of Thompson and co-workers (1965) using the Freireich combination; ten of their 14 patients achieved remissions.

Finally, supportive therapy can carry the leukemic patient through life-threatening situations until drug control can be achieved. Many of these are nonspecific though not available in Osler's day — transfusions for red cell deficits, steroids for hemolytic anemia, antibacterial chemotherapy, and so on. More specific aids have been platelet replacement to prevent hemorrhage from thrombocytopenia, prevention of infection by protecting the depleted patient from the microflora of room air, and treatment of gram-negative septicemia by granulocyte transfusions.

Prognosis

In the chronic leukemias, the improvements have been in the quality of survival rather than its length. The median survival in

299

Leukemia

acute myelocytic leukemia is now about six months. The major advances have been in acute lymphocytic leukemia. In the series of Brubaker and of Zuelzer the median survival is 20 months, and about 10 percent survived 5 years. The 5-year survival in Selawry's series cannot yet be estimated. Burchenal has collected 101 patients with acute myelocytic or lymphocytic leukemia who lived 5 to 14 years after drug therapy. Of these, 64 have no sign of disease.

C. Gordon Zubrod

REFERENCES

Bryan, W.R., Dalton, A.J., and Rauscher, F.J. The Viral Approach to Human Leukemia and Lymphoma: Its Current Status. Progress in Hematology, No. 5. New York, Grune & Stratton, Inc., 1966.

Court Brown, W.M., and Doll, R. Mortality from cancer and other causes after radiotherapy for ankylosing spondylitis. Brit. Med. J., 2:1327, 1965.

Dameshek, W., and Gunz, F. Leukemia, 2nd ed. New York, Grune & Stratton, Inc., 1964.

Frei, E., III, and Freireich, E.J. In Advances in Chemotherapy. Goldin, A., Hawking, F., and Schneitzer, R.J. eds. New York, Academic Press, Inc., 1965, Vol. 2, pp. 269-298.

Galton, D.A.G. Treatment of chronic leukaemias. Brit. Med. Bull., 15:78, 1959.

Symposium: Conference on Obstacles to the Control of Acute Leukemia. Cancer Res., 25:1469, 1965.

Intercurrent infections are not uncommon—influenza, typhoid fever, sepsis—often with remarkable influence, particularly on the leucocytes. In Dock's case within a couple of weeks after an attack of influenza they fell from 367,070 to 7,500 per cmm. Various other conditions influence the disease, and the excess of leucocytes has disappeared after the use of arsenic, quinine, tuberculin, nuclein, and the X-rays.

Prognosis.—Recovery occasionally occurs. A great majority of the cases prove fatal within two or three years. Unfavorable signs are a tendency to hæmorrhage, persistent diarrhœa, early dropsy, and high fever. Remarkable variations are displayed in the course, and a transient improvement may take place for weeks or even months. The pure lymphatic form seems to be of particular malignancy, some cases proving fatal in from three to eight weeks. In one of my cases the leukæmia lasted between eleven and twelve years. The diagnosis was made by the late W. H. Draper, and when I saw the patient, ten years after the onset, the cervical, axillary, and inguinal glands were greatly enlarged; the leucocytes were 242,000 per cubic millimetre, above 90 per cent of them being lymphocytes. The longest course of my hospital series of the lymphatic type was three years, and of the spleno-myelogenous about the same duration.

Treatment.—Fresh air, good diet, and abstention from mental worry and care, are the important general indications. The *indicatio morbi* can not be met. There are certain remedies which have an influence upon the disease. Of these, arsenic, given in large doses, is the best. I have repeatedly seen improvement under its use. On the other hand, there are curious remissions in the disease, as mentioned above, which render therapeutical deductions very fallacious.

Quinine may be given in cases with a malarial history. Iron may be of value in some cases, as may also inhalations of oxygen. Treatment with the X-rays should be tried. Some observers have reported very good results. Personally, I have not seen any very striking improvement.

Excision of the leukæmic spleen has been performed 43 times, with 5 recoveries (J. C. Warren).

Chloroma is a rare form of leukæmia in which there is a tumor-like hyperplasia of the bone-marrow with growths of a greenish color ("green cancer") in the bones, particularly of the head and orbit, and in the organs. There is anæmia and marked leukæmia. Dock has collected 22 cases reported since 1893. The chief symptoms are progressive weakness, pallor, exophthalmos with the tumor formations. Sometimes there are skin eruptions, in Bramwell's case of a greenish color. The cause of the remarkable color is unknown.

III. HODGKIN'S DISEASE.

Definition.—An affection characterized by progressive enlargement of the lymphatic glands (beginning usually on one side of the neck) and spleen, with the formation in the liver, spleen, lungs, and other organs of nodular growths, associated with a secondary anæmia, without leukæmia.

Hodgkin, in 1832, recorded a series of cases of enlargement of the lymphatic glands and spleen. As with Addison's disease, to Wilks we owe a clear conception of the affection with which he associated the name of the distinguished morbid anatomist of Guy's Hospital.*

Clinically the cases resemble certain forms of leukæmia, lympho-sarcoma, and lymphatic tuberculosis; some recent writers even deny the existence of a separate malady, Hodgkin's disease.

Many names have been given to the condition—anæmia lymphatica (Wilks), adénie (Trousseau), pseudo-leukæmia (Cohnheim), and generalized lymphadenoma.

The names malignant lymphoma (Billroth) and lympho-sarcoma have also been given to a form of progressive enlargement of the lymph-glands, but they should be restricted to primary sarcoma of these structures, a very different affection anatomically, though clinically it may resemble Hodgkin's disease.

Etiology.—A majority of the cases occur in young persons. Of 43 cases collected by Mitchell Clark, 37 were in males. Ten occurred below ten years of age and 33 below the fortieth year. Heredity, syphilis, and tuberculosis are doubtful factors. Local irritation about the throat and mouth—regions draining into the cervical glands—often precedes the onset of the swelling (Trousseau). The true nature of the disease is unknown. Certain features suggest that it may be an *acute infection*—the rapidly fatal course of some cases, the frequency with which the disease starts in the cervical glands, and the not infrequent preliminary involvement of the tonsils, the gradual extension from one gland-group to another, and the recurring exacerbations of fever. A possible instance of direct infection is quoted by Murray in Allbutt's system. The results of bacteriological study are as yet uncertain.

RELATION TO MALIGNANT DISEASE.—Much confusion has come from the use of the terms lympho-sarcoma and malignant lymphoma to designate cases of Hodgkin's disease. The two conditions are quite different. We know of no malignant growth the metastases of which occur in one form of tissue only. Sarcoma invades the capsule of the gland and the adjacent textures, and does not limit its extension from one gland-group to another. Histologically there are radical differences between lympho-sarcoma and Hodgkin's disease.

RELATION TO TUBERCULOSIS.—Of late the view has been advanced that Hodgkin's disease is only a peculiar form of lymphatic tuberculosis, a view supported by Sternberg, Crowder, Musser, Sailer, and others. There is an acute tuberculous adenitis and a chronic form (see p. 306), either of which may closely resemble Hodgkin's disease. The statement of the relationship is based upon (1) the presence of tubercle bacilli in the glands in a certain number of cases of Hodgkin's disease, and (2) the successful inoculation of animals, even when the glands did not show tubercle bacilli microscopically. Opposed to this are the facts that (1) in a large majority of all cases bacilli are not present in the glands, and the inoculation experiments are negative (Westphal); (2) the histological changes in the glands in Hodgkin's disease are specific and distinctive (Reed); (3) the tuberculin test in typical cases of the disease is negative (Reed); and (4) the tuberculosis when present is in many cases, at least, a terminal infection.

---

* Students have now easy access to the original account (which appeared in the Transactions of the Royal Med. and Chirur. Society, 1832), in the New Sydenham Society Memoirs, 1902.

Morbid Anatomy.—The superficial lymph-glands are found most extensively involved, and from the cervical groups they form continuous chains uniting the mediastinal and axillary glands. The masses may pass beneath the pectoral muscles and even beneath the scapulæ. Of the internal glands, those of the thorax are most often affected, and the tracheal and bronchial groups may form large masses. The trachea and the aorta with its branches may be completely surrounded; the veins may be compressed, rarely the aorta itself. The masses perforate the sternum and invade the lung deeply. The retroperitoneal glands may form a continuous chain from the diaphragm to the inguinal canals. They may compress the ureters, the lumbar and sacral nerves, and the iliac veins. They may adhere to the broad ligament and the uterus and simulate fibroids. At an early stage the glands are soft and elastic; later they may become firm and hard. Fusion of contiguous glands does not often occur, and they tend to remain discrete, even after attaining a large size. The capsule is not infiltrated, nor are adjacent tissues invaded. On section the gland presents a grayish-white semi-translucent appearance, broken by intersecting strands of fibrous tissue; there is no caseation or necrosis unless a secondary infection has occurred.

The spleen is enlarged in 75 per cent of the cases; in young children the enlargement may be great, but the organ rarely reaches the size of the spleen in ordinary leukæmia. In more than half of the cases lymphoid growths are present.

The marrow of the long bones may be converted into a rich lymphoid tissue. The lymphatic structures of the tonsillar ring and of the intestines may show marked hyperplasia. The liver is often enlarged, and may present scattered nodular tumors, which may also occur in the kidneys.

HISTOLOGY.—The study of D. M. Reed,* from the laboratory of my colleague, Dr. Welch, suggests that there is a specific histological picture in Hodgkin's disease characterized by (1) proliferation of the endothelial and reticular cells; (2) the formation of lymphoid cells (uniform in size and shape) from the mother cells of the lymph-nodes and from the endothelial cells of the reticulum; (3) characteristic giant cells, formed from proliferating endothelial cells, which differ from the giant cells of tuberculosis; (4) great proliferation of the connective-tissue stroma leading to fibrosis; and, lastly, eosinophile cells, which form a marked feature in a large proportion of the cases. The metastatic nodules present the same structure as the glandular growths.

When tuberculosis occurs as a secondary infection the two processes may be readily differentiated in sections of the glands.

Symptoms.—Enlargement of the glands on one side of the neck is usually the first symptom. It is rare that other superficial groups or the deeper glands are first attacked. A chronic tonsillitis may precede the onset. Months, or even several years, may elapse before the glands on the other side of the neck or in the axilla are involved. Usually there is a progressive growth, until quite large groups are formed, in which, however, the individual glands may be felt. There is not often any pain. The inguinal glands may soon be involved and grow rapidly, but in many cases they do not reach the

* Johns Hopkins Hospital Reports, vol. x, 1902.

size of the cervical groups. During what may be called the first stage of the disease the patient's general condition is good. It may be many months before the internal lymph-glands become involved, and they may never enlarge sufficiently to cause symptoms. The spleen enlarges in a majority of cases. In rare instances the lymphoid tumors may be felt on the surface of the enlarged liver and spleen.

As the disease advances the symptoms fall into two groups—those due to pressure of the enlarged glands, and the progressive cachexia. The axillary groups may cause swelling and pain in the hands and arms. The inguinal glands may press on the nerves and cause great pain, with swelling of the feet. Involvement of the mediastinal glands is indicated by paroxysmal cough, attacks of pain, dyspnœa, and sometimes most intense cyanosis of the upper part of the body. Pleural effusion, disturbed heart action, and pupillary changes are rarer events. The cases with paraplegia from invasion of the spine and the cord, are, as a rule, lympho-sarcoma.

The general symptoms of the disease are:

ANÆMIA of a secondary type, not marked at first, and even in the later stages the red corpuscles rarely fall below 2,000,000 per cubic millimetre. The leucocytes may be normal in number or there may be an early leucocytosis, or at any time during the course there may be a transient increase. The small mononuclear forms may be relatively increased. In very rare instances a terminal leukæmia occurs, but, as C. F. Martin suggests, these cases may be true leukæmia from the start.

FEVER.—A majority of the cases present (1) a slight irregular fever; (2) later in the disease there may be a daily rise of three or four degrees, sometimes with a chill and sweat; (3) in a few rare instances Pel has described remarkable periods of fever of ten to fourteen days' duration, alternating with intervals of complete apyrexia. They occurred in two of my cases. Ebstein described it as a form of chronic recurring fever. It is probably due to an intercurrent infection.

CACHEXIA.—A remarkable grade of emaciation ultimately follows, associated with great asthenia, and sometimes anasarca from the anæmia.

Bronzing of the skin may occur, apart from the use of arsenic. An obstinate pruritus and recurring boils may add to the patient's distress.

Diagnosis.—(*a*) TUBERCULOSIS.—It is not sufficiently recognized that there are both acute and chronic forms of general tuberculous adenitis (see p. 306), but such cases do not often present difficulty in diagnosis. In the case of enlargement of the glands on one side of the neck beginning in a young person, it is often not at all easy to determine whether the disease is tuberculosis or beginning Hodgkin's disease. Two points should be decided. First, under cocaine one of the small glands of the affected side should be excised and the structure carefully studied in the light of Dr. Reed's recent observations. The histological changes differ markedly in Hodgkin's disease from those in tuberculosis. Secondly, tuberculin should be used if the patient is afebrile. In early tuberculosis of the glands of the neck the reaction is prompt and decisive. The large experience on this point in the wards of my colleague, Halsted, is conclusive as to the efficiency (and the harmlessness) of the method. In the later stages, when many groups of glands are involved and the cachexia is well advanced, the tuberculin reaction may be present in Hodgkin's disease, but even then the histological changes are distinctive. Other points to be noted are the tendency in the tuberculous adenitis to coalescence of the glands, adhesion to the skin, with suppuration, etc., and the liability to tuberculosis of the lung or pleura.

(*b*) LEUKÆMIA.—As a rule, the blood examination gives the diagnosis at a glance, as Hodgkin's disease presents only a slight leucocytosis. A difficulty arises only in those rare instances of leukæmia, usually the acute lymphatic form, in which the leucocytes gradually decrease or in which the number for a time may become normal. Histologically there are striking differences between the structure of the glands in the two conditions.

(*c*) LYMPHO-SARCOMA.—Clinically the cases may resemble Hodgkin's disease very closely, and in the literature the two diseases have been confounded. The glands, as a rule, form larger masses, the capsules are involved, and adjacent structures are attacked. Pressure signs in the chest and abdomen are much more common in lympho-sarcoma. But the easiest and most satisfactory mode of diagnosis is examination of sections of a gland, as the structure is very different from that seen in Hodgkin's disease. The blood condition, the type of fever, etc., need a more careful study in this group of cases.

Course.—There are acute cases in which the enlargements spread rapidly and death follows in three or four months. As a rule, the disease lasts for two or three years. Remarkable periods of quiescence may occur, in which the glands diminish in size, the fever disappears, and the general condition improves. Even a large group of glands may almost completely disappear, or a tumor mass on one side of the neck may subside while the inguinal glands are enlarging. Usually a cachexia with anæmia and swelling of the feet precedes death. A fatal event may occur early from great enlargement of the mediastinal glands.

Treatment.—When the glands are small and limited to one side of the neck, operation should be advised; even when both sides of the neck are involved, if there are no signs of mediastinal growth, operation is justifiable. The course of the disease may be delayed, even if cure does not follow.

There is a possibility that the X-rays may do good in selected cases. Certainly the glands have been reduced in size, but I know of no case in which complete cure has been reported. Local treatment of the glands seems to do but little good.

Arsenic is the only drug which has a positive value in the disease. In some cases the effects on the glands are striking. It may be given in the form of Fowler's solution in increasing doses. Recoveries have been reported (?). Ill effects from the larger doses are rare. Peripheral neuritis followed the use of ℥ iv, ʒj, ℥ xviij during a period of less than three months. Phosphorus is recommended by Gowers and Broadbent, and may be tried if arsenic is not well borne. Quinine, iron, and cod-liver oil are useful as tonics. For the pressure pains morphia should be given.

IV. PURPURA.

Strictly speaking, purpura is a symptom, not a disease; but under this term are conveniently arranged a number of affections characterized by extravasations of the blood into the skin. In the present state of our knowledge a

hodgkin's disease

Osler's section on Hodgkin's disease, like a Greek temple on a hill, proclaims the greatness of the builder. For example, read his sentence on diagnosis: "under cocaine one of the small glands of the affected side should be excised and the structure carefully studied in the light of Dr. Reed's recent observations." Amen — except for the cocaine. In a large cancer center half the slides submitted as Hodgkin's disease are something else. How many patients today, given the wrong treatment and the wrong prognosis, could have benefited from a careful study of structure?

Etiology

Osler, reserving decision, casts a tentative ballot for acute infection. Today, the question still open, we cast a weak vote for neoplasm. Certainly at the end, Hodgkin's disease has the hallmarks of a malignant tumor. Whatever its causation the initial disease eventually becomes transformed into an invasive and destructive neoplasm, probably because of peculiarities of host response.

Morbid anatomy

Today we share Osler's confidence in Dorothy Reed's observations. The present emphasis is on the wide differences in lymph node histology, their dependence on host response, and their implications for the patient's prognosis. Ewing in 1928 called attention to the neoplastic proliferation of Reed-Sternberg cells. Rosenthal in 1936 pointed out that extensive lymphocytosis in the node was associated with sparsity of Reed-Sternberg cells and indolent clinical progression. Jackson and Parker extended these ideas into the concept of paragranuloma, granuloma, and sarcoma, but these do not correlate with clinical behavior. Rappaport in 1956 called attention to the nodular character of the lymphocytic proliferation. Lukes showed that this nodular form (nodular sclerosis) was associated with collagen formation and a slow progression. In 1950, Vera Peters called attention to the importance of division into clinical stages. She defined four stages, ranging from involvement of a single node area up through many areas including visceral infiltration. The more localized the disease at the time of treatment, the better the prognosis. This has been confirmed by others. Lukes and colleagues in 1963 attempted to correlate prognosis with both histology and staging. Stages I and II are often associated with lymphocytosis, nodular sclerosis, and few histiocytes. Stage III patients show lymphocyte depletion, diffuse fibrosis, eosinophils, and many Reed-Sternberg cells. The ferment in the study of Hodgkin's disease is the understanding of the intense lymphocytosis in the node as perhaps a host response that holds the disease in check. In the absence of lymphocytosis, there is a proliferation of reticular cells, fibrosis, and rapid course.

Pathophysiology

Osler called attention to the negative tuberculin test as a valuable aid in differentiating Hodgkin's disease from tuberculosis. Schier and his colleagues in 1956 showed that loss of delayed skin hypersensitivity to a number of antigens was a common characteristic of Hodgkin's disease. Many other studies have confirmed this skin anergy, and the key question now is its correlation with the histology of the nodes and the aggressiveness of the disease. The anemia of Hodgkin's disease is usually associated with a shortened red cell life span (Berlin). Occasionally there is also underproduction of red cells.

Association with other diseases

Tuberculosis and Hodgkin's disease, often together in Osler's day, are now uncommonly associated. Other common bacterial infections generally become a problem only during the final cachectic phase. Unusual types of infection are frequently seen in Hodgkin's and are probably correlated with the characteristic immune defect. These infections are largely viral (cytomegalovirus, herpes zoster and simplex) and fungal (cryptococcus, histoplasma, and nocardia). Pneumocystis infections are not uncommon, and toxoplasmosis is occasionally seen.

Treatment

Osler was not impressed with the results of therapy — surgical excision of localized disease was sometimes helpful; x-irradiation or arsenic brought some regression. In 1950 Peters published her results with remarkable long-term survivals following the use of tumoricidal doses of x-irradiation in Stages I and II. Easson and Kaplan have now published similar results, and it seems safe to conclude that very long survival and probably cure can be achieved in about 40 percent of patients with early stages of Hodgkin's if 3,500 rads can be delivered to the diseased areas.

Hodgkin's disease

Lymphangiography, inferior vena caval dye studies, and intravenous pyelography add important contributions to the clinical work-up for the extent of disease, since they help define the size of the involved area requiring irradiation. The treatment of choice for Stages I and II is tumoricidal irradiation to all involved areas.

Chemotherapy plays a role in the treatment of the later stages. In 1946 Goodman and Gilman showed that nitrogen mustard caused regression of Hodgkin's disease. This alkylating agent and others (thio-TEPA, cyclophosphamide) have since become extraordinarily useful in managing systemic disease. Other drugs including profound effects on systemic disease are Vinblastine (Hodes and associates, 1960), methyl hydrazine (Mathé, 1963), and streptonigrin (Hackethal and colleagues, 1961). Massive doses of prednisone can cause some regression, but at an unwarranted cost in toxicity. Smaller doses of corticosteroids are useful in interrupting the hemolytic anemia of Hodgkin's.

The best present therapy for Hodgkin's is under intensive study, since presumably the combination of several drugs or of drugs plus x-ray may prove to be of greater benefit than either method alone. Surgical excision cannot be recommended in view of the new information on the curative value of x-ray for localized disease. Splenectomy has been shown by Crosby and Heaton to be valuable for correction of hemolytic anemia.

C. Gordon Zubrod

REFERENCES

Aisenberg, A.C. Hodgkin's disease — prognosis, treatment and etiologic and immunologic considerations. New Eng. J. Med., 270:508, 565, 617, 1964.

Easson, E.C., and Russell, M.H. Cure of Hodgkin's disease. Brit. Med. J., 1:1704, 1963.

Lukes, R.J. Relationship of histologic features to clinical stages in Hodgkin's disease. Amer. J. Roentgen., 90:944, 1963.

Peters, M.V., and Middlemiss, K.C.H. A study of survivals in Hodgkin's disease treated radiologically. Amer. J. Roentgen., 79:114, 1958.

Plattner, P.A., ed. Chemotherapy of Cancer: Proceedings of an International Symposium. New York, Elsevier Publishing Co., 1954.

Symposium: Obstacles to the Control of Hodgkin's Disease. Cancer Res., 26:1045, 1966.

persons in the water, who have fallen in and, though immediately recovered, were dead, or who have died suddenly while bathing, are referred by Paltauf to this condition. And, lastly, there is a large group of cases of sudden death in children without recognizable cause, in whom post mortem the thymus has been found enlarged—the so-called "Thymus Tod" (see under Thymus Gland). It has also been suggested that certain of the sudden deaths during convalescence from the infectious fevers are to be referred to this status lymphaticus. Escherich thinks that certain measures usually harmless, such as hydrotherapy, may have an untoward effect in children in this condition of lymphatism, and adds that tetany and laryngismus may be associated with it.

Two explanations are offered of the sudden death: First, that it is due to mechanical pressure of the enlarged thymus on the trachea. In only one of Blumer's nine cases was there evidence of this. Secondly, that it is caused by a toxæmia, an overproduction of the internal secretion of the thymus. Blumer has extended this view, and suggests that it is a lymphotoxæmia.

VIII. DISEASES OF THE SUPRARENAL BODIES.

1. ADDISON'S DISEASE.

Definition.—A constitutional affection characterized by asthenia, muscular and vascular, irritability of the stomach, and pigmentation of the skin, symptoms due, in all probability, to loss of the internal secretion of the adrenal glands. Tuberculosis of the adrenals is the common anatomical change.

The recognition of the disease is due to Addison, of Guy's Hospital, whose monograph on The Constitutional and Local Effects of Disease of the Suprarenal Capsules was published in 1855.

Etiology.—Males are more frequently attacked than females. In Greenhow's analysis of 183 cases 119 were males and 64 females. A majority of the cases occur between the twentieth and the fortieth year. A congenital case has been described in which the skin had a yellow-gray tint. The child lived for eight weeks, and post mortem the adrenals were found to be large and cystic. Injury such as a blow upon the abdomen or back, and caries of the spine, have in many cases preceded the attack. The disease is rare in America; only 17 cases came under my observation.

Morbid Anatomy and Pathology.—There is rarely emaciation or anæmia. Rolleston thus summarizes the condition of the suprarenal bodies in Addison's disease:

"1. The fibro-caseous lesion due to tuberculosis—far the commonest condition found. 2. Simple atrophy. 3. Chronic interstitial inflammation leading to atrophy. 4. Malignant disease invading the capsules, including Addison's case of malignant nodule compressing the suprarenal vein. 5. Blood extravasated into the suprarenal bodies. 6. No lesion of the suprarenal bodies themselves, but pressure or inflammation involving the semilunar ganglia.

"The first is the only common cause of Addison's disease. The others, with the exception of simple atrophy, may be considered as very rare."

The nerve-cells of the semilunar ganglia have been found degenerated and deeply pigmented, and the nerves sclerotic. The ganglia are not uncommonly entangled in the cicatricial tissue about the adrenals. The spleen has occasionally been found enlarged; a persistent enlarged thymus has been found.

309

The two chief theories which have been advanced to explain the disease are: (*a*) That it depended upon the loss of function of the adrenals. This was the view of Addison. The balance of experimental evidence is in favor of the view that the adrenals are functional glands, which furnish an internal secretion essential to the normal metabolism. Schäfer and Oliver have shown that the human adrenals contain a very powerful extract, which is not to be obtained in cases of Addison's disease; they have also studied the toxic effects on animals of the extracts of the glands. In the cases in which the adrenals have been found involved without the symptoms of Addison's disease, accessory glands may have been present; while in the rare cases in which the symptoms of the disease have been present with healthy adrenals the semilunar ganglia and adjacent tissues have been involved in dense adhesions, which may have interfered readily with the vessels or lymphatics of the glands. On this view Addison's disease is due to an inadequate supply of the adrenal secretion, just as myxœdema is caused by loss of function of the thyroid gland. "Whether the deficiency in this internal secretion leads to a toxic condition of the blood or to a general atony and apathy is a question which must remain open" (Rolleston). (*b*) That it is an affection of the abdominal sympathetic system, induced most commonly by disease of the adrenals, but also by other chronic disorders which involve the solar plexus and its ganglia. According to this view, it is an affection of the nervous system, and the pigmentation has its origin in changes induced through the trophic nerves. The pronounced debility is the outcome of disturbed tissue metabolism, and the circulatory, respiratory, and digestive symptoms are due to implication of the pneumogastric nerves. The changes found in the abdominal sympathetic are held to support this view, and its advocates urge the occurrence of pigmentation of the skin in tuberculosis of the peritonæum, cancer of the pancreas, or aneurism of the abdominal aorta. Bramwell thinks that the symptoms may be in part due to irritation of the sympathetic and in part to adrenal inadequacy.

Symptoms.—In the words of Addison, the characteristic symptoms are "anæmia, general languor or debility, remarkable feebleness of the heart's action, irritability of the stomach, and a peculiar change of color in the skin."

The onset is, as a rule, insidious. The feelings of weakness, as a rule, precede the pigmentation. In other instances the gastro-intestinal symptoms, the weakness, and the pigmentation come on together. There are a few cases in the literature in which the whole process has been acute, following a shock or some special depression. There are three important symptoms:

(1) PIGMENTATION OF THE SKIN.—This, as a rule, first attracts the attention of the patient's friends. The grade of coloration ranges from a light yellow to a deep brown, or even black. In typical cases it is diffuse, but always deeper on the exposed parts and in the regions where the normal pigmentation is more intense, as the areolæ of the nipples and about the genitals; also wherever the skin is compressed or irritated, as by the waistband. At first it may be confined to the face and hands. Occasionally it is absent. Patches showing atrophy of pigment, leucoderma, may occur. The pigmentation is found on the mucous membranes of the mouth, conjunctivæ, and vagina. Pigmentation of the mucous membrane is not distinctive. It has been found in chronic stomach troubles, etc. (Fr. Schultze), and is common in the negro.

310

A patchy pigmentation of the serous membranes has often been found. Over the diffusely pigmented skin there may be little mole-like spots of deeper pigmentation, and upon the trunk, particularly on the lower abdomen, they may be " ribbed " like the sand on the seashore.

(2) GASTRO-INTESTINAL SYMPTOMS.—The disease may set in with attacks of nausea and vomiting, spontaneous in character. Toward the close there may be pain with retraction of the abdomen, and even features suggestive of peritonitis (Ebstein). A marked anorexia may be present. The gastric symptoms are variable throughout the course; occasionally they are absent. Attacks of diarrhœa are frequent and come on without obvious cause.

(3) ASTHENIA, the most characteristic feature of the disease, may be manifested early as a feeling of inability to carry on the ordinary occupation, or the patient may complain constantly of feeling tired. The weakness is specially marked in the muscular and cardio-vascular systems. There may be an extreme degree of muscular prostration in an individual apparently well nourished, whose muscles feel firm and hard. The cardio-vascular asthenia is manifest in a feeble, irregular action of the heart, which may come on in paroxysms, in attacks of vertigo, or of syncope, in one of which the disease may prove fatal. The blood-pressure is low, falling to 70 or 80 mm. of Hg. Headache is a frequent symptom; convulsions occasionally occur. Pain in the back may be an early and important symptom.

Anæmia, a symptom specially referred to by Addison, is not common. In a majority of the patients the blood-count is normal. McMunn has described an increase in the urinary pigments, and a pigment has been isolated of very much the same character as the melanin of the skin.

The mode of termination is either by syncope, which may occur even early in the disease, by gradual progressive asthenia, or by the development of tuberculous lesions. In two cases I have known a noisy delirium with urgent dyspnœa to precede the fatal event.

Diagnosis.—Pigmentation of the skin is not confined to Addison's disease. The following are the conditions which may give rise to an increase in the pigment:

(1) Abdominal growths—tubercle, cancer, or lymphoma. In tuberculosis of the peritonæum pigmentation is not uncommon.

(2) Pregnancy, in which the discoloration is usually limited to the face, the so-called *masque des femmes ençeintes.* Uterine disease is a common cause of a patchy melasma.

(3) *Hæmochromatosis,* associated with hypertrophic cirrhosis, pigmentation of the skin, and diabetes. More commonly in overworked persons of constipated habit and with sluggish livers there is a patchy staining about the face and forehead.

(4) The vagabond's discoloration, caused by the irritation of lice and dirt, which may reach a very high grade, and has sometimes been mistaken for Addison's disease.

(5) In rare instances there is deep discoloration of the skin in melanotic cancer, so deep and general that it has been confounded with *melasma suprarenale.*

(6) In certain cases of exophthalmic goitre abnormal pigmentation occurs, as noted by Drummond and others.

(7) In a few rare instances the pigmentation in scleroderma may be general and deep.

(8) In the face there may be an extraordinary degree of pigmentation due to innumerable small black comedones. If not seen in a very good light, the face may suggest argyria. Pigmentation of an advanced grade may occur in chronic ulcer of the stomach and in dilatation of the organ.

(9) Argyria could scarcely be mistaken, and yet I was consulted in a case in which the diagnosis of Addison's disease had been made by several good observers.

(10) Arsenic when taken for many months may cause a most intense pigmentation of the skin.

(11) With arterio-sclerosis and chronic heart-disease there may be marked melanoderma.

(12) In pernicious anæmia the pigmentation may be extreme, most commonly due to the prolonged administration of arsenic.

(13) There is a form of deep pigmentation, usually in women, which persists for years without change and without any special impairment of health. I have met with two cases; in one the pigmentation was a little more leaden than is usual in Addison's disease; in both the condition had lasted some years.

In any case of unusual pigmentation these various conditions must be sought for; the diagnosis of Addison's disease is scarcely justifiable without the asthenia. In many instances it is difficult early in the disease to arrive at a definite conclusion. The occurrence of fainting fits, of nausea, and gastric irritability are important indications. As the lesion of the capsules is almost always tuberculous, in doubtful cases the tuberculin test may be used. In two of my cases, robust, healthy men with pigmentation and gastric symptoms, the reaction was obtained.

Prognosis.—The disease is usually fatal. The cases in which the bronzing is slight or does not occur run a more rapid course. There are occasionally acute cases which, with great weakness, vomiting, and diarrhœa, prove fatal in a few weeks. In a few cases the disease is much prolonged, even to six or ten years. In rare instances recovery has taken place, and periods of improvement, lasting many months, may occur.

Treatment.—When there is profound asthenia the patient should be confined to bed, as fatal syncope may at any time occur. In three of my cases death was sudden. Arsenic and strychnia are useful tonics. For the diarrhœa large doses of bismuth should be given; for the irritability of the stomach, creasote, hydrocyanic acid, ice, and champagne. The diet should be light and nutritious. Many patients thrive best on a strict milk diet.

Treatment by Suprarenal Extract.—E. W. Adams has analyzed 97 cases. In 7 the condition grew worse, in 3 cases of transplantation death was attributed to the treatment. In 43 there was no effect noticed. In 31 there was temporary improvement; in 16 the relief seemed permanent. In two of our cases there was marked improvement; in one all the severe symptoms disappeared, and the patient died of an acute infection, which apparently had nothing to do with the disease. The adrenals were found sclerotic. The gland may be given raw or partially cooked or in a glycerin extract. Tabloids of the dried extract are given, one grain of which corresponds to fifteen of the gland.

312

Three of the tabloids may be given daily. Operation has been suggested, but has not been carried out on any undoubted case.

2. OTHER DISEASES OF THE SUPRARENAL CAPSULES.

Adrenalitis, Acute Hæmorrhagic.—The lesion resembles that of acute pancreatitis, hæmorrhage and necrosis in varying proportions. The clinical picture is very complex. The onset is sudden with pain and vomiting, profound prostration and death in a few days. In other cases convulsions occur, or there may be a profound myasthenia, acute or subacute. Sudden death has occurred. In children the disease may be associated with purpura, cutaneous and visceral. The symptoms are believed to be due to acute or subacute adrenal insufficiency. The diagnosis is not often made during life. The white line, the anæmic vascular skin reflex, described by Sergent as of diagnostic value, is too common to be of much import.

Hypertrophy.—In chronic nephritis and arterio-sclerosis adenoma or diffuse hyperplasia of the glands has been found, which some have attributed to hyperadrenalism—an overactivity of the antitoxic and angiotonic functions of the gland. In children tumor or hypertrophy has been found associated with remarkable precocity and development of the sexual organs.

Tumors.—Primary growths are rare, secondary are not uncommon. The former are usually mistaken for kidney tumors. There is a special type of malignant growth in children characterized by rapid growth, diffuse infiltration of the liver, and great distention of the abdomen without ascites or jaundice (Pepper tertius); and Robert Hutchison has described a remarkable syndrome in children of adrenal tumor, exophthalmos and cranial tumors.

IX. DISEASES OF THE SPLEEN.

The acute swelling in fever, and the chronic enlargement of the organ in paludism, leukæmia, cirrhosis of the liver, and heart-disease have been fully described, but there remain several conditions to which brief reference may be made.

1. MOVABLE SPLEEN.

Movable or wandering spleen is seen most frequently in women the subjects of enteroptosis. It may be present without signs of displacement of other organs. It may be found accidentally in individuals who present no symptoms whatever. In other cases there are dragging, uneasy feelings in the back and side. All grades are met with, from a spleen that can be felt completely below the margin of the ribs to a condition in which the tumor-mass impinges upon the pelvis; indeed, the organ has been found in an inguinal hernia! In the large majority of all cases the spleen is enlarged. Sometimes it appears that the enlargement has caused relaxation of the ligaments; in other instances the relaxation seems congenital, as movable spleens have been found in different members of the same family. Possibly traumatism may account for some of the cases. Apart from the dragging, uneasy sensations and the worry in nervous patients, wandering spleen causes very few serious symptoms. Torsion of the pedicle may produce a very alarming and serious condition, leading to great swelling of the organ, high fever, or even to

diseases of the suprarenal bodies

During the latter part of the nineteenth century, interest in the endocrine glands and their function attained a high point in clinical medicine. Osler's familiarity with medical literature and his close association with the profession in England undoubtedly added to his interest in disorders of the thyroid as discussed by Gull and in adrenal deficiency as described by Addison. One of Osler's earliest accounts of Addison's disease is to be found in "Pepper's System of Medicine" circa 1885. Comparing the thyroid-deficient state with that of adrenal insufficiency, he comments: "The relation of the affections of the thyroid gland to myxedema and cretinism and the experimental production of these conditions by the removal of the thyroid have widened our view of the importance of the ductless glands. In both there are distinct histological changes in the tissues — in one, an increase in the mucin; in the other, an increase in the pigment — and in both, marked nervous phenomena; mental dullness, progressive dementia in myxedema, profound asthenia in Addison's disease. We regarded the thyroid as unimportant to life until the experience of surgeons and the extirpation in monkeys by Horsley demonstrated that abolition of its function was followed by a serious train of symptoms; and perhaps the experimental removal of the suprarenals in monkeys — so much more closely allied to man than the animals hitherto experimented upon — may demonstrate that these little bodies are also not without their influence upon health."

Ten years later, in 1895, while speaking before the Medico-Chirurgical College in Philadelphia Osler (1896) gave a detailed account of his experience with the use of a glycerin extract of hog adrenals administered three times daily to eight patients with Addison's disease. He reported some temporary improvement in most cases and prolonged improvement in one but stated, "I do not know of any instance in which all the symptoms of the disease have permanently disappeared."

Prior to the publication of the seventh edition of Osler's textbook, Abel in 1897 had isolated epinephrine from the adrenal and Aldrich in 1901 had identified it chemically. It was most disappointing to clinicians of that era to discover that this highly potent extract of adrenal tissue was not effective in mitigating the symptoms of Addison's disease. However, despite this knowledge, the Muirhead treatment of Addison's disease continued to be employed. Muirhead, a physician who suffered from Addison's disease, claimed that dilute epinephrine solutions administered as rectal

314

or colonic enemata were beneficial. The *saline solution* in which the epinephrine was diluted may have been a factor in the reputed temporary benefit!

Subsequently, animal experiments conclusively demonstrated that the total removal of one adrenal, accompanied by destruction of the medulla of the remaining adrenal did not induce the signs and symptoms of adrenal insufficiency. Hence, it seemed evident that the secretion of the "life-maintaining" hormone of the adrenal was limited to the cortex.

In 1927 two groups of investigators (Hartman and his associates and Rogoff and Stewart) reported the preparation of potent extracts of adrenal cortex which were capable of maintaining the life of adrenalectomized animals. Extracts of much greater potency were prepared subsequently in 1930 by Hartman and Brownell and by Swingle and Pfiffner. These extracts were also employed in the treatment of patients with acute Addisonian crises, with striking improvement. The high cost of production of the extract, the limited supply of fresh adrenal glands, and the relatively low yield of hormone restricted the application of this form of therapy to a rather small group of patients.

A milestone in understanding adrenal pathophysiology was the demonstration in 1933 by Loeb in New York and Harrop and associates in Baltimore that adrenalectomized animals and patients with Addison's disease excreted large quantities of sodium in their urine. Administration of sodium salts was shown to be moderately beneficial, and restriction of dietary potassium as a consequence of the studies of Truszkowski and Zwemer and of Wilder and colleagues in 1936 resulted in further improvement. Also in that year, Thorn demonstrated that adrenal cortical extracts were capable of modifying the renal excretion of electrolytes in normal human subjects.

Crystalline substances were first obtained from adrenal cortical extracts by Kendall, Grollman, Wintersteiner, and Reichstein. Subsequently, Thorn and his colleagues demonstrated that Reichstein's 11-deoxycorticosterone and Kendall's Compound E induce biochemical changes in man. The first synthetic adrenal corticoid, 11-deoxycorticosterone, was prepared by Reichstein in Zurich. This substance was shown to be capable of reversing completely the abnormalities in sodium and potassium metabolism which occur in adrenalectomized animals and in patients with Addison's disease. The subcutaneous implantation of pellets of crystalline DOCA (Thorn) which were slowly absorbed over a period of many months provided an economical, efficient, and effective means of replacement therapy. However, this hormonal substance lacked the gluconeogenic or blood sugar-

315

maintaining potency which whole adrenal cortical extracts possessed. Furthermore, although minute quantities of deoxycorticosterone had been isolated from gland extracts, it did not appear that this substance was the principal mineralocorticoid secreted by the adrenal.

Between 1940 and 1950, Kendall and Sarett accomplished the synthesis of several 11-oxygenated adrenal steroids, including the preparation of cortisone and hydrocortisone for therapeutic use. Subsequent achievements in glucocorticoid synthesis resulted in the preparation of much more potent compounds such as prednisone and dexamethasone. These latter differed from hydrocortisone only in their reduced sodium-retaining capacity and in the rate at which they were degraded in the body.

In 1954, aldosterone, the principal salt-retaining hormone of the adrenal was identified by Simpson and Tait in England in collaboration with the Swiss group under Reichstein, and the chemical synthesis of pure d-aldosterone was achieved somewhat later.

Today, in the United States, Addison's disease results predominantly from adrenal atrophy in contrast to the high incidence of tuberculosis as the cause in Osler's day. The etiology of adrenal atrophy is unknown, but the possibility that the changes are the result of an autoimmune process has been suggested. Furthermore, circulating antibodies to adrenal tissue have been reported by several workers. Although spontaneous bilateral hemorrhage into the adrenals is well known in the newborn, it is only recently that an appreciable incidence of hemorrhage into the adrenals in adults has been noted in conjunction with anticoagulant therapy.

With the availability of preparations of ACTH and standardized methods for measuring urinary adrenal steroids, the diagnosis of Addison's disease, as well as conditions of reduced adrenal cortical reserve, has attained a precision rarely matched in modern medicine. The therapy of Addison's disease, in the absence of complicating disease, is highly successful, and the prognosis for life and normal activity is excellent. Present-day maintenance therapy consists essentially of orally administered hydrocortisone, or one of its derivatives, supplemented by a small dose of a synthetic salt-retaining hormone such as α-fluorohydrocortisone. Larger quantities of both hormones are used under conditions of stress.

Thus, in a period of 100 years we have seen a unique clinical disorder described with unusual lucidity and have experienced a tremendous advance in our knowledge of biological function as a consequence of the study of the modifying effects of adrenal insufficiency and replacement therapy on important metabolic processes. We have witnessed

316

the progression of therapy from nonspecific, relatively ineffective procedures to the ready availability of practically unlimited quantities of crystalline, synthetic hormones. We owe a debt of gratitude to William Osler, who from his visits to Europe and his extensive knowledge, made a canny contribution when he prepared an extract from hog adrenals using glycerol as the solvent. Years later, glycerol was shown to be a very effective solvent for adrenal cortical hormones. Subsequently, hog adrenals were shown to contain a much higher concentration of corticoids than adrenals from other commonly used species. In preparing his extract, Osler took the further precautions of insisting on fresh adrenal glands and carrying out the extraction in the cold. It is now known that these conditions are essential for a potent extract! Serendipity?

George W. Thorn

REFERENCES

Abel, J.J., and Crawford, A.D. On the blood-pressure-raising constituent of the suprarenal capsule. Bull. Hopkins Hosp., 8:151, 1897.

Aldrich, J.B. A preliminary report on the active principle of the suprarenal gland. Amer. J. Physiol., 5:457, 1901.

Grollman, A. Physiological and chemical studies on the adrenal cortical hormone. Sympos. Quant. Biol., 5:313, 1937.

Harrop, G.A., Weinstein, A., Soffer, L.J., and Trescher, J.H. Diagnosis and treatment of Addison's disease. J.A.M.A., 100:1850, 1933

Hartman, F.A., MacArthur, C.G., and Hartman, W.E. A substance which prolongs the life of adrenalectomized cats. Proc. Soc. Exp. Biol. Med., 25:69, 1927.

Hartman, F.A., Aaron, A.H., and Culp, J.E. Use of cortin in Addison's disease. Endocrinology, 14:437, 1930.

Kendall, E.C. Chemical and physiological investigation of the suprarenal cortex. Sympos. Quant. Biol., 5:299, 1937.

Loeb, R.F. Effect of sodium chloride in treatment of patient with Addison's disease. Proc. Soc. Exp. Biol. Med., 30:808, 1933.

Muirhead, A.L. An autograph history of a case of Addison's disease. J.A.M.A., 76:652, 1921; 79:556, 1922.

Osler, W. On six cases of Addison's disease, with the report of a case greatly benefited by the use of suprarenal extract. Int. Med. Magazine, 5:3, 1896.

Diseases of the suprarenal bodies

Reichstein, T. Chemie des Cortis und seiner Begleitstoffe. Ergebn. Vitamin Hormonforsch., 1:334, 1938.

Sarett, L.W. Partial synthesis of pregnene-4-triol-17 (β), 20 (β), 21-dione-3, 11 and pregnene-4-diol-17 (β), 21-trione-3, 11, 20 monoacetate. J. Biol. Chem., 162:601, 1946.

Streiger, M., and Reichstein, T. Desoxy-cortico-steron (21-oxy-progesteron) aus 5-3-oxy-atio-cholensaure. Helv. Chim. Acta, 20:1164, 1937.

Swingle, W.W., and Pfiffner, J.J. An aqueous extract of the suprarenal cortex which maintains the life of bilaterally adrenalectomized cats. Science, 71:321, 1930.

Thorn, G.W. Effect of adrenal cortical hormone on renal excretion of electrolytes in normal subject. Proc. Soc. Exp. Biol. Med., 36:361, 1937.

Thorn, G.W., Koepf, G.F., Lewis, R.A., and Olsen, E.F. Carbohydrate metabolism in Addison's disease. J. Clin. Invest. 19:813, 1940.

Thorn, G.W., Dorrance, S.S., and Day, E. Addison's disease; evaluation of synthetic desoxycorticosterone acetate therapy in 158 patients. Ann. Intern. Med., 16:1053, 1942.

Truszkowski, R., and Zwemer, R. Cortico-adrenal insufficiency and potassium metabolism. Biochem. J., 30:1345, 1936.

Wilder, R.M., Kendall, E.C., Snell, A.M., Kepler, E.J., Rynearson, E.H., and Adams, M. Intake of potassium, an important consideration in Addison's disease; a metabolic study. Arch. Intern. Med., 59:367, 1937.

Wintersteiner, O., and Pfiffner, J.J. Chemical studies on the adrenal cortex. III. Isolation of two physiologically inactive compounds. J. Biol. Chem., 116:291, 1936.

5. EXOPHTHALMIC GOITRE.

(*Graves's, Basedow's, or Parry's Disease.*)

Definition.—A disease characterized by exophthalmos, enlargement of the thyroid, and functional disturbance of the vascular system. It is very possibly caused by disturbed function of the thyroid gland (hyperthyroidism).

Historical Note.—In the posthumous writings of Caleb Hillier Parry (1825) is a description of 8 cases of Enlargement of the Thyroid Gland in Connection with Enlargement or Palpitation of the Heart. In the first case, seen in 1786, he also described the exophthalmos: " The eyes were protruded from their sockets, and the countenance exhibited an appearance of agitation and distress, especially in any muscular movement." The Italians claim that Flajani described the disease in 1800. I have not been able to see his original account, but Moebius states that it is meagre and inaccurate, and bears no comparison with that of Parry. If the name of any physician is to be associated with the disease, undoubtedly it should be that of the distinguished old Bath physician. Graves described the disease in 1835 and Basedow in 1840.

Etiology.—The disease is more frequent in women than in men. Of 200 cases tabulated by Eshner, there were 161 females. The age of onset is usually from the twentieth to the thirtieth year. It is sometimes seen in several members of the same family. Worry, fright, and depressing emotions precede the development of the disease in a number of cases.

The disease is regarded by some as a pure neurosis, in favor of which is urged the onset after a profound emotion, the absence of lesions, and the cure which has followed in a few cases after operations upon the nose. Others believe that it is caused by a central lesion in the medulla oblongata. In support of this there is a certain amount of experimental evidence, and in a few autopsies changes have been found in the medulla. Of late years the view has been urged, particularly by Moebius and by Greenfield, that exophthalmic goitre is primarily a disease of the thyroid gland (*hyperthyrea*), in antithesis to myxœdema (*athyrea*). The clinical contrast between these two diseases is most suggestive—the increased excitability of the nervous system, the flushed, moist skin, the vascular erythism in the one; the dull apathy, the low temperature, slow pulse, and dry skin of the other. The changes in the gland in exophthalmic goitre are, as shown by Greenfield, those of an organ in active evolution—viz., increased proliferation, with the production of newly formed tubular spaces and absorption of the colloid material which is replaced by a more mucinous fluid (Bradshaw Lecture, 1893). The thyroid extract given in excess produces symptoms not unlike those of Parry's disease—tachycardia, tremor, headache, sweating, and prostration. Beclère has recently reported a case in which exopthalmos developed after an overdose. Use of the thyroid extract usually aggravates the symptoms of exophthalmic goitre. The most successful line of treatment has been that directed to diminish the bulk of the goitre. These are some of the considerations which favor the view that the symptoms are due to disturbed function of the thyroid gland, probably to hypersecretion of certain materials, which induce a sort of chronic intoxication. Myxœdema may develop in the late stages, and there are transient œdema and in a few cases scleroderma, which indicate that the nutrition

319

of the skin is involved. Persistence of the thymus is almost the rule (Hector Mackenzie), but its significance is unknown.

Symptoms.—Acute and chronic forms may be recognized. In the acute form the disease may arise with great rapidity. In a patient of J. H. Lloyd's, of Philadelphia, a woman, aged thirty-nine, who had been considered perfectly healthy, but whose friends had noticed that for some time her eyes looked rather large, was suddenly seized with intense vomiting and diarrhœa, rapid action of the heart, and great throbbing of the arteries. The eyes were prominent and staring and the thyroid gland was found much enlarged and soft. The gastro-intestinal symptoms continued, the pulse became more rapid, the vomiting was incessant, and the patient died on the third day of the illness. Only the abdominal and thoracic organs could be examined and no changes were found. Two rapidly fatal cases occurred at the Philadelphia Hospital, one of which, under F. P. Henry's care, had marked cerebral symptoms. The acute cases are not always associated with delirium. In a case reported by Sutcliff death occurred within three months from the onset of the symptoms, owing to repeated and uncontrollable vomiting. More frequently the onset is gradual and the disease is chronic. There are four characteristic symptoms of the disease—exophthalmos, tachycardia, enlargement of the thyroid, and tremor.

TACHYCARDIA.—Rapid heart action is only one of a series of remarkable vascular phenomena in the disease. The pulse-rate at first may be not more than 95 or 100, but when the disease is established it may be from 140 to 160, or even higher. Irregularity is not common, except toward the close. In a well-developed case the visible area of cardiac pulsation is much increased, the action is heaving and forcible, and the shock of the heart-sounds is well felt. The large arteries at the root of the neck throb forcibly. There is visible pulsation in the peripheral arteries. The capillary pulse is readily seen, and there are few diseases in which one may see at times with greater distinctness the venous pulse in the veins of the hand. The throbbing pulsation of the arteries may be felt even in the finger tips. Vascular erythema is common—the face and neck are flushed and there may be a wide-spread erythema of the body and limbs. On auscultation murmurs are usually heard over the heart, a loud apex systolic and loud bruits at the base and over the manubrium. The sounds of the heart may be very intense. In rare instances they may be heard at some distance from the patient; according to Graves, as far as four feet. Attacks of acute dilatation of the heart may occur with dyspnœa, cough, and a frothy bloody expectoration.

EXOPHTHALMOS, which may be unilateral, usually follows the vascular disturbance. It is readily recognized by the protrusion of the balls, and partly by the fact that the lids do not completely cover the sclerotics, so that a rim of white is seen above and below the cornea. The protrusion may become very great and the eye may even be dislocated from the socket, or both eyes may be destroyed by panophthalmitis, a condition present in one of Basedow's cases. The vision is normal. Graefe noted that when the eyeball is moved downward the upper lid does not follow it as in health. This is known as Graefe's sign. The palpebral aperture is wider than in health, owing to spasm or retraction of the upper lid (Stellwag's sign). The patient winks less frequently than in health. Moebius has called attention to the lack of convergence of the two eyes. Changes in the pupils and in the optic nerves are rare. Pulsation of the retinal arteries is common.

ENLARGEMENT OF THE THYROID commonly occurs with the exophthalmos. It may be general or in only one lobe, and is rarely so large as in ordinary goitre. The vessels are usually much dilated, and the whole gland may be seen to pulsate. A thrill may be felt on palpation and on auscultation a loud systolic murmur, or more commonly a *bruit de diable*. A double murmur is common and is pathognomonic (Guttmann).

TREMOR is the fourth cardinal symptom, and was really first described by Basedow. It is involuntary, fine, about eight to the second. It is of great importance in the diagnosis of the early cases.

Among other symptoms are anæmia, emaciation, and slight fever. Attacks of vomiting and diarrhœa may occur. The latter may be very severe and distressing, recurring at intervals. The greatest complaint is of the forcible throbbing in the arteries, often accompanied with unpleasant flushes of heat and profuse perspirations.

ERYTHEMATOUS FLUSHING is common. Pruritus may be a severe and persistent symptom. Multiple telangiectases have been described. Solid, infiltrated œdema is not uncommon. It may be transitory. A remarkable myxœdematous state may supervene. Pigmentary changes are very common. They may be patchy or generalized. Hydrocystoma may occur, and the coexistence of scleroderma and Graves's disease has been frequently noticed. Irritability of temper, change in disposition, and great mental depression have been described. An important complication is acute mania, in which the patient may die in a few days. Weakness of the muscles is not uncommon, particularly a feeling of " giving way " of the legs. If the patient holds the head down and is asked to look up without raising the head, the forehead remains smooth and is not wrinkled, as in a normal individual (Joffroy). A feature of interest noted by Charcot is the great diminution in the electrical resistance, which may be due to the saturation of the skin with moisture owing to the vaso-motor dilatation (Hirt). Bryson has noted the fact that the chest expansion may be greatly diminished. The emaciation may be extreme. Glycosuria and albuminuria are not infrequent complications. True diabetes may occur.

The course of the disease is usually chronic, lasting several years. After persisting for six months or a year the symptoms may disappear. There are remarkable instances in which the symptoms have come on with great intensity, following fright, and have disappeared again in a few days. A certain proportion of the cases get well, but when the disease is well advanced recovery is rare.

Diagnosis.—Few diseases are so easily recognized. The difficulty is with the partially developed forms, *formes frustes*, which are not uncommon. The nervous state, the tremor, and tachycardia may be the only features, or there may be slight swelling of the thyroid with tremor alone. The greatest difficulty arises in the cases of hysterical tremor with rapid heart action.

Treatment.—(*a*) The disease is serious enough to warrant strong measures systematically carried out; much valuable time is lost in trying various remedies. The patient should be in bed, at absolute rest, and see very few persons. To quiet the heart's action the ice-bag may be continuously applied through the day, and veratrum viride, aconite, or strophanthus given in full doses.

Ergot, belladonna, phosphate of soda, small doses of opium, and many other remedies are recommended, and in some instances I have seen benefit from the belladonna and the phosphate of soda. Electricity may be helpful.

(*b*) *Serum Therapy.*—Two methods are employed: feeding with the milk of dethyroidized goats, introduced by Lanz, which is obtainable as a substance called rodagen. Good results have been reported by Mackenzie and others. Beebe, on the other hand, uses the serum of animals into which human thyroid extract has been injected. Excellent results have been obtained, but the method has the danger associated with the use of foreign sera.

(*c*) *Surgical Treatment.*—Removal of part of the thyroid gland offers the best hope of permanent cure. It is remarkable with what rapidity all the symptoms may disappear after partial thyroidectomy. A second operation may be necessary in severe cases. The results obtained by the brothers Mayo and by Kocher give a remarkable percentage of recoveries. The operation under cocaine may be done with safety when the condition of the heart and the extreme tachycardia do not contraindicate it. Tying of the arteries and exothyropexia are also recommended. Excision of the superior cervical ganglia of the sympathetic has one beneficial result, viz., the production of slight ptosis, which obviates the staring character of the exophthalmos.

Marked benefit has followed the use of the X-rays in a few cases.

6. MYXŒDEMA (*Athyrea*).

Definition.—A constitutional affection, due to the loss of function of the thyroid gland. The disease, which was described by Sir William Gull as a cretinoid change, and later by Ord, is characterized clinically by a myxœdematous condition of the subcutaneous tissues and mental failure, and anatomically by atrophy of the thyroid gland.

Clinical Forms.—Three groups of cases may be recognized—cretinism, myxœdema proper, and operative myxœdema. To Felix Semon is due the credit of recognizing that these were one and the same condition and all due to loss of function of the thyroid.

CRETINISM.—This remarkable impairment of nutrition follows absence or loss of function of the thyroid gland, either congenital or appearing at any time before puberty. There is remarkable retardation of development, retention of the infantile state, and an extraordinary disproportion between the different parts of the body. Two forms are recognized, the *sporadic* and the *endemic*. In the sporadic form the gland may be congenitally absent, it may be atrophied after one of the specific fevers, or the condition may develop with goitre. Since we have learned to recognize the disease it is surprising how many cases have been reported. In Great Britain the disease is not uncommon, and many cases have been reported.

The condition is rarely recognized before the infant is six or seven months old. Then it is noticed that the child does not grow so rapidly and is not bright mentally. The tongue looks large and hangs out of the mouth. The hair may be thin and the skin very dry. Usually by the end of the first year and during the second year the signs become very marked. The face is large, looks bloated, the eyelids are puffy and swollen; the alæ nasi are thick, the nose looks depressed and flat. Dentition is delayed, and the teeth which appear decay early. The abdomen is swollen, the legs are thick and short, and the hands and feet are undeveloped and pudgy. The face is pale and sometimes has a waxy, sallow tint. The fontanelles remain open; there is much muscular weakness, and the child can not support itself. In the supraclavicular regions there are large pads of fat. The child does not develop mentally; there are various grades of idiocy and imbecility.

A very interesting form is that in which, after the child has thriven and developed until its fourth or fifth year, or even later, the symptoms begin after a fever, in consequence of an atrophy of the gland. Parker suggests for this variety the name juvenile myxœdema.

Endemic cretinism occurs under local conditions, as yet unknown, in association with goitre. It is met with chiefly in Switzerland and parts of Italy and France.

The *diagnosis* is very easy after one has seen a case or good illustrations. Infants a year or so old sometimes become flabby, lose their vivacity, or show a protuberant abdomen and lax skin with slight cretinoid appearance. These milder forms, as they have been termed, are probably due to transient functional disturbance in the gland. There is rarely any difficulty in recognizing the different other types of idiocy. The condition known as *fœtal rickets, achondroplasia,* or *chondrodystrophia fœtalis,* is more likely to be mistaken for cretinism. The children which survive birth grow up as a remarkable form of dwarfs, characterized by shortness of the limbs (micromelia) and enormous enlargement of the articulations, due to hyperplasia of the cartilaginous ends of the bones. *Infantilism*—the condition characterized by a preservation in the adult of the exterior form of infancy with the non-appearance of the secondary sexual characters—could scarcely be mistaken for cretinism.

MYXŒDEMA OF ADULTS (*Gull's Disease*).—In this, women are very much more frequently affected than men—in a ratio of 6 to 1. The disease may affect several members of a family, and it may be transmitted through the mother. In some instances there has been first the appearance of exophthalmic goitre. Though occurring most commonly in women, it seems to have no special relation to the catamenia or to pregnancy; the symptoms of myxœdema may disappear during pregnancy or may develop post partum. Myxœdema and exophthalmic goitre may occur in sisters. It is not so common in America as in England. In sixteen years I saw only 10 cases in Baltimore, 7 of which were in the hospital. C. P. Howard has collected 100 American cases, of which 86 were in women. The symptoms of this form, as given by Ord, are marked increase in the general bulk of the body, a firm, inelastic swelling of the skin, which does not pit on pressure; dryness and roughness, which tend, with the swelling, to obliterate in the face the lines of expression; imperfect nutrition of the hair; local tumefaction of the skin and subcutaneous tissues, particularly in the supraclavicular region. The physiognomy is altered in a remarkable way: the features are coarse and broad, the lips thick, the nostrils broad and thick, and the mouth is enlarged. Over the cheeks, sometimes the nose, there is a reddish patch. There is a striking slowness of thought and of movement. The memory becomes defective, the patients grow irritable and suspicious, and there may be headache. In some instances there are delusions and hallucinations, leading to a final condition of dementia. The gait is heavy and slow. The temperature may be below normal. The functions of the heart, lungs, and abdominal organs are normal. Hæmorrhage sometimes occurs. Albuminuria is sometimes present, more rarely glycosuria. Death is usually due to some intercurrent disease, most frequently tuberculosis (Greenfield). The thyroid gland is diminished in size and may become completely atrophied and converted into a fibrous mass. The subcutaneous fat is abundant, and in one or two instances a great increase in the mucin has been found. The larynx is also involved.

The course of the disease is slow but progressive, and extends over ten or fifteen years. A condition of acute and temporary myxœdema may develop in connection with enlargement of the thyroid in young persons. Myxœdema may follow exophthalmic goitre. In other instances the symptoms of the two diseases have been combined. I have reported a case in which a young man became bloated and increased in weight enormously during three months, then had tachycardia with tremor and active delirium, and died within six months of the onset of the symptoms.

OPERATIVE MYXŒDEMA; CACHEXIA STRUMIPRIVA.—Horsley, in a series of interesting experiments, showed that complete removal of the thyroid in monkeys was followed by the production of a condition similar to that of myxœdema and often associated with spasms or tetanoid contractures, and followed by apathy and coma. When the monkeys were kept warm myxœdema was averted, and, instead of an acute myxœdema, the animals had a condition which closely resembled cretinism. An identical condition may follow extirpation of the thyroid in man. Kocher, of Bern, found that after complete extirpation a cachectic condition followed in many cases, the symptoms of which are practically identical with those of myxœdema. The disease follows only a certain number of total and a much smaller proportion of partial removals of the thyroid gland. Of 408 cases, in 69 the operative myxœdema occurred. It has been thought that if a small fragment of the thyroid remains, or if there are accessory glands, which in animals are very common, these symptoms do not develop. It is possible that in men, in the cases of complete removal, the accessory fragments subserve the function of the gland. Operative myxœdema is very rare in America. A few years ago I was able to find only two cases, one of which, McGraw's, referred to in previous editions of this work, has since been cured.

The *diagnosis* of myxœdema is easy, as a rule. The general aspect of the patient—the subcutaneous swelling and the pallor—suggests Bright's disease, which may be strengthened by the discovery of tube-casts and of albumin in the urine; but the solid character of the swelling, the exceeding dryness of the skin, the yellowish-white color, the low temperature, the loss of hair, and the dull, listless mental state should suffice to differentiate the two conditions. In dubious cases not too much stress should be laid upon the supraclavicular swellings. There may be marked fibro-fatty enlargements in this situation in healthy persons, the supraclavicular pseudo-lipomata of Verneuil.

Treatment.—The patients suffer in cold and improve greatly in warm weather. They should therefore be kept at an even temperature, and should, if possible, move to a warm climate during the winter months. Repeated warm baths with shampooing are useful. Our art has made no more brilliant advance than in the cure of these disorders due to disturbed function of the thyroid gland. That we can to-day rescue children otherwise doomed to helpless idiocy—that we can restore to life the hopeless victims of myxœdema—is a triumph of experimental medicine for which we are indebted very largely to Victor Horsley and to his pupil Murray. Transplantation of the gland was first tried; then Murray used an extract subcutaneously. Hector Mackenzie in London and Howitz in Copenhagen introduced the method of feeding. We now know that the gland, taken either fresh, or as the watery or glycerin extract, or dried and powdered, is equally efficacious in a majority of all the cases of myxœdema in infants or adults. Many preparations are now on the market, but it makes little difference how the gland is administered. The dried powdered gland and the glycerin extract are most convenient. It is well to begin with the powdered gland, 1 grain three times a day, of the Parke-Davis preparation, or one of the Burroughs and Welcome tablets. The dose may be increased gradually until the patient takes 10 or 15 grains in the day. In many cases there are no unpleasant symptoms; in others there are irritation of the skin, restlessness, rapid pulse, and delirium; in rare instances tonic spasms, the condition to which the term *thyroidism* is applied. The results, as a rule, are most astounding—unparalleled by anything in the whole range of curative measures. Within six weeks a poor, feeble-minded, toad-like caricature of humanity may be restored to mental and bodily health. Loss of weight is one of the first and most striking effects; one of my patients lost over 30 pounds within six weeks. The skin becomes moist, the urine is increased, the perspiration returns, the temperature rises, the pulse-rate quickens, and the mental torpor lessens. Ill effects are rare. Two or three cases with old heart lesions have died during or after the treatment; in one instance a temporary condition of Graves' disease was induced.

The treatment, as Murray suggests, must be carried out in two stages—one, early, in which full doses are given until the cure is effected; the other, the permanent use of small doses sufficient to preserve the normal metabolism. In the cases of cretinism it seems to be necessary to keep up the treatment indefinitely. I have seen several instances of remarkable relapse follow the cessation of the use of the extract.

XI. DISEASES OF THE THYMUS GLAND.

The functions of this gland are unknown. It is a suggestive fact that Baumann found in it minute quantities of a compound containing iodine. It has been thought that its internal secretion has an influence in combating infective agents. Friedleben's estimate of the weight of the organ at birth—13 grammes—is stated by Dudgeon to be too high. He puts it at 7.10 grammes. The largest in his series occurred in a child aged five months, 47 grammes. At the ninth month the gland weighs 20 grammes, and at the second year 25 to 30.

The organ, after reaching its largest size about the end of the second year, gradually wastes, until at the time of puberty it is a mere fatty remnant, in which, however, there are "traces of its original structure in the form of small masses of thymus corpuscles, and even of concentric corpuscles" (Quain). A complete consideration of the affections of this gland is to be

diseases of the thyroid gland

Exophthalmic goiter

Today we accept readily the thought that hyperthyroidism is due to overproduction of hormone by the thyroid gland, but in Osler's day the nature of the disorder was unclear. Osler prefaced his remarks on hyperthyroidism by stating, "It is very possibly caused by disturbed function of the thyroid gland." MacCallum, the pathologist, in 1907 clearly set forth the reservations which he and clinicians held on the cause of toxic goiter, namely that organs hypertrophy only to meet a need of the body, not to insult it. For example, hypertrophy of the left ventricle in aortic stenosis was readily understood to result from an increased work load upon the heart, whereas hypertrophy of the thyroid gland producing a detrimental effect upon the body was not so readily conceded.

Dr. Osler noted the similarity of the symptoms of thyrotoxicosis to those of overdosage of thyroid extract and concluded: "These are some of the considerations which favor the view that the symptoms are due to disturbed function of the thyroid gland, probably to hypersecretion of certain materials, which induce a sort of chronic intoxication." That exophthalmic goiter is, indeed, a hyperfunctioning hypertrophy of the thyroid working to harm the patient was finally accepted within a few years when it was widely recognized, as Osler had stated, that either the removal of the thyroid gland by surgery or its reduction in function by x-ray treatment resulted in improvement or correction of the disorder.

Osler wrote of "exophthalmic goitre," using eponyms such as Graves', Basedow's, and Parry's disease. In only three and a half pages he gave a lucid clinical description of hyperthyroidism (hyperthyrea) and contrasted it with hypothyroidism (athyrea). The exophthalmic component of hyperthyroidism was stressed. We know today, however, that some patients with diffuse goiter and hyperthyroidism may have no proptosis, and conversely that exophthalmos may occur without overt hyperthyroidism. We know, furthermore, that either single or multinodular adenomatous goiter may also cause hyperthyroidism, and that in these patients there is little likelihood of exophthalmos.

Of the cause of exophthalmos we have learned little in the past 57 years. While some experimental work points to a pituitary factor, exophthalmos has been described in hypopituitarism. Pituitary thyrotropic

326

hormone (TSH) is clearly not the cause, yet the serum of some exophthalmic subjects contains a substance called Long Acting Thyroid Stimulator (LATS), which has delayed TSH-like properties and is carried with the gamma globulins. Moreover, no progress in specific therapy of exophthalmos has occurred, and the treatment in use at present, both medical and surgical, is directed at alleviating the symptoms associated with this distressing disorder.

Osler described scleroderma and "solid, infiltrated oedema" in some patients with exophthalmic goiter; it is uncertain as to whether or not he was describing so-called pretibial myxedema. This lesion, which has now been thoroughly detailed, occurs in some patients with exophthalmos with or without hyperthyroidism and is probably caused by the same unknown factor(s) which produce exophthalmos. Titers of LATS are uniformly increased in such patients.

We are no better informed on the cause of hyperthyroidism today than was Dr. Osler. The mechanisms which induce the thyroid gland to hyperfunction are truly an enigma. Osler wrote, "Worry, fright, and depressing emotions precede the development of the disease in a number of cases." The importance of worry and fright as etiological factors is less highly regarded now than formerly. Evaluating the psychiatric aspects of hyperthyroidism, Lidz and Whitehorn have pointed toward the frequency in which patients are seen who develop hyperthyroidism when they have lost confidence in someone, usually a close relation whom they love.

Tachycardia remains one of the hallmarks of thyrotoxicosis. "Irregularity is not common, except toward the close" was Osler's recognition of the fact that cardiac arrhythmias may occur in briskly thyrotoxic patients. Atrial fibrillation complicating this disorder was fully discussed by Thomas (1931) and by Andrus (1932). Osler's description of "loud bruits at the base and over the manubrium" is likely the murmur now called the Means-Lerman scratch.

In his text Osler seldom employed the adverb *very* and it can be assumed that his occasional use of the word should lend true emphasis. When writing "The sounds of the heart may be very intense," he led physiologists and clinicians later to appreciate the increased cardiac work in hyperthyroidism and to recognize that heart failure is associated with high cardiac output.

The Thyroid Hormones

While E. C. Kendall first isolated the crystalline hormone from the thyroid gland and named it thyroxine, it remained for Harington (now Sir Charles Harington) of Great Britain to identify its correct chemical structure and to synthesize the compound in the laboratory. Harington also synthesized numerous analogues of thyroxine, none of which had greater metabolic potency than its parent. He did not, however, synthesize triiodothyronine, a compound now known to have significance in metabolism, a probable important role in thyroid physiology, and striking metabolic properties in comparison to thyroxine.

The existence of triiodothyronine was postulated by Trikojus, who suspected its presence in iodinated casein. Its presence in the serum of patients with hyperthyroidism was also suspected by Gross and Pitt-Rivers, who later identified the hormone accurately and established its thyroid hormone-like properties. Numerous investigators have now shown that triiodothyronine works rapidly in comparison to thyroxine and has approximately three times the potency of thyroxine. Its exact role in thyroid physiology is unknown, although it is clear that the mammalian thyroid does produce small amounts of triiodothyronine in health and larger amounts when the gland is hyperfunctioning, as in endemic goiter or hyperthyroidism or when stimulated by exogenous administration of TSH. Rates of turnover and distribution of the thyroid hormones are well known; the turnover of both hormones is accelerated in hyperthyroidism and diminished in hypothyroidism.

Treatment As previously mentioned, Osler accepted the benefits of either x-ray therapy or subtotal thyroidectomy in hyperthyroidism. While Dr. Osler did not refer to the mortality of this disease, he considered carefully its striking morbidity. He recognized, as has been stressed in recent publications, that a late consequence of hyperthyroidism is often the development of hypothyroidism.

In 1922, it was recognized by Plummer that iodine produces involution of the thyroid gland and a diminution in the manifestations of Graves' disease. Preoperative therapy with iodine permitted surgeons to remove the gland with greater facility, since its vascularity was lessened and the hazard of postoperative thyroid storm reduced. Thus from 1922 until the advent of the antithyroid drugs in the early 1940s, this was the therapy of choice.

The antithyroid drugs provided a tremendous forward step in the therapy of hyperthyroidism (Astwood, 1945). These drugs (in the United States, chiefly propylthiouracil and methimazole) block the synthesis of the thyroid hormones, thus making it possible to restore to euthyroidism those hyperthyroid patients who tolerate the medication satisfactorily, as fortunately most of them do. Accordingly, the antithyroid drugs are now used to prepare such patients for thyroidectomy, with iodine also given a few days before operation. The drugs are also used in the long-term therapy of hyperthyroidism in which approximately one half of those treated for one or two

328

years have a diminution in the size of the goiter and a return to euthyroidism which persists after the drug is withdrawn. They are also used to lessen thyrotoxicity prior to the therapeutic administration of radioactive iodine.

Radioactive iodine is a third form of treatment developed since Osler's day. In adequate amounts it destroys thyroid tissue, and the thyroid gland cannot secrete an excess quantity of thyroid hormone.

Myxedema (athyrea)

Osler recognized three types of clinical hypothyroidism: "cretinism, myxoedema proper and operative myxoedema." Since Osler's remarks of 1909 on myxedema little of importance has been added, nor is there need of subtraction. His clinical description of the disease is as lucid as those of Gull, Ord, Fagge, and other clinical stalwarts of his era.

Despite much work, only limited advancement has been made in understanding the mechanisms by which thyroxine, the principal thyroid hormone, brings about an acceleration of the metabolism of cells. Some progress in our knowledge of myxedema has been made since Osler's day, chiefly in the extension of the clinical description of hypothyroidism, in recognition of certain goitrogenic foodstuffs and drugs, in immunology of the thyroid gland, in improved methods of laboratory diagnosis of thyroid disorders and in a modicum of improvement in therapy.

Clinical Forms   Osler recognized that cretinism "follows absence or loss of function of the thyroid gland, either congenital or appearing at any time before puberty." Two types were defined, *sporadic* and *endemic*. In the sporadic form Osler stated that the gland was likely congenitally absent or atrophied, whereas in the *endemic* form the patient was often goitrous.

Extensive work has now been done by a number of investigators on goitrous cretinism. Some forms are endemic, due to iodine deficiency. Others, however, result from a congenital enzymatic defect in synthesis of thyroxine. The parents of goitrous cretins are often related. Six types of defects of synthesis of thyroid hormone have now been described in goitrous cretinism; in one form severe nerve deafness occurs.

Goitrogenic Foodstuffs and Drugs   The late Alan D. Chesney and his associates were among the first to recognize that some foodstuffs contain goitrogens. Noting goiter in rabbits fed raw cabbage, Chesney related the goiter to the diet and could prevent its occurrence by giving the animals iodine. A complete review of antithyroid compounds has been published recently by Greer.

329

Diseases of the thyroid gland

Surprisingly, in some individuals iodine produces goiter and hypothyroidism. Moreover, goiter in infants born of mothers who took iodine during pregnancy has also been described.

Immunology of the Thyroid Gland and the Thyroid Hormones

It is now clearly recognized that Hashimoto's struma (lymphadenoid goiter, struma lymphomatosa) is frequently associated with the presence in the serum of antibody to thyroglobulin and that the disease often ends in hypothyroidism. An extensive knowledge has been built up in recent years concerning the development of autoantibodies to thyroglobulin and in some instances to thyroid cells as well. The subject has been concisely reviewed by Belyavin.

It is to be recalled that in the Oslerian period adult myxedema was associated only with destruction, either surgically or pathologically, of the gland. Perhaps Osler was describing Hashimoto's struma when he wrote, "A condition of acute and temporary myxoedema may develop in connection with enlargement of the thyroid in young persons," but against such an interpretation is the fact that this type of thyroid failure is usually permanent.

Clinical Features   The clinical aspects of myxedema have been further elucidated since Osler's description of the disease. In the tissues he noted a "great increase in mucin"; the nitrogenous content of myxedema fluid, as revealed in studies of myxedematous patients before and during replacement therapy with thyroid hormone, has since been defined. The "yellowish-white color" of the skin is due to the accumulation in the tissues of carotene which can be converted to vitamin A only in the presence of the thyroid hormone. "Striking slowness of movement" has been elaborated upon to include delayed relaxation phases of the reflexes, especially the ankle jerks, in myxedematous subjects. What has been described by Ascher as "myxedematous madness" was earlier portrayed by Osler as "delusions and hallucinations, leading to a final condition of dementia."

Extensions of our clinical knowledge of myxedema also include recognition in some patients of pericardial effusion which may be asymptomatic or occasionally produce manifestations of obstruction to cardiac filling. Also recognized are coma, severe hypothermia, restricted pulmonary ventilation, megacolon, and an increased tendency toward phlebothrombosis and pulmonary embolism and, lastly, marked atherosclerosis in untreated patients.

Diagnostic Procedures   Within a few years following the publication of Dr. Osler's first edition two tests of thyroid function became available. Shortly after Abel's isolation of epinephrine it was recognized that this hormone has an exaggerated effect in hyperthyroid subjects and little or none in hypothyroid subjects. Goetsch measured the response in pulse rate of patients with myxedema or hyperthyroidism to the administration of epinephrine. The Goetsch test was soon supplanted, however, by the measurement of the basal metabolic rate. Although subject to technical limitations, the basal metabolic rate remains the single quantitative measurement of effect of the thyroid hormones upon the whole organism.

The advent of radioactive iodine, which can be used to ascertain the avidity of the thyroid gland for this precursor of its hormones, and of methods for the accurate chemical measurement of iodine in blood have led in the first instance to the radioactive iodine tracer test and in the second to the serum protein-bound iodine test. Each of these tests is now well standardized not only for use in patients with suspected hypothyroidism but with hyperthyroidism as well. The tyrosine tolerance test, as described by Rivlin, also appears to be taking its place as a diagnostic test.

Treatment   In Osler's day the term "thyroid extract" was applied to preparations used in the treatment of myxedema. This term was appropriate, since the preparation consisted of a glycerine extract of crude thyroid tissue. Shortly thereafter, however, it was appreciated that whole dried thyroid was as effective therapeutically as the extract, and the commercially available preparation was designated "desiccated thyroid." Yet physicians were slow to give up use of the term "thyroid extract," and continued to use it even though the preparations they prescribed were of whole thyroid.

Problems of standardization of desiccated thyroid have long plagued the pharmaceutical and medical professions. The preparations are standardized on the basis of their iodine content, rather than of thyroxine content. In recent years they have also been standardized on their ability to promote oxygen consumption in thyroidectomized animals. Despite these improvements physicians appear to be turning toward the use of the crystalline hormones, chiefly thyroxine, prepared either as an extract of thyroid tissue or by synthesis. While Harington earlier held that thyroxine was inadequately absorbed from the gastrointestinal tract, it is now accepted that this absorption is adequate for successful replacement therapy.

Osler stressed two aspects of treatment: selection of proper dosage and the need for continuous replacement. An interesting description of the value of long-term replacement therapy has been presented

Diseases of the thyroid gland

by MacGregor, who reported the successful lifelong therapy of one of the first patients with myxedema given thyroid extract.

The late Lawson Wilkins stressed the importance of early treatment of cretinism, for those athyreotic infants whose therapy is delayed develop permanent defects in intelligence. Osler was fully aware of this when he wrote, "we can to-day rescue children otherwise doomed to helpless idiocy." The satisfaction which Osler felt toward the treatment of myxedema is expressed as "Our art has made no more brilliant advance . . . a triumph of experimental medicine."

J. Howard Means

REFERENCES

Aikawa, J.K. Myxedema. Springfield, Ill., Charles C Thomas, 1961. (The history of various aspects of thyroid physiology and pathology is usefully reviewed.)

Andrus, F.C. Heart in hyperthyroidism; clinical and experimental study. Amer. Heart J., 8:66, 1932.

Astwood, E.B. Chemotherapy of hyperthyroidism. Harvey Lect., 40:195, 1945.

Belyavin, G. Immunological aspects of thyroid disease. In The Thyroid Gland, Pitt-Rivers, R., and Trotter, W.R., eds., London, Butterworths, 1963, Vol. 2, Ch. 13.

Chesney, A.M., Clawson, T.A., and Webster, B. Endemic goiter in rabbits. I. Incidence and characteristics. Bull. Hopkins Hosp., 43:261, 1928.

Greer, M.A., Kendall, J.W., and Smith, M. Antithyroid compounds. In The Thyroid Gland, Pitt-Rivers, R., and Trotter, W.R. eds. London, Butterworths, 1964, Vol. 1, Ch. 14.

Gross, J., and Pitt-Rivers, R. Identification of 3,5:3'-e-triiodo-thyronine in human plasma. Lancet,1:439, 1952.

Harington, C.R., and Barger, G. Chemistry of thyroxine. III. Constitution and synthesis of thyroxine. Biochem. J., 21:169, 1927.

Kendall, E.C. The isolation in crystalline form of the compound containing iodine which occurs in the thyroid. J.A.M.A., 64:2042, 1915.

Lidz, T., and Whitehorn, J.C. Psychiatric problems in a thyroid clinic. J.A.M.A., 139:698, 1949.

MacCallum, W.G. The Pathology of exophthalmic goiter. J.A.M.A., 49:1158, 1907.

Means, J.H., De Groot, L.J., and Stanbury, J.B. The Thyroid and Its Diseases, 3rd ed. New York, Blakiston Div., McGraw-Hill Book Company, 1963, p. 189.

Plummer, H.S. Results of administering iodine to patients having exophthalmic goiter. J.A.M.A., 80:1955, 1923.

Rivlin, R.S., Melmon, K.L., and Sjoerdsma, A. An oral tyrosine tolerance test in thyrotoxicosis and myxedema. New Eng. J. Med., 272:1134, 1965.

Thomas, H.M., Jr. The heart in hyperthyroidism. Ann. Intern. Med., 5:184, 1931.

Wilkins, L., Blizzard, R.M., and Migeon, C.J. The Diagnosis and Treatment of Endocrine Disorders in Childhood and Adolescence, 3rd ed. Springfield, Ill., Charles C Thomas, 1965.

Very little good is obtained from the smaller quantities. It should be given freely, 20 minims three times a day.

If there is great rapidity of action, aconite may be tried or veratrum viride. There are cases associated with sleeplessness and restlessness which are greatly benefited by bromide of potassium. Digitalis is very rarely indicated, but in obstinate cases it may be tried with the nux vomica.

Cases of heart hurry are often extremely obstinate, as may be judged from the case of the physician reported by H. C. Wood, in whom the condition persisted in spite of all measures for fifty years. The bromides are sometimes useful; the general condition of neurasthenia should be treated, and during the paroxysm an ice-bag may be placed upon the heart, or Leiter's coil, through which ice-water may be passed. Electricity, in the form of galvanism, is sometimes serviceable, and for its mental effect the Franklinic current. For the condition of slow pulse but little can be done. A great majority of the cases are not dangerous.

IX. ANGINA PECTORIS.

Stenocardia, or the breast-pang, described by Heberden, is not an independent affection, but a symptom associated with a number of morbid conditions of the heart and vessels, more particularly with sclerosis of the root of the aorta and changes in the coronary arteries. True angina is characterized by paroxysms of agonizing pain in the region of the heart, extending into the arms and neck. In violent attacks there is a sensation of impending death.

Etiology.—It is a disease of adult life and occurs almost exclusively in men. In Huchard's statistics of 237 cases only 42 were in women. In my first series of 40 cases there was only one woman. It may occur through several generations, as in the Arnold family. Gout and diabetes are important factors. A number of cases of angina pectoris have followed influenza. Attacks are not infrequent in certain forms of heart-disease, particularly aortic insufficiency and adherent pericardium. It is much less common in disease of the mitral valve. Almost without exception the subjects of angina have arterio-sclerosis, either general or localized at the root of the aorta, with changes in the coronary arteries and in the myocardium. Severe attacks may occur in the early period of the growth of aortic aneurism. In men under thirty-five syphilitic aortitis is an important factor.

PHENOMENA OF THE ATTACK.—The exciting cause is in a majority of all cases well defined. In only rare instances do the patients have attacks when quiet. They come on during exertion most frequently, as in walking up hill or doing something entailing sudden muscular effort; occasionally even the effort of dressing or of stooping to lace the shoes may bring on a paroxysm. Mental emotion is a second very potent cause. John Hunter appreciated this when he said that " his life was in the hands of any rascal who chose to annoy and tease him." In his case a fatal attack occurred during a fit of anger. A third, and in many instances the most important, factor is flatulent distention of the stomach. Another common exciting cause is cold; even the chill of getting out of bed in the morning or on bathing may bring on a paroxysm.

333

Usually during exertion or intense mental emotion the patient is seized with an agonizing pain in the region of the heart and a sense of constriction, as if the heart had been seized in a vice. The pains radiate to the neck and down the arm, and there may be numbness of the fingers or in the cardiac region. The face is usually pallid and may assume an ashy-gray tint, and not infrequently a profuse sweat breaks out over the surface. The paroxysm lasts from several seconds to a minute or two, during which, in severe attacks, the patient feels as if death were imminent. As pointed out by Latham, there are two elements in it, the pain—*dolor pectoris*—and the indescribable feeling of anguish and sense of imminent dissolution—*angor animi*. There are great restlessness and anxiety, and the patient may drop dead at the height of the attack or faint and pass away in syncope. The condition of the heart during the attack is variable; the pulsations may be uniform and regular. The pulse tension, however, is usually increased, but it is surprising, even in cases of extreme severity, how slightly the character of the pulse may be altered. After the attack there may be eructations, or the passage of a large quantity of clear urine. The patient usually feels exhausted, and for a day or two may be badly shaken; in other instances in an hour or two the patient feels himself again. While dyspnœa is not a constant feature, the paroxysm is not infrequently associated with a form of asthma; there is wheezing in the bronchial tubes, which may come on very rapidly, and the patient gets short of breath. Many patients the subjects of angina die suddenly without warning and not in a paroxysm. In other instances death follows in the first well-marked paroxysm, as in the case of Thomas Arnold. In a third group there are recurring attacks over long periods of years, as in John Hunter's case; while in a fourth group of cases there are rapidly recurring attacks for several days in succession, with progressive and increasing weakness of the heart.

With reference to the radiation of pain in angina, the studies of Mackenzie and of Head are of great interest. Head concludes that (1) in diseases of the heart, and more particularly in aortic disease, the pain is referred along the first, second, third, and fourth dorsal areas; (2) in angina pectoris the pain may be referred in addition along the fifth, sixth, and seventh, and even the eighth and ninth dorsal areas, and is always accompanied by pain in certain cervical areas. A remarkable fact is the early localization of the pain in distant parts, not infrequently in the left arm; in one of my cases in the left testis, and in another in the jaw.

Theories of Angina Pectoris.—(1) That it is a neuralgia of the cardiac nerves, but the agonizing cramp-like character of the pain, the suddenness of the onset, and the associated features, are unlike any neuralgic affection. The pain, however, is undoubtedly in the cardiac plexus and radiates to adjacent nerves. It is interesting to note, in connection with the almost constant sclerosis of the coronary arteries in angina, that Thoma has found marked sclerosis of the temporal artery in migraine and Dana has met with local thickening of the arteries in some cases of neuralgia. (2) Heberden believed that it was a cramp of the heart-muscle itself. Cramp of certain muscular territories would better explain the attack. (3) That it is due to the extreme tension of the ventricular walls, in consequence of an acute dilatation associated, in the majority of cases, with affection of the coronary arteries. Traube, who supported this view, held that the agonizing pain resulted from the great stretching and tension of the nerves in the muscular substance. A modified form of this view is that there is a spasm of the coronary arteries with great increase of the intracardiac pressure.

(4) The theory of Allan Burns, revived by Potain and others, that the condition is one of transient ischæmia of the heart-muscle in consequence of disease, or spasm, of the coronary arteries. The condition known as intermittent claudication illustrates what may take place. In man (and in the horse), in consequence of thrombosis of the abdominal aorta or iliacs, transient paraplegia and spasm may follow exertion. The collateral circulation, ample when the limbs are at rest, is insufficient after the muscles are actively used, and a state of relative ischæmia is induced with loss of power, which disappears in a short time. This " intermittent claudication " theory best explains the angina paroxysm. A heart the coronary arteries of which are sclerotic or calcified, is in an analogous state, and any extra exertion is likely to be followed by a relative ischæmia and spasm. In Allan Burns's work on The Heart (1809) the theory is discussed at length, but he does not think that spasm is a necessary accompaniment of the ischæmia.

In fatal cases of angina the coronary arteries are almost invariably diseased either in their main divisions, or there is chronic endarteritis with great narrowing of the orifices at the root of the aorta. Experimentally, occlusion of the coronary arteries produces slowing of the heart's action, gradual dilatation, and death within a very few minutes. Cohnheim has shown that in the dog ligation of one of the large coronary branches produces within a minute a condition of arrhythmia, and within two minutes the heart ceases in diastole. These experiments, however, do not throw much light upon the etiology of angina pectoris. Extreme sclerosis of the coronary arteries is common, and a large majority of the cases present no symptoms of angina. Even in the cases of sudden death due to blocking of an artery, particularly the anterior branch of the coronary artery, there is usually no great pain either before or during the attack.

Diagnosis.—There are many grades of true angina. A man may have slight præcordial pain, a sense of distress and uneasiness, and radiation of the pains to the arm and neck. Such attacks following slight exertion, an indiscretion in diet, or a disturbing emotion, may alternate with attacks of much greater severity, or they may occur in connection with a pulse of increased tension and signs of general arterio-sclerosis. In the milder grades the diagnosis can not rest upon the symptoms of the attack itself, since they may be simulated by what is known as the neurotic or functional variety; but the diagnosis should be based upon the examination of the heart and arteries and a careful consideration of the mode of onset and symptoms. The cases of neurotic angina pectoris in women call for the greatest care in the diagnosis, and attention to the points given in the table of Huchard will be of the greatest aid. The existence of a marked increase in the blood-pressure is confirmatory evidence of organic disease.

FUNCTIONAL ANGINA PECTORIS.—There are two main groups, the neurotic and the toxic. The former embraces the hysterical and neurasthenic cases, which are very common in women. Huchard has given an excellent differential table between the two forms.

TRUE ANGINA.	NEUROTIC FORM.
Most common between the ages of forty and fifty years.	At every age, even six years.
More common in men. Attacks brought on by exertion.	More common in women. Attacks spontaneous.
Attacks rarely periodical or nocturnal.	Often periodical and nocturnal.
Not associated with other symptoms.	Associated with nervous symptoms.
Vaso-motor form rare. Agonizing pain and sensation of compression by a vice.	Vaso-motor form common. Pain less severe; sensation of distention.
Pain of short duration. Attitude: silence, immobility.	Pain lasts one or two hours. Agitation and activity.
Lesions: sclerosis of coronary artery.	Neuralgia of nerves and cardio-plexus.
Prognosis grave, often fatal.	Never fatal.
Arterial medication.	Antineuralgic medication.

Nothnagel has described as *vaso-motor angina* a form in which the symptoms set in with coldness and numbness in the extremities, followed by great præcordial pain and feelings of faintness. Some have recognized also a reflex variety.

Toxic Angina.—This embraces cases due to the abuse of tea, coffee, and tobacco. There are three groups of cases of so-called tobacco heart: First, the irritable heart of smokers, seen particularly in young lads, in which the symptoms are palpitation, irregularity, and rapid action; secondly, heart pain of a sharp, shooting character, which may be very severe; and, thirdly, attacks of such severity that they deserve the name of angina.

Prognosis.—Cardiac pain without evidence of arterio-sclerosis or valve-disease is not of much moment. Angina in men is almost invariably associated with marked cardio-vascular lesions, in which the prognosis is always grave. With judicious treatment the attacks, however, may be long deferred, and a few instances recover completely. The prognosis is naturally more serious with aortic insufficiency and advanced arterio-sclerosis. Patients who have had well-marked attacks may live for many years, but much depends upon the care with which they regulate their daily life.

Treatment.—Patients subject to this affection should live a quiet life, avoiding particularly excitement and sudden muscular exertion. During the attack nitrite of amyl should be inhaled, as advised by Lauder Brunton. From 2 to 5 drops may be placed upon cotton-wool in a tumbler or upon the handkerchief. This is frequently of great service in the attack, relieving the agonizing pain and distress. Subjects of the disease should carry the *perles* of the nitrite of amyl with them, and use them on the first indication of an attack. In some instances the nitrite of amyl is quite powerless, though given freely. If within a minute or two relief is not obtained in this way, chloroform should at once be given. A few inhalations act promptly and give great

336

relief. Should the pains continue, a hypodermic of morphia may be administered. In severe and repeated paroxysms a patient may display remarkable resistance to the action of this drug.

In the intervals, nitroglycerin may be given in full doses, as recommended by Murrell, or the nitrite of sodium (Matthew Hay). The nitroglycerin should be used for a long time and in increasing doses, beginning with 1 minim three times a day of the 1-per-cent solution, and increasing the dose 1 minim every five or six days until the patient complains of flushing or headache. The fluid extract of English hawthorn—*Crategus oxycantha*—has been strongly recommended by Jennings, Clements, and others.

Huchard recommends the iodides, believing that their prolonged use influences the arterio-sclerosis. Twenty grains three times a day may be given for several years, omitting the medicine for about ten days in each month. In some instances this treatment is most beneficial, particularly in middle-aged men with a history of syphilis.

For the neurotic, the treatment must be directed to the general nervous condition. Electricity is sometimes very beneficial, particularly the Franklinic form.

X. CONGENITAL AFFECTIONS OF THE HEART.

These have only a limited clinical interest, as in a large proportion of the cases the anomaly is not compatible with life, and in others nothing can be done to remedy the defect or even to relieve the symptoms.

The congenital affections result from interruption of the normal course of development or from inflammatory processes—endocarditis; sometimes from a combination of both.

(*a*) **General Anomalies.**—Of *general anomalies* of development the following conditions may be mentioned: *Acardia*, absence of the heart, which has been met with in the monstrosity known by the same name; *double heart*, which has occasionally been found in extreme grades of fœtal deformity; *dextrocardia*, in which the heart is on the right side, either alone or as part of a general transposition of the viscera; *ectopia cordis*, a condition associated with fission of the chest wall and of the abdomen. The heart may be situated in the cervical, pectoral, or abdominal regions. Except in the abdominal variety the condition is very rarely compatible with extra-uterine life. Occasionally, as in a case reported by Holt, the child lives for some months, and the heart may be seen and felt beating beneath the skin in the epigastric region. This infant was five months old at the date of examination.

(*b*) **Anomalies of the Cardiac Septa.**—The septa of both auricles and ventricles may be defective, in which case the heart consists of but two chambers, the *cor biloculare* or reptilian heart. In the septum of the auricles there is a very common defect, owing to the fact that the membrane closing the foramen ovale has failed at one point to become attached to the ring, and leaves a valvular slit which may be large enough to admit the handle of a scalpel. Neither this nor the small cribriform perforations of the membrane are of any significance.

The foramen ovale may be patent without a trace of membrane closing it. In some instances this exists with other serious defects, such as stenosis

337

angina pectoris

Just as Osler, between the second and third editions, changed his reference to pneumonia as "the special enemy of old age" to "the friend of the aged," so between 1896 and 1909 he changed his emphasis in treatment of angina from the physiological to the pharmacological. In his lectures to Hopkins students in 1896, published in the *New York State Medical Journal* and in the monograph "Angina Pectoris and Allied States," he had said: *Diet* is in many cases the central point in the treatment. . . . There is 'death in the pot' for angina patients." Also he had advised that "steady, quiet exercise should be encouraged." But in 1909 his only therapeutic advice is the use of nitrites, iodides, and fluid extract of English hawthorn, for he had come to realize that people who have angina will rarely change their diet or their sedentary life.

What had concerned Osler about diet was the precipitation of attacks, or of sudden death, by large meals of rich food. In 1916 the *Journal of Experimental Medicine* published confirmation by American pathologists of the Russian experiments showing that arterial disease could be produced in animals by feeding diets rich in animal fat, or even pure cholesterol. Ignatovsky had been led to the experiments by observing the difference in incidence of vascular disease in the rich and the poor, a difference Osler also had noted. The first Russian report had emphasized protein rather than fat in the diet of egg yolk and milk which elicited atheromatous lesions. Heart specialists, in leading textbooks, recommended custard, milk, and eggs as the diet for acute coronary occlusion as late as 1958. The effect of diet in accelerating coagulation, increasing platelet stickiness, and retarding fibrinolysis had been repeatedly demonstrated, and atherosclerosis had been evoked in thousands of mammals and birds by dietary manipulation. The geographical and social distribution of coronary disease now seems best explained by the animal fat and sucrose content of the diets of various populations. The American Heart Association, in 1965, recommended a low animal fat, low calorie diet in prophylaxis and management of vascular disease. Diet, early ambulation, and after convalescence "steady, quiet exercise" again, as in 1896, are stressed in discussions of myocardial infarction and angina pectoris. No really effective substitutes for the nitrites Osler recommended have been found among the many drugs which have been tried.

In spite of René Marie's splendid monograph on myocardial infarction in 1896 and a series of case histories published in America, Russia, and Germany in the subsequent 20 years; in spite of Herrick's Pardee's, and Levine's reports (1918–1924) of electrocardiographic signs of acute and healed infarction, professors of medicine knew less about that form of coronary disease in 1926 than Osler and his pupils had known 30 years before. Infarction occurring in a famous electrocardiographer, 1n 1926, was diagnosed acute indigestion by the victim and confirmed by a world-renowned London professor of medicine. The amplifier tube, making possible portable substitutes for the ponderous string galvonmeter, made coronary disease — and six weeks total bed rest as its therapy — familiar to most laymen by 1940. The test for rise in plasma enzyme levels, the use of antiprothrombin agents and of heparin, and early ambulation were equally commonplace by 1960.

Many operative attacks on angina, all "very effective," were reported between 1924 (Wenckebach-Hofer, "depressor nerve" section) and the mammary artery ligation of 1960. Cervical, upper thoracic, and preaortic sympathetic fibers were severed; coronary veins plicated; the epicardium was stripped, powdered, and sheathed in plastic foam; coronary occlusions were removed; and mammary arteries were implanted in the left ventricular wall. With cineangiography and selective coronary or mammary artery visualization, objective data now are available to compare preoperative and postoperative vascularization. Such studies have confirmed the necropsy-based conclusion that severe diffuse coronary obstruction may fail to cause angina, and single lesions, partially obstructing, may cause disabling disease. By and large most anginal patients show what Jenner predicted and found in John Hunter — numerous partial or complete obstructions. And in spite of stress tests and smoking tests for altered electrical or mechanical function of the heart, a carefully elicited history remains the best basis for the diagnosis.

Clinicians, finding in a few patients with angina gallop rhythm or pulsus alternans, present only during attacks, suspected that the ventricular muscle was significantly embarrassed. Catheter studies show that the end diastolic pressure in the left ventricle does rise, even before pain comes on, and falls when nitrites give relief. Osler ignored the Widal Clinic's claim for marked benefit from the "low chloride" diet and Sir Clifford Allbutt's belief in the efficacy of six weeks complete bed rest. However, in 1896 (but not 1909), he advised: "In severe recurring attacks a period of absolute rest should be enjoined." We now know that sodium depletion or prolonged recumbency lead to a reduced blood volume. This is especially effective, like the nitrites, in preventing a high venous return and overloading of the ischemic ventricle. In favoring Allan Burns' theory that angina is analogous to intermittent claudication, Osler chose wisely in his discussion of theories

Angina pectoris

of causation. "The collateral circulation, ample when the limbs are at rest, is insufficient after the muscles are actively used, and a state of relative ischaemia is induced with loss of power [of the left ventricle]."

William Dock

REFERENCES

Andrus, E.C., and Maxwell, C.H. The Heart and Circulation. Second National Conference of Cardiovascular Diseases, Washington, D.C., 1963. Washington, Fed. Amer. Soc. Exp. Biol., 1965.

Herrick, J.B. A Short History of Cardiology. Springfield, Ill., Charles C Thomas, 1942.

Willius F.A., and Dry, T.J. A History of the Heart and the Circulation. Philadelphia, W.B. Saunders Co., 1948.

Willius, F.A., and Keys, T.E. Cardiac Classics. St. Louis, The C.V. Mosby Co., 1941.

why a disease should be limited to a definite system of neurones. One view is based upon the idea that in certain individuals one or the other of these systems has an innate tendency to undergo degeneration; another assumes that neurones with a similar function have a similar chemical construction (which differs from that of neurones with a different function), and this is taken to explain why a poison circulating in the blood should show a selective action for a single functional system of neurones.

In the afferent tract locomotor ataxia stands alone as a system disease, and we now believe that herpes zoster is an inflammation of the dorsal root ganglia and stands in the same relation to tabes that acute anterior poliomyelitis does to chronic progressive muscular atrophy. In the efferent tract progressive (central) muscular atrophy is the chief representative, as in it the whole motor path is more or less involved. Theoretically, primary lateral sclerosis is a disease confined to the upper segment of the efferent tract, while chronic anterior poliomyelitis involves the lower segment of the tract.

In connection with locomotor ataxia, general paralysis is considered on account of their frequent association and of the possibility of their being different expressions of one and the same morbid process; and with progressive (central) muscular atrophy, the other forms of muscular atrophy are considered as a matter of convenience. In other instances, too, diseases are arranged in positions to which they might not be entitled, had a rigid classification of system diseases been maintained.

II. DISEASES OF THE AFFERENT OR SENSORY SYSTEM.

LOCOMOTOR ATAXIA.

(*Tabes Dorsalis; Posterior Spinal Sclerosis.*)

Definition.—An affection characterized clinically by sensory disturbances, incoördination, trophic changes, and involvement of the special senses, particularly the eyes. Anatomically there are found degenerations of the root fibres of the dorsal columns of the cord, of the dorsal roots, and at times of the spinal ganglia and peripheral nerves. Degenerations have been described in the brain, particularly the cortex cerebri, in the ganglion cells of the cord, and in the endogenous fibres of the dorsal columns.

Etiology.—It is a wide-spread disease, more frequent in cities than in the country. The relative proportion may be judged from the fact that of 16,562 cases in the neurological dispensary of the Johns Hopkins Hospital, there were 201 cases of locomotor ataxia. Males are attacked more frequently than females, the proportion being nearly 10 to 1. The disease, although uncommon in the negro, is seen in them more frequently than some authors state. It is a disease of adult life, the great majority of cases occurring between the thirtieth and fiftieth years. Occasionally cases are seen in young men, and it may occur in children with hereditary syphilis. Of special causes syphilis is the most important. According to the figures of Erb, Fournier, Gowers, Starr, and others, in from 50 to 90 per cent of all cases there is a history of this disease. In the Johns Hopkins Hospital the percentage, as found by Thomas, was 63.1. Erb's recent figures are most striking—of 300 cases of tabes in private practice, 89 per cent had had syphilis. Moebius goes so far as to say, " The longer I reflect upon it, the more firmly I believe that tabes never originates without syphilis."

Excessive fatigue, overexertion, injury, exposure to cold and wet, and sexual excesses are all assigned as causes. There are instances in which the disease has closely followed severe exposure. James Stewart has noted that the Ottawa lumbermen, who live a very hard life in the camps during the winter months, are frequently the subjects of locomotor ataxia. Trauma has been noted in a few cases. Alcoholic excess does not seem to predispose to the disease. Among patients in the better classes of life I do not remember one in which there had been a previous history of prolonged drunkenness. There are now a good many cases on record of the existence of the disease in both husband and wife, and a few where the children are also affected.

Morbid Anatomy and Pathology.—With a fuller knowledge of the anatomy of the nervous system, our conception of *tabes dorsalis* has undergone many changes. Posterior spinal sclerosis, although the most obvious gross change, is now no longer, as in Romberg's time, an adequate description of the condition, for we know that the dorsal columns are composed of definite fibre systems, and many attempts have been made to determine which of these are affected in tabes, and where the primary lesion is situated. The dorsal fibres are of two kinds, those with their cell bodies outside the cord in the spinal ganglia, the so-called exogenous, or root fibres, and those which arise from cells within the cord, the endogenous fibres. These two sets occupy fairly well-determined regions of the dorsal columns and a study of early cases of tabes has shown that it is the exogenous or root fibres that are first affected. The fibres of the dorsal roots enter the cord in two divisions, an external and an internal; the former is composed of fibres of small calibre, which, in the cord, make up Lissauer's tract, and occupy the space between the apex of the dorsal cornua and the periphery of the cord, and really do not form part of the dorsal columns. They are short, soon entering the gray matter, and do not seem to be affected, or only slightly so, in early cases (Mott, and Orr and Rowe).

The larger fibres enter the cord by the internal division, just medial to the cornua, in what is known as the root entry zone. Some enter the gray matter of the spinal cord almost directly and others after a longer course, while still others run in the cord to the medulla, to end in the nuclei of the dorsal columns. As the fibres of every spinal nerve enter the cord between the dorsal cornua and the nerve fibres which have entered lower down, the fibres from each root are successively pushed more and more toward the median line, and so in the cervical cord the fasciculi of Goll are largely composed of long fibres derived from the sacral and lumbar roots.

That it is the coarse dorsal root fibres which are first affected in tabes is generally admitted, but there is much divergence of opinion as to the character and location of the initial process.

Certain observers believe that the morbid agent, syphilis, for instance, acts primarily on extra-nervous tissues, and that change in the root fibres is a secondary degeneration. Nageotte calls attention to the frequency of a transverse, interstitial neuritis of the dorsal roots just after they have left the ganglia and are still surrounded by the dura, and he believes that it is this neuritis which is the primary lesion in tabes. Obersteiner and Redlich have laid great stress on the presence of an inflammation of the pia mater over the dorsal aspect of the cord, which involves the root fibres as they pass through. They point out that it is just here that the dorsal roots are most vulnerable, for at this point—that is, while surrounded by the pia—they are almost completely devoid of their myelin sheaths. Changes in the blood-vessels of the cord, of the pia, and of the nerve roots have been described in early tabes, and very lately Marie and Guillain have advanced the belief that the changes in the cord are due to an affection (syphilis) of the posterior lymphatic system which is confined to the dorsal columns of the cord, the pia mater over them, and the dorsal roots. For them the changes in the nervous system are only apparently radicular or systemic. Other observers regard the primary change as an interstitial myelitis of the dorsal columns accompanied by secondary changes.

In the belief of most authors, tabes is a systemic disease, at least it starts as such; but here again there is much dispute as to just which part of the sensory neurones is first affected. The peripheral nerves, the dorsal ganglia, the dorsal roots, and the intermedullary portions of the neurones have all been pointed out as starting places of the disease.

Flechsig, Trepinsky, and others hold that the disease is so truly systemic that the degeneration in the dorsal columns follows closely the embryological systems as determined by the time of their myelinization. Orr and Rowe, in cases of general paresis, have described in detail what appear to be the earliest tabetic changes in the dorsal columns, corresponding closely to the description given by Mott in certain of his cases of tabo-paralysis.

With Marchi stain, degeneration of the root fibres in the root entry zone was a constant finding. This change was radicular in the sense that it varied in intensity with the different roots and was most marked in the sacral and lumbar regions. The degeneration was not found in the dorsal roots, but began within the cord just beyond where the root fibres had lost their neurolemma and their myelin sheaths, and the authors believe that it is here that the fibres are exposed to the action of poisons. They found no meningitis to account for it. Degenerated fibres could be traced into the dorsal gray matter and among the ganglion cells of the columns of Clarke. The long columns which ascend the cord also degenerated.

In a study of more advanced cases, Mott found, in addition to the lesion described above, degeneration of the dorsal roots and some alteration of the cells in the spinal ganglia. The fibres distal to the ganglia were practically normal, although at times the sensory fibres, at the periphery of a limb, showed degeneration. Within the cord, the exogenous fibres were diseased as already described, but he also found degeneration in the endogenous system of fibres. This was in advanced cases with marked ataxia. He thinks the process shows both a systemic and a segmental election, and in this he is in agreement with a number of other observers. In some cases the cells of Clarke's columns were found diseased with secondary changes in the cerebellar tracts.

Mott found optic atrophy quite frequently, and believes that had he examined the optic nerves of all the cases changes would have been found in 60 per cent. The other cranial nerves, especially the fifth with its ganglion, have been found degenerated.

The disease occasionally spreads beyond the sensory system in the cord, and in advanced cases the cells in the ventral horns may be degenerated in association with muscular atrophy. In his asylum cases, Mott very generally found more or less marked changes in the pyramidal fibres; these he believed to be evidence of changes in the cerebral cortex. Degeneration of the cortex was to be expected in his cases of tabo-paralysis, but even in cases where the mental symptoms were absent, or very mild, similar though slight changes have been described, just as in general paralysis, without marked tabetic symptoms, there may be degeneration of the dorsal columns. The close association, or even identity, of tabes and general paralysis will be considered later.

Symptoms.—These are best considered under three stages—the incipient stage, the ataxic stage, and the paralytic stage.

The Incipient Stage.—This is sometimes called the pre-ataxic stage. The manner in which tabes makes its onset differs very widely in the different cases, and mistakes in diagnosis are often made early in the disease. The following are the most characteristic initial symptoms:

Pains, usually of a sharp stabbing character; hence the term lightning pains. They last for only a second or two and are most common in the legs or about the trunk, and tend to follow dorsal root areas. They dart from place to place. At times they are associated with a hot burning feeling and often leave the affected area painful to pressure, and occasionally herpes may follow. The intensity of the pain varies from a sore, burning feeling of the skin to a pain so intense that were it not for its momentary duration it would exceed human endurance. They occur at irregular intervals, and are prone to follow excesses or to come on when health is impaired. When typical, these pains are practically pathognomonic of the condition. (See Sir William Gowers' clinical lecture.) The gastric crises and other crises may occur. Paræsthesia may also be among the first symptoms,—numbness of the feet, tingling, etc., and at times a sense of constriction about the body.

Ocular Symptoms.—(*a*) Optic atrophy. This occurs in about 10 per cent of the cases, and is often an early and even the first symptom. There is a gradual loss of vision, which in a large majority of cases leads to total blindness. (*b*) Ptosis, which may be double or single. (*c*) Paralysis of the external muscles of the eye. This may be of a single muscle or occasionally of all the muscles of the eye. The paralysis is often transient, the patient merely complaining that he saw double for a certain period. (*d*) Argyll Robertson pupil, in which there is loss of the iris reflex to light but contraction during accommodation. The pupils are often very small—spinal myosis.

Bladder Symptoms.—The first warning of the disease which the patient has may be a certain difficulty in emptying the bladder. Incontinence of urine occurs only at a later stage of the disease. Decrease in sexual desire and power may also be an early symptom.

Trophic Disturbances.—These usually occur later in the disease, but at times they are very early symptoms and it is not very infrequent to have one's attention called to the trouble by the presence of a perforating ulcer or of a characteristic Charcot's joint.

Loss of the Deep Reflexes.—This early and most important symptom may occur years before the development of ataxia. Even alone it is of great mo-

58

ment, since it is very rare to meet with individuals in whom the knee and ankle jerks are normally absent.   The combination of loss of either of these with one or more of the symptoms mentioned above, especially with the lightning pains and ptosis or Argyll Robertson pupil, is practically diagnostic. These reflexes gradually decrease, and one may be lost before the other, or disappear first in one leg.

These are the most common symptoms of the initial stage of tabes and may persist for years without the development of incoördination.   The patient may look well and feel well, and be troubled only by occasional attacks of lightning pains or of one of the other subjective symptoms.   Moebius goes so far as to state that the typical Argyll Robertson pupil means either tabes or general paralysis, and that paralysis of the external muscles of the eye developing in adults is of almost equal importance, especially if it develops painlessly.

The time between the syphilitic infection and the occurrence of the first symptoms of locomotor ataxia varies within wide limits.   About one-half the cases occur between the sixth and fifteenth year, but many begin even later than this.

The disease may never progress beyond this stage, and when optic atrophy develops early and leads to blindness, ataxia rarely, if ever, supervenes, but the mental symptoms of paresis not infrequently follow, a sequence which must be kept in mind.   There is a sort of antagonism between the ocular symptoms and the progress of the ataxia.   Charcot laid considerable stress upon this, and both Dejerine and Spiller have since emphasized the point.

ATAXIC STAGE.—*Motor Symptoms.*—The ataxia is believed to be due to a disturbance or loss of the afferent impulses from the muscles, joints, and deep tissues, and a disturbance of the muscle sense itself can usually be demonstrated.   It develops gradually.   One of the first indications to the patient is inability to get about readily in the dark or to maintain his equilibrium when washing his face with the eyes shut.   When the patient stands with the feet together and the eyes closed, he sways and has difficulty in maintaining his position (Romberg's symptom), and he may be quite unable to stand on one leg.   He does not start off promptly at the word of command.   On turning quickly he is apt to fall.   He descends stairs with more difficulty than he ascends them.   Gradually the characteristic ataxic gait develops.   The patient, as a rule, walks with a stick, the eyes are directed to the ground, the body is thrown forward, and the legs are wide apart.   In walking, the leg is thrown out violently, the foot is raised too high and is brought down in a stamping manner with the heel first, or the whole sole comes in contact with the ground. Ultimately the patient may be unable to walk without the assistance of two canes.   This gait is very characteristic, and unlike that seen in any other disease.   The incoördination is not only in walking, but in the performance of other movements.   If the patient is asked, when in the recumbent posture, to touch one knee with the other foot, the irregularity of the movement is very evident.   Incoördination of the arms is less common, but usually develops in some grade.   It may in rare instances exist before the incoördination of the legs.   It may be tested by asking the patient to close his eyes and to touch the tip of the nose or the tip of the ear with the finger, or with the arms thrust out to bring the tips of the fingers together.   The incoördination may early be noticed by a difficulty which the patient experiences in buttoning his collar or in performing one of the ordinary routine acts of dressing.

One of the most striking features of the disease is that with marked incoordination there is but little loss of muscular power. The grip of the hands may be strong and firm, the power of the legs, tested by trying to flex them, may be unimpaired, and their nutrition, except toward the close, may be unaffected.

There is a remarkable muscular relaxation which enables the joints to be placed in positions of hyperextension and hyperflexion. It gives sometimes a marked backward curve to the legs. Fränkel, who calls the condition hypotonia, says it may be an early symptom.

Sensory Symptoms.—The lightning pains may persist. They vary greatly in different cases. Some patients are rendered miserable by the frequent occurrence of the attacks; others escape altogether. In addition, common symptoms are tingling, pins and needles, particularly in the feet, and areas of hyperæsthesia or of anæsthesia. The patient may complain of a change in the sensation in the soles of the feet, as if cotton was interposed between the floor and the skin. Sensory disturbances occur less frequently in the hands. Objective sensory disturbances can usually be demonstrated, and indeed almost every variety of sensory disturbance has been described. They have been carefully studied in America by Knapp and by Patrick, and in Europe by many observers. Bands about the chest of a moderate grade of anæsthesia are not uncommon; they are apt to follow the distribution of spinal segments. The most marked disturbances are usually found on the legs. Retardation of the sense of pain is common, and a pin-prick on the foot is first felt as a simple tactile impression, and the sense of pain is not perceived for a second or two or may be delayed for as much as ten seconds. The pain felt may persist. A curious phenomenon is the loss of the power of localizing the pain. For instance, if the patient is pricked on one limb he may say that he feels it on the other (allocheiria), or a pin-prick on the foot may be felt on both feet. The muscular sense which is usually affected early, becomes much impaired and the patient no longer recognizes the position in which his limbs are placed. This may be present in the pre-ataxic stage.

Reflexes.—As mentioned, the loss of the knee and ankle jerks is one of the earliest symptoms of the disease. Occasionally a case is found in which they are retained. The skin reflexes may at first be increased, but later are usually involved with the deep reflexes.

Special Senses.—The eye symptoms noted above may be present, but, as mentioned, ataxia is rare with atrophy of the optic nerve.

Deafness may develop, due to lesion of the auditory nerve. There may also be attacks of vertigo. Olfactory symptoms are rare.

Visceral Symptoms.—Among the most remarkable sensory disturbances are the tabetic crises, severe paroxysms of pain referred to various viscera; thus laryngeal, gastric, nephric, rectal, urethral, and clitoral crises have been described. The most common are the gastric and laryngeal. In the former there are intense pains in the stomach, vomiting, and a secretion of hyperacid gastric juice. The attack may last for several days or even longer. There may be severe pain without any vomiting. The attacks are of variable intensity and usually require morphia. Paroxysms of rectal pain and tenesmus are

346

described. They have not been common in my experience. Laryngeal crises also are rare. There may be true spasm with dyspnœa and noisy inspiration. In one instance at least the patient has died in the attack. There are also nasal crises, associated with sneezing fits.

The sphincters are frequently involved. Early in the disease there may be a retardation or hesitancy in making water. Later there is retention, and cystitis may occur. Unless great care is taken the inflammation may extend to the kidneys. Constipation is extremely common. Late in the disease the sphincter ani is weakened. The sexual power is usually lost in the ataxic stage.

Trophic Changes.—Skin rashes may develop in the course of the lightning pains, such as herpes, œdema, or local sweating. Alteration in the nails may occur. A perforating ulcer may develop on the foot, usually beneath the great toe. A perforating buccal ulcer has also been described. Onychia may prove very troublesome.

Arthropathies (Charcot's Joints).—Anatomically there are: (1) enlargement of the capsule with thickening of the synovial membranes and increase in the fluids; (2) slight enlargement of the ends of the bones, with slight exostoses; (3) a dull velvety appearance of the cartilages, with atrophy in places (V. E. Henderson). The knees are most frequently involved. The spine is affected in rare instances. Recurring trauma is an important element in the causation, but trophic disturbances have a strong influence in the etiology. A striking feature is the absence of pain. Suppuration may occur, also spontaneous fractures. Among other trophic disturbances may be mentioned atrophy of the muscles, which is usually a late manifestation, but may be localized and associated with neuritis. In any very large collection of cases many instances of atrophy are found, due either to involvement of the ventral horns or to peripheral neuritis.

Cerebral Symptoms.—Hemiplegia may develop at any stage of the disease, more commonly when it is well advanced. It may be due to hæmorrhagic softening in consequence of disease of the vessels or to progressive cortical changes. Hemianæsthesia is sometimes present. Very rarely the hemiplegia is due to coarse syphilitic disease.

Dementia paralytica frequently exists with tabes; indeed we have come to regard these two diseases as simply different localizations of the same morbid process. In other instances melancholia, dementia, or paranoia occur.

PARALYTIC STAGE.—After persisting for an indefinite number of years the patient gradually loses the power of walking and becomes bedridden or paralyzed. In this condition he is very likely to be carried off by some intercurrent affection, such as pyelo-nephritis, pneumonia, or tuberculosis.

The Course of the Disease.—A patient may remain in the pre-ataxic stage for an indefinite period; and the loss of knee-jerk and the gray atrophy of the optic nerves may be the sole indication of the true nature of the disease. In such cases incoördination rarely develops. In a majority of cases the progress is slow, and after six or eight years, sometimes less, the ataxia is well developed. The symptoms may vary a good deal; thus the pains, which may have been excessive at first, often lessen. The disease may remain stationary for years; then exacerbations occur and it makes rapid progress. Occasionally the process seems to be arrested. There are instances of what may be called acute ataxia, in which, within a year or even less, the incoördination is marked, and the paralytic stage may develop within a few months. The disease itself rarely causes death, and after becoming bedridden the patient may live for fifteen or twenty years.

Diagnosis.—In the initial stage the lightning pains are almost distinctive, and when combined with any of the other signs are quite so. The association of progressive atrophy of the optic nerves with loss of knee-jerk is also characteristic. The early ocular palsies are of the greatest importance. A squint, ptosis, or the Argyll Robertson pupil may be the first symptom, and may exist with the loss only of the knee-jerk. Loss of the knee-jerk alone, however, does occasionally occur in healthy individuals. A history of preceding syphilis lends added weight to the symptoms, and its presence or absence may be of the utmost importance in determining the diagnosis. If the possibility of syphilitic infection can be excluded, a circumstance but too rarely met with, only the most unequivocal combination of symptoms can justify the diagnosis of locomotor ataxia. Cytodiagnosis may be a help in doubtful cases (see General Paresis), and Wassermann's reaction may be present.

The diseases most likely to be confounded with locotomor ataxia are: (1) PERIPHERAL NEURITIS.—The steppage gait of arsenical, alcoholic, or diabetic paralysis is quite unlike that of locomotor ataxia. In these forms there is a paralysis of the feet, and the leg is lifted high in order that the toes may clear the floor. The use of the word ataxia in this connection should no longer be continued. In the rare cases in which the muscle sense nerves are particularly affected and in which there is true ataxia, the absence of the lightning pains and eye symptoms and the history will suffice in a majority of cases to make the diagnosis clear. In diphtheritic paralysis the early loss of the knee-jerk and the associated eye symptoms may suggest tabes, but the history, the existence of paralysis of the throat, and the absence of pains render a diagnosis easy.

(2) ATAXIC PARAPLEGIA.—Marked incoördination with spastic paralysis is characteristic of the condition which Gowers has termed ataxic paraplegia. In a majority of the cases this affection is distinguished also by the absence of pains and of eye symptoms, but it may be a manifestation of the cord lesions in tabo-paralysis.

(3) CEREBRAL DISEASE.—In diseases of the brain involving the afferent tracts ataxia is at times a prominent symptom. It is usually unilateral or limited to one limb; this, with the history and the associated symptoms, excludes tabes.

(4) CEREBELLAR DISEASE.—The cerebellar incoördination has only a superficial resemblance to that of locomotor ataxia, and is more a disturbance of equilibrium than a true ataxia; the knee-jerk is usually present, there are no lightning pains, no sensory disturbances; while, on the other hand, there are headache, optic neuritis, and vomiting.

(5) Some ACUTE AFFECTIONS involving the dorsal columns of the cord may be followed by incoördination and resemble tabes very closely. In a case under my care, the gait was characteristic and Romberg's symptom was present. The knee-jerk, however, was retained and there were no ocular symptoms. The condition had developed within three or four months, and there was a well-marked history of syphilis. Under large doses of iodide of potassium the ataxia and other symptoms completely disappeared.

348

(6) GENERAL PARESIS.—Even though these two diseases are so nearly allied and often associated, it is of very great practical importance to determine, when possible, whether the type is to be spinal or cerebral, for, in the great majority of cases, when this is established, it does not change. The difficulty arises in the premonitory stage, when ocular changes and abnormalities of sensation and the deep reflexes may be the only symptoms. At this stage any alteration in the mental characteristics is of the utmost significance. (See General Paresis.) Loss of the deep reflexes and lightning pains speak for tabes; active reflexes, with ocular changes, especially optic atrophy, are suggestive of paresis.

(7) VISCERAL CRISES and NEURALGIC SYMPTOMS may lead to error, and in middle-aged men with severe, recurring attacks of gastralgia it is always well to bear in mind the possibility of tabes, and to make a careful examination of the eyes and of the knee-jerk.

Prognosis.—Complete recovery can not be expected, but arrest of the process is not uncommon and a marked amelioration of the symptoms is frequent. Optic-nerve atrophy, one of the most serious events in the disease, has this hopeful aspect—that incoördination rarely follows and the progress of the spinal symptoms may be arrested. On the other hand, mental symptoms are more likely to follow. The optic atrophy itself is occasionally checked. On the whole, the prognosis in tabes is bad. The experience of such men as Weir Mitchell, Charcot, and Gowers is distinctly opposed to the belief that locomotor ataxia is ever completely cured. No such case has come under my personal observation.

Treatment.—To arrest the progress and to relieve, if possible, the symptoms are the objects which the practitioner should have in view. A quiet, well-regulated method of life is essential. It is not well, as a rule, for a patient to give up his occupation so long as he is able to keep about and perform ordinary work, provided there is no evident mental change. I know tabetics who have for years conducted large businesses, and there have been several notable instances in our profession of men who have risen to distinction in spite of the existence of this disease. Excesses of all sorts, more particularly *in baccho et venere,* should be carefully avoided. A man in the pre-ataxic stage should not marry.

Care should be taken in the diet, particularly if gastric crises have occurred. To secure arrest of the disease many remedies have been employed. Although syphilis plays such an important *rôle* in the etiology, it is universally acknowledged that neither mercury nor the iodide of potassium have anything like the same influence over the tabetic lesions that they have over the ordinary syphilitic processes. However, when the syphilis is comparatively recent, when symptoms develop within two years of the primary infection, the disease may be arrested by mercury and iodide of potassium. The French authors have recently spoken much more hopefully of the benefit of anti-syphilitic treatment in early cases of tabes, and it is well to give the patient the benefit of at least one thorough course of mercurial inunctions and iodide of potassium. Of remedies which may be tried and are believed by some writers to retard the progress, the following are recommended: Arsenic in full doses, nitrate of silver in quarter-grain doses, Calabar bean, ergot, and the preparations of gold.

349

For the pains, complete rest in bed, as advised by Weir Mitchell, and counter-irritation to the spine (either blisters or the thermo-cautery) may be employed. The severe spells which come on particularly after excesses of any kind are often promptly relieved by a hot bath or by a Turkish bath. For the severe recurring attacks of lightning pains spinal cocainization may be tried. In an instance reported to me by Dr. George Goodfellow, of San Francisco, excellent results followed. A prolonged course of nitrate of silver seems in some cases to allay the pains and lessen the liability to the attacks. I have never seen ill effects from its use in spinal sclerosis. Antipyrin and antifebrin may be employed, and occasionally do good, but their analgesic powers in this disease have been greatly overrated. Cannabis indica is sometimes useful. In the severe paroxysms of pain hypodermics of morphia or of cocaine must be used. The use of morphia should be postponed as long as possible. Electricity is of very little benefit. For the severe attacks of gastralgia, morphia is also required. The laryngeal crises are rarely dangerous. An application of cocaine may be made during the spasm, or a few whiffs of chloroform may be given, or nitrate of amyl. In all cases of tabes with increased arterial tension the prolonged use of nitroglycerin, given in increasing doses until the physiological effect is produced, is of great service in allaying the neuralgic pains and diminishing the frequency of the crises. Its use must be guarded when there is aortic insufficiency. The special indication is increased tension. The bladder symptoms demand constant care. When the organ can not be perfectly emptied the catheter should be used, and the patient may be taught its use and how to keep it thoroughly sterilized.

Frenkel's method of re-education often helps the patient to regain to a considerable extent the control of the voluntary movements which he has lost. (English translation of his work by P. Blakiston's Son & Co.) By this method the patient is first taught, by repeated systematic efforts, to perform simple movements; from this he goes to more and more complex movements. The treatment should be directed and supervised by a trained teacher, as the result depends upon the skill of the teacher quite as much as upon the perseverance of the patient.

GENERAL PARALYSIS OF THE INSANE AND TABO-PARALYSIS

(*Dementia Paralytica; General Paresis*).

As has been said in the last section, the belief in the essential identity of general paralysis and tabes has gained more and more ground and has much in its favor. Mott says: " I maintain that etiologically and pathogenetically there is *one tabes* which may begin in the brain (especially in certain regions), or in the spinal cord in certain regions, or in the peripheral nervous structures connected with vision, or in nervous structures connected with the viscera, constituting, therefore, different types, any of which may be present or be associated with one or all of the others." Fournier has taken practically the same view and describes them together under the heading *Les Affections Parasyphilitiques.* Moebius, Shaffer, and others are equally positive in their statements.

It is undoubted that most cases of tabes run their course with practically no mental symptoms, and that cases of general paralysis may never present symptoms that suggest tabes. For practical purposes we are forced to keep the distinction clearly in mind, and for this reason it seems best, at least for the present, to consider them separately.

There is, however, a group of cases in which the symptoms of the two diseases are associated in every combination. The name "tabo-paralysis" has been given to these cases.

(a) General Paralysis.

Definition.—A chronic, progressive disease of the brain and its meninges, associated with psychical and motor disturbances, finally leading to dementia and paralysis.

Etiology.—As in tabes, the most important individual factor is syphilis, which is antecedent in both conditions in from 70 to 90 per cent of all cases. Males are affected much more frequently than females. It occurs chiefly between the ages of thirty and fifty-five, although it may begin in childhood as the result of congenital syphilis. An overwhelming majority of the cases are in married people, and not infrequently both husband and wife are affected, or one has paresis and the other tabes. Statistics show that it is more common in the lower classes of society, but in America in general medical practice the disease is certainly more common in the well-to-do classes. Heredity is a more important factor here than in tabes, although its influence is not great. An important predisposing cause is "a life absorbed in ambitious projects with all its strongest mental efforts, its long-sustained anxieties, deferred hopes, and straining expectation" (Mickle). The habits of life so frequently seen in active business men in our large cities, and well expressed by the phrase "burning the candle at both ends," strongly predispose to the disease.

Morbid Anatomy.—The dura is often thickened, and its inner surface may show the various forms of hypertrophic pachymeningitis. The pia is cloudy, thickened, and adherent to the cortex. The cerebro-spinal fluid is increased in the meningeal spaces, especially in the meshes of the pia, and at times to such an extent as to resemble cysts. The brain is small, and weighs less than normal. The convolutions are atrophied, especially in the anterior and middle lobes. In acute cases the brain may be swollen, hyperæmic, and œdematous. The brain cortex is usually red, and, except in advanced cases, it may not be atrophied, the atrophy of the hemispheres being at the expense of the white matter. The lateral ventricles are dilated to compensate for the atrophy of the brain, and the ependyma may be granular. The fourth ventricle is more constantly dilated, with granulations of its floor covering the calamus scriptorius, a condition seldom seen in any other affection.

Histologically there is atrophy of the nerve fibres, especially the tangental and supra-radial, degeneration of the nerve cells of the cortex, and a great overgrowth of the neuroglia, with the presence of numerous giant spider cells. In the dilated adventitial spaces of the blood-vessels there is a great accumulation of cells—plasma cells with a few lymphocytes and an occasional mast cell. In the tissue itself are found the curious rod-shaped structures, which are derived from the vessel walls. Compound granular corpuscles are also found near necrotic areas. There is often a very great increase in the small blood-vessels, and various kinds of alterations of the vessel walls have been described. The improved methods of staining the neuro-fibrils (Cajal and

351

Pielschowsky) are beginning to throw light upon the essential cellular changes.

The disease process is diffuse, and affects practically all parts of the brain, but its intensity varies greatly, even in adjoining areas. As a rule the cortex of the frontal and central convolutions and the gray matter about the ventricles are mòst affected.

In many cases changes are present in the spinal cord and peripheral nerves. There are the typical tabetic changes described in the preceding section. There may be degeneration of the pyramidal systems of fibres secondary to the cortical changes. Most commonly there is a combination of these two processes. Foci of hæmorrhages, and softening dependent upon coarse vascular changes, are not infrequently found, but are not typical of the disease.

There are various views as to the nature of the changes. The vascular theory is that from an inflammatory process starting in the sheaths of the arterioles there is a diffuse parenchymatous degeneration with atrophic changes in the nerve cells and neuroglia. The most generally accepted view is that some unknown toxin causes degeneration in the nervous tissues with secondary changes in the neuroglia and vascular systems.

Symptoms.—PRODROMAL STAGE.—This is of variable duration, and is characterized by a general mental state which finds expression in symptoms trivial in themselves but important in connection with others. Irritability, inattention to business amounting sometimes to indifference or apathy, and sometimes a *change in character,* marked by acts which may astonish the friends and relatives, may be the first indications. There may be unaccountable fatigue after moderate physical or mental exertion. Instead of apathy or indifference there may be an extraordinary degree of physical and mental restlessness. The patient is continually planning and scheming, or may launch into extravagances and speculation of the wildest character. A common feature at this period is the display of an unbounded egoism. He boasts of his personal attainments, his property, his position in life, or of his wife and children. Following these features are important indications of moral perversion, manifested in offences against decency or the law, many of which acts have about them a suspicious effrontery. Forgetfulness is common, and may be shown in inattention to business details and in the minor courtesies of life. At this period there may be no motor phenomena. The onset of the disease is usually insidious, although cases are reported in which epileptiform or apoplectiform seizures were the first symptoms. Among the early motor features are tremor of the tongue and lips in speaking, slowness of speech and hesitancy. Inequality of the pupils, the Argyll Robertson pupil, optic atrophy, and changes in the deep reflexes may precede the occurrence of mental symptoms for years.

SECOND STAGE.—This is characterized in brief by mental exaltation or excitement and a progress in the motor symptoms. " The intensity of the excitement is often extreme, acute maniacal states are frequent; incessant restlessness, obstinate sleeplessness, noisy, boisterous excitement, and blind, uncalculating violence especially characterize such states " (Lewis). It is at this stage that the delusion of grandeur becomes marked and the patient believes himself to be possessed of countless millions or to have reached the most exalted sphere possible in profession or occupation. This expansive delirium, as it is called, is, however, not characteristic, as was formerly supposed, of paralytic dementia. Besides, it does not always occur, but in its stead there may be marked melancholia or hypochondriasis, or, in other instances, alternate attacks of delirium and depression.

The facies has a peculiar stolidity, and in speaking there is marked tremulousness of the lips and facial muscles. The tongue is also tremulous, and may be protruded with difficulty. The speech is slow, interrupted, and blurred. Writing becomes difficult on account of unsteadiness of the hand. Letters, syllables, and words may be omitted. The subject matter of the patient's letters gives valuable indications of the mental condition. In many instances the pupils are unequal, irregular, sluggish, sometimes large. Important symptoms in this stage are apoplectiform seizures and paralysis. There may be slight syncopal attacks in which the patient turns pale and may fall. Some of these are *petit mal*. In the true apoplectiform seizure the patient falls suddenly, becomes unconscious, the limbs are relaxed, the face is flushed, the breathing stertorous, the temperature increased, and death may occur. Epileptic seizures are more common than the apoplectiform. There may be a definite aura. The attack usually begins on one side and may not spread. There may be twitchings either in the facial or brachial muscles. Typical Jacksonian epilepsy may occur. In a case which died recently under my care, these seizures were among the early symptoms and the disease was regarded as cerebral syphilis. Recurring attacks of aphasia are not uncommon, and paralysis, either monoplegic or hemiplegic, may follow these epileptic seizures, or may come on with great suddenness and be transient. In this stage the gait becomes impaired, the patient trips readily, has difficulty in going up or down stairs, and the walk may be spastic or occasionally tabetic. This paresis may be progressive. The deep reflexes are usually increased, but may be lost. Bladder or rectal symptoms gradually develop. The patient becomes helpless, bedridden, and completely demented, and unless care is taken may suffer from bedsores. Death occurs from exhaustion or from some intercurrent affection. The spinal-cord features of dementia paralytica may come on with or precede the mental troubles. There are cases in which one is in doubt for a time whether the symptoms indicate tabes or dementia paralytica, and it is well to bear in mind that every feature of preataxic tabes may exist in the early stage of general paresis.

(b) Tabo-paralysis.

Emphasis has been laid on the probable identity of the processes underlying tabes and dementia paralytica, the spinal cord in the first case receiving the full force of the attack, and the brain in the second. It has been thought that stress is the factor which determines the location of the process, and that men whose occupations require much bodily exercise would be apt to have tabes, while those whose activities are largely mental would suffer from paresis. Usually when the cord symptoms are pronounced the symptoms from the brain remain in abeyance, and the reverse is also true. There are exceptions to this, and cases of well marked tabes may later show the typical symptoms of paresis, but even then the ataxia, if it is not of too high a grade, often improves.

353

Optic atrophy, when it occurs in the pre-ataxic stage of tabes, usually indicates that the ataxia will never be pronounced, but unfortunately it is frequently followed by the occurrence of mental symptoms. Mott believes that about 50 per cent of his asylum cases of tabo-paralysis had had preceding optic atrophy. Its occurrence is therefore of grave significance. The mental symptoms may be delayed for many years.

The *symptom complex* of tabo-paralysis is made up of a combination of the symptoms of the two conditions, and varies greatly. It may begin as tabes with lightning pains, bladder symptoms, Argyll Robertson pupil, loss of the deep reflexes, etc., to have the mental symptoms added later; or, on the other hand, cord symptoms may come on after the patient has shown marked mental changes. In a number of cases the symptoms are from the first so combined that the name tabo-paralysis is at once applicable. Absent knee-jerks, ocular palsies, or pupillary symptoms may precede the breakdown for many years, but none of them have so grave a significance in regard to the mental state as has optic atrophy. Other types of alienation may interrupt the course of tabes, and the mistake must not be made of regarding them all as general paralysis. In such instances the mind may become clear and remain so to the end.

Diagnosis.—The recognition of general paralysis in the earliest stage is extremely difficult, as it is often impossible to decide that the slight alteration in conduct is anything more than one of the moods or phases to which most men are at times subject. The following description by Folsom is an admirable presentation of the diagnostic characters of the early stage of the disease: " It should arouse suspicion if, for instance, a strong, healthy man, in or near the prime of life, distinctly not of the ' nervous,' neurotic, or neurasthenic type, shows some loss of interest in his affairs or impaired faculty of attending to them; if he becomes varyingly absent-minded, heedless, indifferent, negligent, apathetic, inconsiderate, and, although able to follow his routine duties, his ability to take up new work is, no matter how little, diminished; if he can less well command mental attention and concentration, conception, perception, reflection, judgment; if there is an unwonted lack of initiative, and if exertion causes unwonted mental and physical fatigue; if the emotions are intensified and easily change, or are excited readily from trifling causes; if the sexual instinct is not reasonably controlled; if the finer feelings are even slightly blunted; if the person in question regards with a placid apathy his own acts of indifference and irritability and their consequences, and especially if at times he sees himself in his true light and suddenly fails again to do so; if any symptoms of cerebral vaso-motor disturbances are noticed, however vague or variable."

There are cases of cerebral syphilis which closely simulate dementia paralytica. The mode of onset is important, particularly since paralytic symptoms are usually early in syphilis. The affection of the speech and tongue is not present. Epileptic seizures are more common and more liable to be cortical or Jacksonian in character. The expansive delirium is rare. While symptoms of general paresis are not common in connection with the development of gummata or definite gummatous meningitis, there are, on the other hand, instances of paresis following closely upon the syphilitic infection. Post mortem in such cases there may be nothing more than a general arterio-sclerosis and diffuse meningo-encephalitis, which may present nothing distinctive, but the lesions, nevertheless, may be caused by the syphilitic virus. Cases also occur in which typical syphilitic lesions are combined with the ordinary lesions of dementia paralytica. There are certain forms of lead encephalopathy which resemble general paresis, and, considering the association of plumbism with arterio-sclerosis, it is not unlikely that the anatomical substratum of the disease may result from this poison. Tumor may sometimes simulate progressive paresis, but in the former the signs of general increase of the intracranial pressure are usually present. The Wassermann reaction (see Syphilis) is present in a majority of cases.

Cytodiagnosis.—The study of the cellular elements suspended in the cerebro-spinal fluid, first instituted by Widal and Ravaut (1900) in cases of dementia paralytica, has come to be an important diagnostic measure, particularly in tabes and paresis. In both of these affections spinal lymphocytosis is the rule and is usually associated with a marked albumin reaction—the normal fluid containing no albumin, or at most minute traces, and a negligible number of formed elements. It is simply the expression of a subacute or chronic inflammatory process, just as polymorphonuclear leukocytosis is characteristic of an acute process. It is, however, first and foremost the syphilitic triad—tabes, paresis, and cerebro-spinal lues—which is suggested by lymphocytosis in the spinal fluid. Positive reactions, cytological and chemical, are among the earliest somatic symptoms, and may therefore clear up obscure cases of tabes and paresis, just at the time when diagnosis is most difficult.

Prognosis.—The disease rarely ends in recovery. As a rule the progress is slowly downward and the case terminates in a few years, although it is occasionally prolonged ten or fifteen years.

Treatment.—The only hope of permanent relief is in the cases following syphilis, which should be placed upon large doses of iodide of potassium, and given a mercurial course. Careful nursing and the orderly life of an asylum are the only measures necessary in a great majority of the cases. For sleeplessness and the epileptic seizures bromides may be used. Prolonged remissions, which are not uncommon, are often erroneously attributed to the action of remedies. Active treatment in the early stage by wet-packs, cold to the head, and systematic massage have been followed by temporary improvement.

HERPES ZOSTER

(Zona; Acute Hæmorrhagic Inflammation of the Dorsal Root Ganglia).

Zoster is an acute specific disease of the nervous system with a localization in the ganglia of the posterior roots (Head and Campbell). There are hæmorrhages and inflammatory foci, with destruction of certain of the ganglion cells, leading to degeneration of their axis-cylinder processes. W. T. Howard has shown, even in the herpes facialis such as accompanies pneumonia, that hæmorrhagic lesions akin to those of true zoster are demonstrable in the Gasserian ganglion. The two conditions, however, are etiologically quite distinct.

Chauffard reports cases which indicate an extension of the process from the posterior ganglia to the neighboring meninges. There may be pains down the spine, girdle pains, and exaggerated knee jerks with marked lymphocytosis. Herpes auricularis is associated with lesions in the otic ganglion (Ramsay

tabes and paresis

When William Osler prepared the 1909 edition of his textbook, syphilis was a disease with four centuries of recorded history. General paresis and tabes dorsalis were less venerable, their recognition belonging, like Osler himself, to the nineteenth century. John Haslam had reported the first identifiable case of paresis in 1798, and the name "general paralysis of the insane," later modified to general paresis, dementia paralytica, of the familiar GPI dates to the 1820s and derives principally from Calmeil. Osler's own birth in 1849 almost coincided with Romberg's classic description of tabes dorsalis, and he was already a practicing physician when Romberg died.

The impact of the discoveries of paresis and tabes on the infant neurology and psychiatry of the time is difficult to appreciate today. The concept of a specific disease of the brain, causing progressive sensori-motor paralysis and dementia, and ending in insanity and death, with obvious and consistent changes in meninges and brain, is commonplace enough to us. To the neurology and psychiatry of the early nineteenth century, it was revolutionary. It removed mental illness forever from the exclusive realm of misty speculation. It demanded a consideration of the brain as the organ of mind and emotion, and of their effective expression, which was to survive even the assault of psychoanalysis in the twentieth century. And it served as prototype and inspiration for those careful clinical, physiological, and pathological studies of human brain disease which graced the neurology and psychiatry Osler know. Similarly, the description of tabes dorsalis by Romberg, Todd, and Duchenne was not only the initial step in the clarification of spinal cord disease; it was also a major achievement in spinal cord anatomy and physiology and a landmark in the developing doctrine of localization of function in the nervous system.

Effective medical knowledge of paresis and tabes in 1909 was limited principally to their signs, symptoms, and pathological anatomy. In these it was complete. Succeeding decades have added little to Osler's accounts. Only one major therapeutic advance — the use of mercury — antedated this period, and only one major descriptive feat — the demonstration of treponemes in the brain in paresis — was to follow it. The great years of clinical and pathoanatomical description were over. But the dozen years surrounding the 1909 edition saw discoveries coming from laboratories of medical sciences which were to change neurosyphilis, and indeed all of medical thought, just as Haslam, Calmeil, and Romberg had changed it in their day.

356

Osler was keenly aware of the enormous importance of Metchnikoff and Rous' transmission of human syphilis to apes, of Wassermann's application of Bordet and Gengou's studies on complement fixation to the serodiagnosis of syphilis, and of Schaudinn and Hoffman's discovery of *Treponema pallidum.* He could not know that 1909 was to see Ehrlich's announcement of arsphenamine, the most potent antisyphilitic drug yet to be developed, and one of the first great triumphs of chemotherapy. He probably knew of, but did not comment on, Wagner-Jauregg's early papers on fever therapy of paresis. He certainly could not know that as he wrote, a young Scot, who was one day to discover penicillin, was beginning his duties as assistant bacteriologist at St. Mary's Hospital.

Pathology of neurosyphilis since Osler

Though few great contributions to the pathological anatomy of tabes and paresis remained to be made, several long-standing arguments were gradually resolved. Nageotte's descriptions of the principal lesion of tabes as a spinal radiculitis, involving the root just central to the ganglion, came slowly to be accepted over such alternatives as subpial demyelinization, or lymphatic stasis of the dorsal surface of the cord. Syphilitic optic atrophy was recognized as a chronic constrictive inflammation of the optic nerve sheaths, rather than the result of an obscure neurotoxin of syphilis. Much careful histological work was done on iron deposits in the paretic cortex, and the changes produced by arsenical, malarial, or penicillin treatment. Arsenical treatment, in particular, produced a series of neurotoxic sequelae of its own: accelerated Herxheimer reactions, hemorrhagic encephalopathy, tryparsamide optic atrophy, transverse myelitis, and arsenical neuritis, each interesting in its own right and each receiving its share of study. The great post-Oslerian pathological feat, however, was the demonstration of spirochetes in the brain in paresis, achieved by Noguchi and Moore in 1913.

Curiously, one of the commonest and best known signs of neurosyphilis remains inadequately understood to this day. The pathological anatomy of the Argyll Robertson pupil is still the source of argument. Lesions placed in the pregeniculate gray matter abolish the pupillary light response while preserving the response to accommodation, but the small, irregular, and excentric pupil of tabes is not reproduced. The suggestion that syphilitic scarring of the oculomotor nerve or the geniculate region is responsible seems hardly tenable. Iridial atrophy, a common feature of the tabetic pupil, implies an autonomic injury, but convincing proof for such a lesion is wanting.

Diagnosis of neurosyphilis since Osler

No diagnosis of an infection is as satisfying as that won by isolating the offender. This is seldom possible in neurosyphilis. *Treponema pallidum* cannot be cultured in vitro, accessible fresh lesions are rare, and demonstration of spirochetes in a peripheral lesion does not prove involvement of the nervous system. Brain biopsy was too formidable for serious consideration. The task was to prove, by other than isolation methods, the presence of both syphilis and syphilitic brain disease.

The two essential techniques were at hand in 1909. Quincke's lumbar puncture, introduced in 1891 as a treatment for hydrocephalus, was a therapeutic disaster, but, as Quincke realized, it made cerebrospinal fluid, and in a sense the internal environment of brain and cord, readily and repeatably available for study. Wassermann's complement-fixation reaction became popular soon after 1906 and, interestingly enough, was never supplanted in study of the CSF. Precipitation reactions became more popular for peripheral blood and so numerous that today they are known generically as VDRL or STS, rather than eponymically.

By 1909, Osler could draw on a considerable body of experience with the CSF changes in neurosyphilis. Pleocytosis, increased protein, and presence of reagin were clearly established, and he could with justification comment that spinal fluid examinations "may clear up obscure cases of tabes and paresis just at the time when diagnosis is most difficult."

Nonne had begun, and in 1912 Lange completed, the demonstration of increased CSF globulin fractions in neurosyphilis. The various tests, beginning with Pandy's phenol precipitation and ending with the colloidal-precipitation reactions of which Lange's gold-sol curves were the prototypes, added the last important tool for the spinal fluid diagnosis of neurosyphilis.

Therapy of neurosyphilis since Osler

Drug treatment of syphilis is as old as the disease itself. Mercury, almost certainly used in the Neapolitan epidemic, remained the only effective agent until Wallace introduced iodides in 1835. These two, together with bismuth which Levaditi popularized after Osler's death, were the only chemotherapeutic agents worthy of mention until Ehrlich brought forward the most effective of all — the arsenicals. Salvarsan, Ehrlich's 606 which he announced definitively in 1909, rapidly proved the prime antisyphilitic drug of its time, and new arsenical compounds at once more treponemicidal and less toxic soon followed. Among them, neoarsphenamine (Ehrlich's 914), tryparsamide, considered the most effective against paresis, but a potent cause of optic atrophy, and silver-salvarsan, notorious for the argyria it caused, are all remembered. With mercury, bismuth, and iodides, the arsenicals remained the mainstay of drug therapy until penicillin.

The arsenicals brought their own problems with them. Jarisch, and later Herxheimer, had noted the worsening of the symptoms of syphilis on overvigorous treatment with mercury and had distinguished this from mercurial poisoning, itself common to such therapy. Arsenicals, besides being much more treponemicidal that mercury, proved also a much more potent source of Jarisch-Herxheimer reactions, and severe or even fatal ones rapidly became fairly familiar, until their origins in the massive release of dead treponemal protoplasm was recognized and their control by gradual initiation of therapy was practiced.

The arsenicals, however carefully used, were never completely free of toxic side effects. In combination with mercury, iodides, and later bismuth, they were fairly effective against primary and secondary syphilis and prevented most congenital syphilis. But their value in general paresis proved distressingly small, and on the symptoms of tabes dorsalis they had really no material effect at all. Syphilologists were in a receptive mood when Wagner-Jauregg published his definitive account of the malarial therapy of paresis. Like most discoveries this was not new. Ruy Diaz in the sixteenth century, had noted improvement of syphilis during malarial attacks. Wagner-Jauregg, himself, had first experimented with malarial treatment in 1887, but then abandoned it and tried fevers induced with Koch's Old Tuberculin. Finding these artificially induced fevers prophetically ineffective, he returned to malaria. In 1917 he was able to report a cure rate for paresis of one third, with another third greatly improved. Such statistics, though unimpressive today, were unparalleled in 1917, and for the next 30 years, malaria alone and in combination with other antisyphilitic drugs was the treatment of general paresis.

To avoid the many difficulties and hazards of malarial infections, other forms of induction of fever were tried, usually with diathermy, heating cabinets, or hot baths. Wagner-Jauregg's early experiences with tuberculin were borne out. These artificial fevers proved less effective, and until well into the penicillin era, the paresis room, screened to exclude adventurous mosquitoes and harboring the paretic in his malarial rigors, was a familiar sight in all hospitals where neurosyphilis was treated.

The real advance in treatment went initially unheralded. In 1928, Alexander Fleming announced the discovery of penicillin. Not until 15 years later — in 1943 — Mahoney tried the new drug on syphilis with gratifying results. In 1945, its powerful effect on paresis was described, and

Tabes and paresis

the treatment of all forms of syphilis but one was assured. Tabes alone remains, as always, resistant, though corticosteroids have some small effect against tabetic pains.

Penicillin will apparenty prevent the development of paresis or tabes, even if given intermittently and at intervals. It has reduced these illnesses to the status of medical curiosities. It cannot, of course, restore damaged brain to advanced paretics, especially the juvenile variety, though recovery is often surprisingly good. Jarisch-Herxheimer reactions are rare and seldom severe. As yet there is no evidence for development of resistant strains of treponemata, and for the rare patient sensitive to the drug, other antibiotics, especially tetracyclines, have proven adequate.

David B. Clark

REFERENCES

Dennie, C.C. A History of Syphilis. Springfield, Ill., Charles C Thomas, 1962.

Dreyfus, G.L. Die Methoden der Untersuchung des Liquor cerebrospinalis bei Syphilis. Munchen. Med. Wschr., 59:2576, 1912.

Hahn, R.D. Penicillin treatment of general paresis (dementia paralytica). Arch. Neurol. (Chicago), 81:557, 1959.

Lange, Carl. Uber die Ausflockung von Goldsol durch Liquor cerebrospinalis. Berlin. Klin. Wschr., 19:897, 1912.

Langworthy, O.R., and Ortega, L. The iris. Innervation of the iris of the albino rabbit. Medicine, 22:298, 1943.

Levaditi, C. Bismuth dans le syphilis. Presse Med., 30:633, 1922.

Magoun, H.W., and Ranson, S.W. The central path of the light reflex. A study of the effect of lesions. Arch. Ophthal. (Chicago), 13:791, 1935.

Noguchi, H., and Moore, J.W. A demonstration of Treponema pallidum in the brain in cases of general paralysis. J. Exp. Med., 17:232, 1913.

Olansky, S., and Garson, W. The treatment of syphilis with antibiotics other than penicillin. Arch. Derm. (Chicago), 77:648, 1958.

Robertson, G.M. The discovery of general paralysis. J. Ment. Sci., 69:1, 1923.

Wagner-Juaregg, J. Ueber die Infektionsbehandlung der progressiven Paralyse. Munchen. Med. Wschr., 78:4, 1931.

Wallace, W. Treatment of the venereal disease by the hydriodate of potash, or iodide of potassium. Lancet, 2:5, 1836.

epilogue

A comment cogent to all the sections reviewed here is that at the level of clinical and pathological description of the natural history of disease nothing substantial has been added since Osler's résumé of 1909. What has been added in our understanding is mainly in the realms of etiology, pathogenesis, and therapy.

The important, although indirect, contribution which Osler's textbook made to the progress of medical science through its influence on philanthropists has been surveyed in the Introduction. It is worth pointing out that it also contributed heavily to medical progress through its influence on physicians and clinical investigators. Two generations of medical students in all parts of the world, the same medical students who were responsible for many of the advances of the last half-century outlined in the commentaries, were introduced to medicine by Osler's text. Assembling and presenting the knowledge of medicine in a coherent manner which preserves the excitement of discovery and the urgency of unsolved problems is an important aid to research.

Indeed, teaching and research are the warp and woof of the fabric of medical progress. Each is dependent on the other. The importance of both is now well recognized by medical schools and research institutes alike. In his autobiography James B. Herrick* (1861–1954), the discoverer of sickle cell anemia and an early student of acute coronary occlusion, expressed the same view:

"I have no desire to debate the question of the comparative merits of research as opposed to textbook authorship. If I were to attempt it, I fear I should make a poor showing in trying to prove that any textbook has benefited mankind as have the researches of a Galileo, a Harvey, a Newton, a Pasteur, a Koch, a Roentgen. But a strong case can be made out for the claim that most honorable mention may justly be accorded the author of a good textbook. And I would call in as a supporting witness William Rainey Harper, who, many years ago, said to me that though he himself was a devotee of research and the president of a university the major activity of which was original investigation, he was unwilling to say that the contribution of the one who sought for the new was of greater value than that of the competent teacher or the writer of a genuinely good textbook who made known and interpreted the old. As I see it, such a service was rendered by the textbook of William Osler."

A.M.H.
V.A.M.

*Herrick, J.B. *Memories of Eighty Years*. Chicago, University of Chicago Press, 1949.